Atlas
Effectors of Anti-Tumor Immunity

Atlas
Effectors of Anti-Tumor Immunity

Editor

Mikhail V. Kiselevsky
NN Blokhin Russian Cancer Research Center RAMS, Moscow, Russia

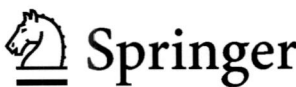 Springer

Editor

Mikhail V. Kiselevsky
Laboratory of Cell Immunity
NN Blokhin Russian Cancer
Research Center
Russian Academy of Medical Sciences
Kashirskoe shosse 24
Moscow
Russia 115478

ISBN: 978-1-4020-6930-7   e-ISBN: 978-1-4020-6931-4

Library of Congress Control Number: 2007939885

Printed on acid-free paper.

9 8 7 6 5 4 3 2 1

springer.com

Table of Contents

Preface

Traditional understanding of anti-tumor immunity is based on the theory of immunological surveillance and it suggests function of cytotoxic lymphocytes that can recognize tumor-specific antigens and lyse malignantly transformed cells. However tumor development is not the direct result of immune system disorders and even in case of marked immuno-deficiencies, in particular, in patients – transplant recipients, immune dysfunction does not always lead to higher cancer incidence comparing with total population. This phenomenon may be explained by the concept of immuno-editing, which suggests that anti-tumor immunity effectors can not only protect the organism from tumor development, but also select low immunogenic clones of transformed cells that can escape from immuno-biological surveillance. Mechanism of avoiding the immune attack is primarily due to the lack of specific antigens on tumor cell surface and loss or down-regulation of expression rate of molecules of major histocompatibility complex, which are necessary factors for initiation of adaptive immune response and generation of antigen-specific T-lymphocytes. Therefore recent data have more often given evidence in favor of innate immunity being the main weapon of immune surveillance over tumor development. And NKs play the crucial role as they can recognize and lyse transformed cells in MHC and antigen independent manner. An important part in realization of anti-tumor defense is assigned to other effectors of innate immunity as well, first of all, as potential NK activators, such as dendritic cells and natural killer T-cells. Along with the mentioned functions innate immunity effectors can have a negative regulatory effect on anti-tumor immuno-biological surveillance by secreting Th2 cytokines. Contemporary standpoints in understanding mechanisms of innate and adaptive immunity are the basis for development and improvement various methods of adoptive immunotherapy.

Anti-tumor immunity has been subject of most thorough interest and detailed investigation over the last decades. Nowadays more and more specialists in medicine and adjacent areas face the problem of immuno-biological surveillance function. Research data on this issue are diverse and extensive. In numerous monographs, educational books and scientific papers a keen reader can find practically any material concerning the questions of interest. The purpose of the present publication is to convey considerably full and up-to-date information to the reader in a reasonably comprehensible format. To make the material easy for perception the Atlas has a large number of illustrative pictures, which also help to track interrelations between morphological features of anti-tumor immunity effectors and their phenotype and functional characteristics. The Atlas is aimed at a wide audience of students and teachers of medical and biology faculties, specialists of research laboratories and diagnostics centers, practicing oncologists and immunologists, as well as physicians of different specializations.

The Atlas comprises over 200 figures and schemes referring to effectors of anti-tumor immunity and methods of anti-cancer adoptive immunotherapy.

List of Contributors

Vyacheslav M. Abramov
Institute Immunological Engineering Moscow Region, Russia

Nelly K. Akchmatova
II Metchnikov Research Institute of Vaccines and Serums, Laboratory of Therapeutic Vaccines, Moscow, Russia

Nathalie Yu. Anisimova
NN Blokhin Russian Cancer Research Center RAMS, Laboratory of Cell Immunity, Moscow, Russia

Gianfranco Baronzio
Family Medicine Area ASL1 Legnano (Mi) and Radiotherapy, Hyperthermia Service, Policlinico di Monza, Monza, Italy

Irina O. Chikileva
NN Blokhin Russian Cancer Research Center RAMS, Laboratory of Cell Immunity, Moscow, Russia

Lev V. Demidov
NN Blokhin Russian Cancer Research Center RAMS, Department of Biotherapy, Moscow, Russia

Isabel Freitas
University of Pavia, Department of Animal Biology and IGM-CNR Center for Histochemistry and Cytometry, Pavia, Italy

Evgenia O. Khalturina
I.M. Setchenov Medical Academy, Departtament of Microbiology, Virusology and Immunology Moscow, Russia

Mikhail V. Kiselevsky
NN Blokhin Russian Cancer Research Center RAMS, Laboratory of Cell Immunity, Moscow, Russia

Olga V. Lebedinskaya
EAVagner Perm Medical Academy, Departtament of Histology, Embryology and Cytology Perm, Russia

María I. Sada-Ovalle
Research Unit, Biochemistry Department, National Institute of Respiratory Diseases, Calzada de Tlalpan 4502, Col. Sección XVI, Delegación Tlalpan, México D.F., Mexico

Irina Zh. Shubina
NN Blokhin Russian Cancer Research Center RAMS, Moscow, Russia

Joseph G. Sinkovics
St. Joseph's Hospital's Cancer Institute Affiliated with the H. L. Moffitt Comprehensive Cancer Center at the University of South Florida College of Medicine; Department of Medical Microbiology & Immunology, the University of South Florida College of Medicine, Tampa FL, USA

Nadezhda P. Velizheva
NN Blokhin Russian Cancer Research Center RAMS, Moscow, Russia

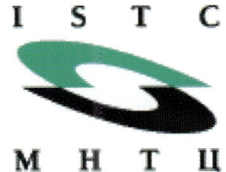

The *Atlas Effectors of Anti-Tumor Immunity* was published with the financial support of The International Science and Technology Center (ISTC). Chapters 3–8 have been written by the participants of ISTC-supported projects. This publication has been produced with the financial assistance of the European Union as a Funding Party to the Agreement establishing the ISTC.

The International Science and Technology Center is an intergovernmental organization holding diplomatic status, created to prevent nuclear weapons proliferation, contribute to global security, and to link the demands of international markets with the exceptional pool of scientific talent available in Russian and other Commonwealth of Independent States (CIS) institutes. The ISTC was established in 1992 by the European Union, Japan, the Russian Federation, and the United States of America on the basis of a multinational agreement. Canada joined as a full Governing Board member in 2004. The ISTC's core activity is associated with the development of international science projects. Since 1994, the ISTC has managed financial support exceeding USD 769M to 2500 projects, encompassing over 70,000 scientists and technicians at more than 700 institutes in Russia and CIS. The ISTC also provides a tax and customs-duty exempt mechanism for its 370 commercial and governmental agency Partners to fund research with ISTC beneficiary institutes. Biotechnology is the most dynamically evolving direction of the ISTC activity, with over 640 projects totaling USD 202M.

The ISTC has established strategic partnerships with Russian and CIS innovation foundations and organizations, has engaged in technology transfer using its internationally agreed procedures, and has assisted a broad range of other international institutions, government organizations, universities, and the scientific community as a whole, to deliver their R&D and commercialization objectives.

Contact details
Steve Bourne
Communications Manager
Krasnoproletarskaya ul. 32-34, ISTC
P.O. Box 20, 127473 Moscow,
Russian Federation
Email: bourne@istc.ru
Office: (7-495) 982 3141
Web site www.istc.ru

1. Adoptive immunotherapy for human cancers: Flagmen signal first "open road" then "roadblocks." A narrative synopsis

JOSEPH G. SINKOVICS

St. Joseph's Hospital's Cancer Institute Affiliated with the H. L. Moffitt Comprehensive Cancer Center at the University of South Florida College of Medicine
Department of Medical Microbiology & Immunology, the University of South Florida College of Medicine, Tampa FL
USA

Keywords: Immune T cells, NK cells, T_{REG} cancer vaccines, codon CUG

Abstract

There was overwhelming evidence documented *in vitro* in the early 1970s for lymphocyte-mediated cytotoxicity to autologous cancer cells. Cancer-bearing patients circulated small compact lymphocytes in their blood that promptly killed their tumor cells *in vitro*. These lymphocytes were identified later as $CD8^+$ immune T cells. Tumor cells were killed by cytoplasmic lysis with perforins and granzymes, or by nuclear clumping by Fas ligand and related ligands. With the discovery of T cell growth factor (interleukin-2), the road for lymphocyte therapy of human cancers appeared wide open. Then emerged the "large granular lymphocytes". These cells occurred not only in patients with cancer, but in healthy cancer-free individuals. The author of this article served as "negative (healthy) control" in the cytotoxicity assays in the late 1960s and early 1970s. Some project site visitors of the National Cancer Institute could not comprehend that "immune reactions could exist without pre-immunization" and referred to the phenomenon as an "*in vitro* artifact" (worse than that: they canceled grant support for its study). It was years later, that first in mice and then in human patients the "large granular lymphocytes" were recognized as natural killer cells. Then emerged the "suppressor/regulatory T cells" (TREG). This lymphocyte population is responsible for curtailing autoimmune reactions against "self". Tumor cells masquerading as "self" are protected by TREG against cytotoxicity executed by immune T cells, and even by NK cells. Adoptive immune lymphocyte therapy of human cancer will be effectively resolved when technology develops for the neutralization of the TREG population.

1.1. Flagmen Signaling: "The Road Is Clear!"

1.1.1. "Starry Sky"

In the 1960s monocytes and macrophages were given the credit for being the major defensive cells by engulfing and digesting cancer cells. In the "starry sky" histologically viewed phenomenon, antibody-coated lymphoma cells were phagocytosed and digested by macrophages. These phenomena occurred in human Burkitt's lymphoma and in a retrovirally induced mouse lymphoma

1

M.V. Kiselevsky (ed.), Atlas Effectors of Anti-tumor Immunity, 1–23.

(reviewed in references [86, 87]). This event may result in antigen-presentation by the macrophage to CD4 lymphocytes (*vide infra*).

1.1.2. Cytotoxic Lymphocytes

By the early 1970s it has become abundantly documented that autologous lymphocytes killed various types of human malignant cells *in vitro*. In the chamber-slide assay, it was actually visualized that small compact lymphocytes promptly surrounded and lysed autologous tumor cells, and large granular lymphocytes attacked and killed allogeneic tumor cells (reviewed in references [82, 90, 93, 97, 98]). In radioisotope assays, these events were not actually seen, but the radioisotopes released from disintegrating tumor cells exposed to purified lymphocyte preparations were readily detectable (reviewed in reference [93]). Figures 1.1–1.3 show

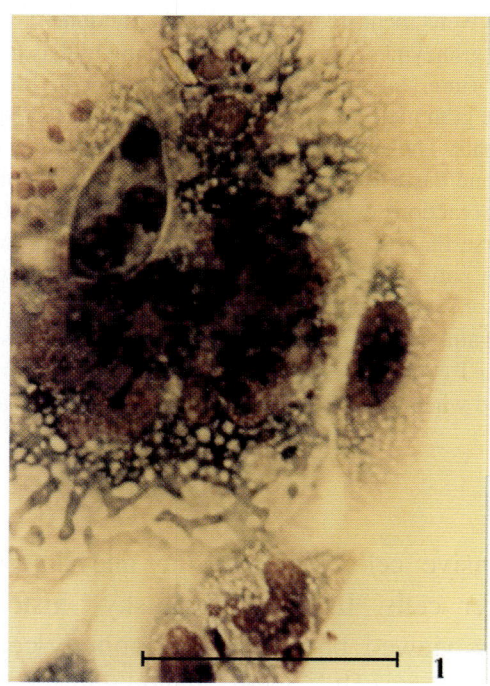

Figure 1.1. Chondrosarcoma cells established in permanent culture in 1968–9 (cell line #1459) of male patient (MDAH #73587). Scale bar: 20 μm

microphotographs of historical value: in 1969 the author serving as "healthy negative control" yielded large granular lymphocytes from his blood that killed allogeneic cancer (chondrosarcoma) cells *in vitro*. Figure 1.2 show the patient's autologous small compact lymphocytes (later recognized to be immune T cells) surrounding and attacking autologous chondrosarcoma cells. Figure 1.3 shows the healthy control's (JGS, author of this article) large granular lymphocytes (later recognized to be natural killer cells) attaching firmly to the allogeneic chondrosarcoma cell. Figure 1.4 displays a morphological comparison of small compact (immune T cell) and large granular (NK cells) human lymphocytes reacting to a sarcoma cell. Figure 1.5 depicts large granular lymphocytes (NK cells) mobilized after immunotherapy of the patient with a viral oncolysate vaccine. The patient with metastatic liposarcoma was in remission; his NK cells release their cytoplasmic granules as they react to an allogeneic sarcoma cell; his immune T cells are in the minority of the reactive lymphocyte population [93]. Figure 1.6 compare lymphocyte-mediated cytolysis and nuclear lysis of the targeted malignant cells.

1.1.3. Death by Design

Cancer cell death was seen to occur either by cytoplasmic lysis or by nuclear clumping. Perforins or granzymes released by cytotoxic T lymphocytes caused the cytoplasmic lysis (reviewed in reference [82, 93]). The complement-related perforins [66] punctured holes in the cancer cells' cytoplasm; through these holes the cytoplasm poured out. Fas ligand (FasL) and related death domain ligands-to-receptors processes (FasL-to-CD95Fas; tumor necrosis factor-related apoptosis-inducing ligand, TRAIL) induced a cascade terminating in the activation of caspases and

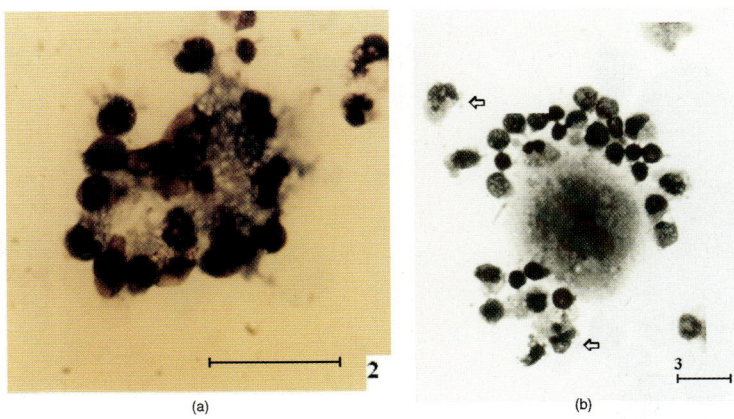

(a)   (b)

Figure 1.2. The patient's (MDAH #73587) "small compact lymphocytes" (later recognized to be immune T cells) purified from his blood, immediately surround and lyse his autologous tumor (chondrosarcoma) cell *in vitro*. In **a**: The tumor cell targeted by the lymphocytes succumbs to cytolysis. Scale bar: 20 μm. In **b** (in black and white), the tumor cell withstands the attack of the autologous small compact lymphocytes: some of the lymphocytes undergo nuclear clumping (arrow), other lymphocytes show fine cytoplasmic vacuolizations. These pictures were taken on September 8, 1969. Scale bar: 10 μm

nucleases clumping and cutting the cells chromosomes and the DNA strands within in a ladder-like fashion (reviewed in reference [85, 92]). Thus, the phenomena of externally induced programmed cell death (apoptosis) were re-discovered: the processes known to have occurred in the ontogenesis of worms (*Caenorhabditis*) and insects (*Drosophila*) became applicable to the host- tumor relationships, even though physiologically, during ontogenesis, the mitochondria-initiated endogenous apoptosis might have been more frequent, than the exogenous forms of programmed cell death [92].

1.1.4. *"No Immunity May Exist Without Pre-immunization." The Story of NK Cells*

In observing *in vitro* the phenomena of lymphoid cell-induced tumor cell death, a major controversy had arisen, when it was found that healthy (tumor-free) individuals yielded from their blood samples lymphoid-like cells that killed allogeneic tumor cells (reviewed in reference [93]). Representatives

of a major granting agency considered the phenomenon an "*in vitro* artifact," occurring in the chamber-slide assays, inasmuch as immune reactions without pre-immunization were not supposed to have developed in a healthy host. Healthy donors of those "large granular lymphoid cells" that killed allogeneic tumor cells *in vitro* were considered to be survivors of latent cancers; this notion was withdrawn when male donors of these lymphoid cells (first of them the author of this article) killed female ovarian, uterine and breast cancer cells *in vitro*. Graph 1.1 shows an early experiment, in which the author's lymphoid cells (the "large granular lymphoid cells") suppressed the growth of allogeneic tumor cells; the reaction to this phenomenon was reviewed in reference [93]. From the first observation of these large granular lympho-cytes of healthy donors killing allogeneic tumor cells *in vitro* (1969) to the acceptance that natural killer cells existed (1974–1975) almost five years went by [42]. The ancestors of the innate NK cells were recognized in the ascidian protochordate, the *Botryllus*,

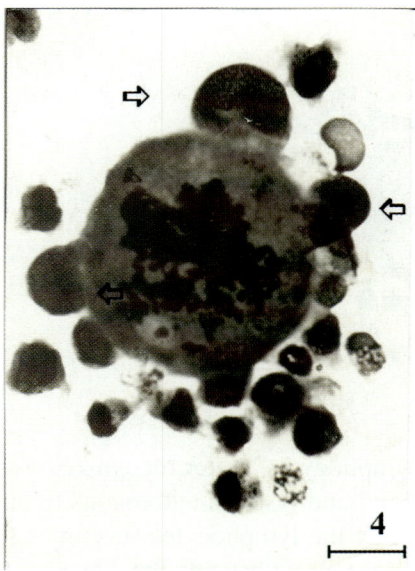

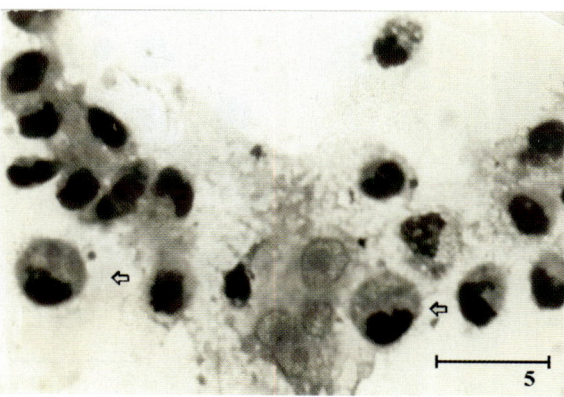

Figure 1.4. For comparison, in the center, a large lymphocyte with granular cytoplasm (arrow), later recognized to be an NK cell and a small compact lymphocyte, later recognized to be immune T cells, are positioned next to a multinuclear sarcoma cell showing early signs of cytoplasmic lysis. Scale bar: 10 μm

Figure 1.3. Lymphoid cells taken from the blood of the healthy control donor (JGS (the author of this article)) surround, but do not immediately attack the patient's (MDAH #73587) chondrosarcoma cell; the small compact allogeneic lymphocytes refrain from attacking the patient's tumor cell, but the "large lymphoid cells with granular cytoplasm" (later recognized to be natural killer cells) firmly attach to the patient's tumor cell (arrows). Some 36–48 hours later the "large granular lymphocytes" of the healthy donor will kill the patient's tumor cells, either by nuclear clumping (apoptosis in the pre-apoptosis era), or by cytolysis. These photographs, taken on December 3, 1969, are the first pictures showing human natural killer (NK) cells attacking an allogeneic human tumor (chondrosarcoma) cell. Scale bar: 10 μm

monocytes-macrophages and NK cells were activated to kill tumor cells, either by perforin release or by apoptosis induction [101].

1.1.6. Tumor Cells Armed with FasL Are Killed by Leukocytes

When tumor cells acquire FasL expression to kill those immune Fas$^+$ host lymphocytes [62, 85, 92], which express the Fas receptor (CD95), granulocytes (polymorphonuclear leukocytes) attack and kill (enzymatically digest) such tumor cells [29, 62, 111]. In Epstein-Barr virus-carrier nasopharyngeal carcinoma cells, FasL expression by tumor cells correlated with IL-10 secretion, and with latent membrane protein -2 (LMP) formation [62]. These events immortalize the tumor and suppress Th1-type immune reactions in the host in favor of a Th2-type immune environment in which the tumor prevails.

emerging during the Cambrian explosion (cited in reference [93]).

1.1.5. The Contribution of the B-Cell Compartment

Antibody- and complement-induced tumor cell death was documented after the discovery and clinical administration of monoclonal antibodies. Even better, in the ADCC-reaction, the Fc receptor-possessing

1.1.7. Cancer Vaccines Induce Th1-Type Host Immune Response

The innate and adaptive immune systems are not well united in their anticancer reactions.

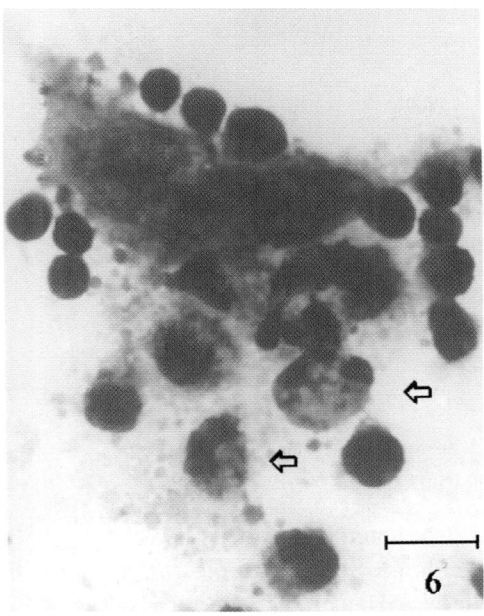

Figure 1.5. Male patient (MDAH #90641) with liposarcoma in remission received immunotherapy with sarcoma "viral oncolysates" in the mid-1970s; he mobilized a great number of large granular lymphocytes (later recognized to be NK cells) releasing their solubilized cytoplasmic granules (arrows), and small compact lymphocytes (later recognized to be immune T cells). The lymphocytes attack a sarcoma cells (from established cell line #3743), from which sarcoma cell line, the viral oncolysate vaccine was prepared. Scale bar: 10 μm

Disintegrating tumor cells, fused with, or engulfed by and within macrophages and dendritic cells (DC), release their tumor antigens for the expression of these peptides on the surface of these professional antigen-presenting (PAP) cells. Major histocompatibility (MHC) class I molecules ascend from the endoplasmic reticulum, passing through the Golgi system, to the cell surface. From the cell's proteasomes, transporter proteins (TAP) move exogenous antigenic peptides into the antigen-presenting sites (groves) of the MHC molecules. The class I MHC molecules present antigenic peptides to CD8$^+$ T lymphocytes. Endogenous antigenic peptides synthesized in the endoplasmic reticulum are expressed by MHC class II molecules, and are presented to CD4$^+$ T lymphocytes. The T cell receptor (TCR) makes contact with the antigenic peptide, but the T cell initiates its activation processes only after the binding of its CD28 ligand to the costimulatory receptor B7 of the PAP. If the expanding reactive (immune) T cell clone secretes interferon-gamma (INFγ), the host will create a Th1 immune environment characterized by high IL-2 and tumor necrosis factor-alpha (TNFα) levels, and by lymphocyte-mediated cytotoxicity carried out against tumor cells. If the expanding reactive (immune) T cell clone secretes IL-4, the host will create a Th2 immune environment characterized by high IL-10 and high antibody levels and very low, if any, lymphocyte-mediated cytotoxicity directed at tumor cells. The placenta of the fetus and tumor cells alike, thrive to induce a Th2-type host immune environment. Many pathogens, from viruses (HIV-1), through intracellular bacteria and single-celled pathogens (plasmodia, leishmania), to helminths prevail in a Th2-type immune environment of the host, but may perish (become rejected) in a Th1-type immune environment.

Many cancer vaccines (irradiated tumor cells; tumor cell lysates) of the past failed to induce Th1-type immune response in the host. Viral oncolysates (VOs) mobilized NK cells (and some immune T cells) (reviewed in references [91, 94]), and exerted protection against micrometastases left behind after surgical removal of gross tumors. VOs were used as vaccines to prevent relapses in malignant melanoma [17]. Even when a VO vaccine failed to induce a remission (in patients with metastatic sarcoma), it rendered tumor cells in vaccinated patients more susceptible to co-administered or subsequent chemotherapy [91, 95].

Dendritic cell (DC) vaccines are prepared from DCs and autologous irradiated tumor cell chimeras, or from DCs loaded (pulsed) with

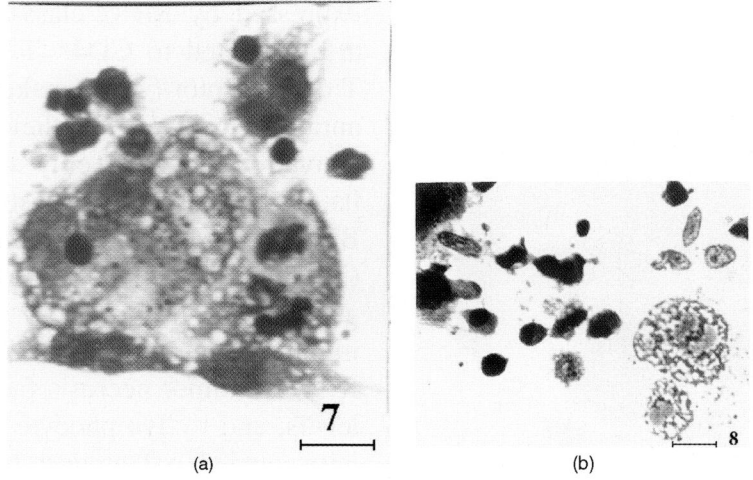

Figure 1.6. Comparison of cytoplasmic and nuclear lysis of targeted tumor cells by autologous small compact lymphocytes (later recognized to be immune T cells). **a** Shows cytoplasmic lysis, **b** shows nuclear lysis of the targeted autologous tumor cells. Scale bar: 10 μm. The author (JGS) applied to Professor József Tímár, editor of the journal Pathology Oncology Research (Budapest, Hungary) for permission to be granted for the reproduction of these figures from the journal's volume 19(3):174–187, 2004

tumor antigen peptides [57]. DC vaccines are expected to break the host's tolerance toward its cancer and mobilize immune CD8$^+$ T cells. On occasion, DC vaccines are able to mobilize immune responses strong enough to induce remissions of established tumors. Long stabilizations of partially remitted tumors are the most common responses to currently used DC cancer vaccines. Patients receiving vaccinations against cancer yield immune lymphocyte clones for adoptive immunotherapy (*vide infra*). For patients with metastatic prostate cancer, a vaccine is being licensed; the vaccine consists of antigen-presenting cells (APC) loaded with a fusion protein; the fusion protein is formed by the enzyme prostate-specific acid phosphatase and granulocyte-monocyte colony-stimulating factor (GM-CSF). Vaccinated patients experience tumor size reductions and significantly prolonged survival [7].

The graft-*versus*-leukemia reaction was discovered in mice [84]; it benefited human bone marrow transplant recipients mightily for decades, especially when the anti-leukemia effects could be separated from the anti-recipient attack [100]. A DC vaccine potentiates the graft-*versus*-leukemia reaction [76]. DCs transfected with tumor antigen mRNA and co-expressing IL-12 generate anti-tumor cytotoxic T cell clones [12]. Genetically engineered cancer vaccines express cytokines-chemokines for T cell (INFγ or IL-2), or for DC (GM-CSF) stimulation [35, 70]. A DC breast cancer vaccine targets the amplified oncogene HER-2/*neu* by releasing bursts of IL-12 driving the host to create a Th1-type immunological environment, in which cytotoxic lymphocytes attack the target [22].

1.1.8. Costimulatory Lymphokines

The efficacy of cancer vaccines or adoptively re-infused immune T cells/LAK cells (*vide infra*) is often potentiated by the co-administration of IL-2 or IL-12. It is medical history that metastatic melanoma and kidney carcinoma responded best to IFNα and IL-2 (early results reviewed in reference [83]). Osteogenic sarcoma, Ph$^+$

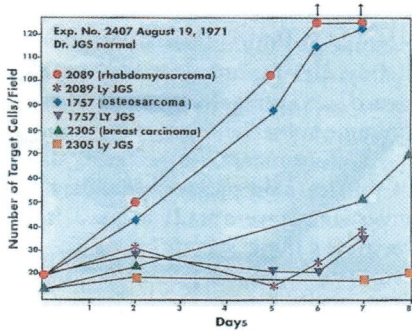

My buffy coat lymphocytes as tested on 8/19/71 strongly inhibit the growth of allogeneic sarcoma and breast carcinoma cell lines. When this phenomenon was observed in 1971, we referred to it as "immune surveillance at work," and wondered if a medical oncologist could develop "immunity" to some cancers to which he is repeatedly exposed in his professional life. This observation sharply contradicted the doctrine emanating from Seattle according to which patients with cancer circulated lymphocytes cytotoxic only to their tumor cells and healthy donors served as negative controls. It was at the NCI where the lymphocyte population responsible for this type of cytotoxicity was later called that of "natural killer cells." (Herberman RB, Djeu JK, Kay HD, et al: Immunol Rev 1979;44:43).

From: Sinkovics JG: On the Threshold of the Door of "No Admittance," in Szentivanyi A, Friedman H, eds: Immunologic Revolution, 1994, CRC Press, Boca Raton, FL, pp 241-286 (reprinted with permission).

Graph 1.1. The lymphoid cells (Ly) of the healthy donor (JGS (the author of this article)) taken from his blood, consisted of small compact (in the majority) and large granular (in the minority) lymphocytes. In August 1971, the existence of natural killer (NK) cells was far from being recognized. The author (JGS) and his associates (Drs. H. David Kay and H. Thota reviewing this experiment soon thereafter) presumed that the large granular lymphoid cell population was responsible for the suppression of growth of the allogeneic tumor cell lines, as shown in the growth curves, in contrast to the sharp growth of control cell lines not exposed to the lymphocytes: cell line #2089, rhabdomyosarcoma; cell line #1757, osteosarcoma; and cell line #2305, female breast carcinoma. These cell lines were characterized in the reference "Growth of human tumor cells in established cultures" by J. G. Sinkovics et al, Methods in Cancer Research, Academic Press, volume XIV, pp 243–323, 1978. The original 1971 graph was re-drawn by an artist for the Oncology Times (in volume XVIII/7 pp 2–3, 1996) with faithful reproduction of the growth curves of the targeted tumor cell lines. The issue of the Oncology Times which published the graph was edited by editor S. Stockwell; the graph is reprinted here without her objections

chronic myelogenous leukemia and hairy cell leukemia responded to IFNα, but somewhat less successfully. This author predicts that the era of targeted cancer therapy will be followed by a second phase, when inhibitors of oncogenic kinase pathways will be combined with biologicals and immunogens (oncolytic viral therapy; cancer vaccines; interferons and interleukins and immune lymphocytes). This combined approach will probably be applied first to the now incurable glioblastoma multiforme. For this tumor, vaccination with a viral oncolysate of the autologous tumor followed by adoptive lymphocyte therapy has been proposed in a protocol that adds immunotherapy to the standard (but ineffective) therapy of surgical (incomplete) removal of the tumor, radiotherapy to the brain and chemotherapy with temozolomide [96].

1.1.9. Adoptive Lymphocyte Therapy

Expanded *ex vivo*, autologous lymphocytes cytotoxic to the patient's own tumor cells are re-infused intravenously and continued to be expanded *in vivo* by the co-administration of low doses of IL-2. Again, metastatic melanoma and kidney carcinoma respond the best [71]; however, durable complete responses are rare outside the NIH/NCI clinics; instead, durable minor and partial responses are commonly observed [93]. Joseph C. Horvath and the author reported complete remissions induced by adoptive lymphocyte therapy: in one patient with ovarian carcinoma showing resolution of intra-abdominal tumors (cited in reference [93]), and in one patient with relapsed Hodgkin's disease showing Reed-Sternberg cells in the bone marrow undergoing apoptotic deaths upon close encounter with *ex vivo* expanded and intravenously and repeatedly reinfused autologous lymphocytes (cited in reference [92]).

1.1.10. Immune Gene Therapy

Transduction by retrolenti- or adenoviral vectors of the genes that encode the receptors of immunoreactive T cells directed at tumor cell peptide epitopes, into naïve lymphocytes of the host (or a healthy donor) creates a population of specifically immunoreactive T cells, which when expanded *in vitro* and then *in vivo*, can secure an attacker (effector, T_{eff}) and memory T cell population, that would secure permanent immunity against the targeted tumor cells [31, 45]. The main targets of this new technology are metastatic melanoma and renal cell carcinoma.

1.2. Flagmen Signaling: "Roadblocks Ahead!"

1.2.1. The Tumor Cell Expropriates the Host's Immune Defense Reactions for its Own Promotion

Human melanoma cells have been recognized to use IL-2 and its receptor (IL-2R) in an autocrine growth loop for self-propagation [1, 39]. Other human melanoma cells converted the FasL-to-Fas "death domain" into an autocrine growth loop. For the mechanism of this activity, the melanoma cell might have utilized some misaligned broken chromosomes leaving the Fas receptor expressed on the cell surface, but uniting its intracellular domain with that of the G-CSF pathway; this way, the captured FasL would induce cell mitoses. Indeed, the two chromosomes that harbor the genes for the Fas receptor (10q23–26) and G-CSF (1p32–34) frequently suffer breaks in melanoma cells. The broken chromosomes misaligned may function as a fusion oncoprotein: t(1;10)(p32–34;q23–26) [85, 92]. Indeed, fragments of these two chromosomes could be united *ex vivo* [104]. Glioblastoma cells were shown to utilize the FasL-to-Fas reaction as an autocrine growth circuit [79]. Neuroblastoma

cells utilize TNFα for their own growth stimulation [36]. B-lineage chronic lymphocytic leukemia cells are driven by IFNγ to grow and are protected from apoptotic death by stromal-derived factor-1 (SDF-1) [14, 15, 92]. Sèzary cells use IL-7 and IL-15 as their growth factors [68].

Kaposi's sarcoma (KS) cells harboring their causative virus HHV-2, utilize growth factors produced by the host: these are IFNγ, TNFα, IL-6 and nerve growth factor; but a KSHV/HHV-8 gene also encodes an IL-6-like molecule. The virally encoded kaposin protein (*vide infra*) induces malignant transformation in heterologous (murine) cells. KS cells induce the host to provide neoangiogenic factors (vascular endothelial growth factor, VEGF) and produce their own neoangiogenesis-inducer growth factor, basic fibroblast growth factor, bFGF. KS cells harbor and express an endogenous retrovirus (reviewed in references [88, 89]). It is proposed that either a retrovirally encoded and intranuclearly translocated DNA-binding protein, or the insertion of the retroviral proviral DNA next to the bFGF gene at the locus 11q13 induces bFGF overproduction in KS cells [99].

1.2.2. Regulatory T Cells. Immature Tolerogenic DCs

The host must be protected against autoimmunity, and successfully accomplished immune reactions must be terminated. The healthy host generates a population of T cells (T_{REG}) in the fetal thymus and in the periphery that accomplishes these tasks. Immature DCs in the immunological synapse established with T cells, induce tolerance. The $CD4^+CD25^+FoxP3^+$ T_{REG} cells expand under the effect of IL-2 and terminate $CD8^+$ T cell-mediated immune reactions. Tumor cells mobilize the chemokines (*vide infra*) that attract T_{REG} cells into the tumor's microenvironment. There, T_{REG} cells eliminate immune

T cells and exempt the tumor from a Th1-type immune attack. Immature DCs and T_{REG} cells by secreting IL-10 and TGFβ, tolerize γδTCR$^+$ CD8$^+$ T cells, which abstain from attacking tumor cells; veto T cells express FasL and kill Fas receptor-expressor CD8$^+$ immune T cells [64].

1.2.3. Subversion of Innate Chemokines

Notoriously, it is stromal-derived factor (SDF-1, CXCL-12) expressed by tumor cells (for example, by ovarian carcinoma cells) that attracts the T_{REG} cells expressing its receptor, CCR4, to the tumor bed, where the CD3$^+$CD4$^+$CD25$^{+(IL-2R)}$ forkhead box FoxP3$^+$ T_{REG} cells attack and kill CD8$^+$ immune T cells, thus eliminating a potentially effective anti-tumor immune reaction of the host [78].

1.2.4. Fusions of Tumor Cells with Macrophages, Lymphocytes or with other Tumor Cells

Fusion of an antibody-producer plasma cell, or a cytokine-secretory T cell with a malignant lymphoid (myeloma) cell in the laboratory created the B cell and T cell hybridomas of Kohler and Milstein, and gave rise to the industrial production of monoclonal antibodies (reviewed in reference [86]). This author (JGS) observed already in the 1960s "natural hybridoma" formation *in vivo* in a case of a retrovirally induced mouse lymphoma [86, 87]. The lymphoma cells fused with a mouse leukemia virus-specific antibody-producer plasma cell. The fused cell gained increased virulence and pathogenicity and resisted lymphocyte- and antibody-mediated immune reactions of the host, but succumbed to macrophages engulfing antibody-coated lymphoma cells, thus creating the "starry sky" phenomena [87]. Since then, many other cases of cell fusions between a malignant cell and a host lymphocyte, or

macrophage, have been observed. In these unions, it is usually the defensive cell that is subverted to serve the malignant cell.

Malignant cell populations are heterogeneous. Individual malignant cells fused by a fusogenic virus, may create multinucleated tumor cell chimaeras with increased malignancy [110]. In these chimaeras, two or more oncogenic pathways, that functioned separately in the individual tumor cells, now operate in unison in the fused "multikaryons". Fusogenic viruses may infect a tumor-bearing host naturally, or may be introduced into a tumor-bearing host with the intention of viral therapy of cancer, since many fusogenic viruses are also oncolytic (like the vesicular stomatitis virus, VSV). If the fused cancer cells eventually succumb to oncolysis, as in the case of VSV (reviewed in reference [95]), the tumor-bearing host was served well. However, if the fused tumor cells resist viral oncolysis, the host may succumb to a tumor of increased virulence (unless the virally fused tumor cells display increased susceptibility to targeted- or chemotherapy).

1.2.5. Subversion of the Tumor Stroma

The tumor stroma frequently supports the tumor by providing growth factor chemo-, lympho-, and cytokines, and provides the ingrowth of newly formed blood vessels. It is the tumor that evokes these reactions by releasing the proper inducing factors and the subverted stroma readily obliges the tumor (reviewed in reference [94]).

1.2.6. Induction of Blocking Antibodies

In the Th2-type host environment, antibodies are produced that cover antigenic tumor cell epitopes, thus "blinding" immune T cells, which see "self" immunoglobulins, instead a tumor antigen. These T cells will refrain from an attack on a "self" structure. Experiments carried out *in vitro* in the early 1970s in the author's laboratory and expressed as growth curves in graphs, showed that the anti-tumor cell cytotoxicity of "large granular lymphoid cells" (later recognized to be NK cells) was frequently enhanced by antibody-pretreatment of the tumor cells, whereas the cytotoxicity of "small compact lymphocytes" (later recognized to be immune T cells) was frequently blocked by antibody-pretreatment of the tumor cells (cited in reference [93]). The explanation was revealed by the discovery of the antibody-directed cell-mediated cytotoxiciy (ADCC) reaction later; NK cells do, immune T cells do not, possess Fc receptors for the capture of the heavy chain end of immunoglobulin molecules. This contact, the antibody's light chain end on its specific antigenic target and the antibody's heavy chain fitted into the FcR of a macrophage or NK cell, triggers the release of cytolytic molecules (perforins; granzymes) from the attacker cell that lyses the target cell. Fortuitously, nonspecific antibodies may cover epitopes on the melanoma cell surface and inhibit the access of disialoganglioside-recognizing immune T cells to their target [48].

1.2.7. Tumor Target Antigen Withdrawal

If a tumor cell can survive without the expression of a cell surface antigen, if the structure is not essential for the tumor cell's survival, under immunological attack, the tumor cell will withdraw the expression of that antigen, and thus exempt itself from being subjected to an attack by a killer lymphocyte specifically directed to that antigen. The phenomenon is best observed when antigens targeted by monoclonal antibodies (CD20 targeted by rituximab) disappear from the lymphoma cells; and the expression of tumor antigens targeted by immune lymphocytes could be cancelled just the same. Cancer cells readily shed their "carcinoembryonic antigens (CA-125, CA-15-3, CEA, PSA); ovarian carcinoma cells treated with erlotinib

and/or cetuximab release CA-125 excessively [53]; such a reaction is not a sign of failure to respond to the treatment. Antigenic epitopes shed from the cell surface may react with their specific antibodies extracellularly, with no consequences to the cell [11, 53].

1.2.8. The Codon CUG versus the Codon AUG

Major shock waves shook up cell biologists in 1979 and again in 1981, when human mitochondria decoded the isoleucine code AUA as methionine and some yeast cells defied the immutable universal genetic code further by decoding the leucine codon CUG as serine [37, 56, 73]. The codon AUA was used for the initiation of protein synthesis (translation) in the ancient Archaea [50]. Certain proteins are synthesized (initiate translation) not from the standard initiator, methionine codon AUG, but from the leucine codon CUG, therefore in the protein product, leucine can be replaced by serine. The consequences are biological-functional for the protein, and immunological for the host, as the changed protein structures may escape recognition by immune T cells, since proteins derived from translation initiation at CUG are "unanticipated proteins" [77]. Some cell surface proteins encoded by a mouse leukemia (Moloney) retrovirus derived from CUG [67]. The Tat protein of the equine anemia retrovirus is initiated at the CUG codon [61, 75]. The Tax protein of the human lymphotropic retrovirus type I uses CUG as an additional initiation codon [19]. Kaposi sarcoma cells (vide supra) encode the neoangiogenic bFGF both from AUG and CUG initiator codons; the two products differ in biological behavior (and presumably in antigenicity). The CUG product localizes in the nucleus; the AUG product localizes in the endoplasmic reticulum's secretory pathways and induces cell growth in colonies in soft agar [3, 4, 20, 108]. The

ORF K12 of the KS-associated herpes virus, HHV-8, encodes the kaposin proteins. The kaposin proteins derive from variant translational initiation at the CUG codons [58, 72]. The human proto-oncogene c-*myc* encodes its proteins Myc1 and Myc2 from two initiation codons, CUG and AUG. If targeted therapy suppresses AUG, the tumor cell will produce Myc proteins from CUG [9]. The *pim* gene is the locus for the insertion site of retroviral DNA provirus in T cell leukemias; the human Pim protein is a serine/threonine kinase regulating Ca^{++}/calmodulin metabolism and it is over expressed in hematolymphoid malignancies. The *pim* mRNA alternately initiates Pim protein translation from initiator codons AUG or CUG. The standard AUG-derived Pim protein is induced by cytokines and it functions as a positive ("booster") immunomodulatory molecule [6, 52, 74]. How about the CUG-derived Pim? The Wilms tumor suppressor protein WT may derive from initiator codon AUG, or CUG [16]; would the CUG-derived WT protein function as a tumor suppressor? The tumor stroma may produce AUG-derived and CUG-derived VEGF [44]; would the CUG-derived VEGF be suppressed by bevacizumab as well as the AUG-derived VEGF?

Defiance of the universal genetic code has apparently been practiced widely by some ancient plant cells (*Arabidopsis*) [24, 38], plant viruses (wheat mosaic virus) [80], viruses of mammalian cells (Sendai virus) [55], and healthy cells (archaea; prokaryota; single-celled eukaryota), both in nuclear and in mitochondrial genes [65, 113]. HeLa cells practice unconventional translation initiation of the enzyme trypsinogen 4 isoform B at leucine codon CUG (not at the conventional methionine codon AUG); thus the enzyme is expressed with a leucine N terminus [60]. When oncogenic viruses and tumor cells assume this practice, it may serve them well in their escape of host control. It is the TCRs that recognize the peptides of oncogenic kinases,

and a changed amino acid in the strand could mean non-recognition.

1.2.9. Incapacitation of Lymphocytes

It is a common observation that circulating lymphocytes in a tumor-bearing host are malfunctioning and are not capable to activate their cytotoxic pathways. The "activation-induced T cell death" sets in as the antigen-engaged $CD4^+$ T cells intrinsically activate their own FasL-to-Fas death domain. Myeloma cell-derived glycolipids incapacitate NK cells, which fail to respond with IFNγ production in a ligand-dependent manner [26]. Gangliosides/glycosphingolipids are shed from tumor cells. Kidney carcinoma cell-derived gangliosides induce apoptotic deaths in host immune T cells; it is TNFα that promotes the release of these lymphotoxic substances from the tumors cells [54, 69, 107]. Not only cytotoxic chemotherapy, but some agents of the new targeted therapeuticals also damage lymphocyte function. The proteasome inhibitor bortezomib: it can induce remission of multiple myeloma, but it incapacitates DCs. It inhibits $CD4^+$ T cell and NK cell activation by DCs; DCs fail to produce TNFα or IL-12 [102].

1.2.10. Induction of Neoangiogenesis. Tumor Cells Become Endothelial-Like Cells

Tumor cells either induce the stroma to produce VEGF, and VEGF-R^+ endothelial cells respond with proliferation, or the tumor cell itself will produce VEGF to induce neo-angiogenesis. In a most bizarre manner, tumor cells may transform into endothelial-like cells and form channels for the influx of more blood into the tumor bed. The phenomena of "vascular mimicry" are practiced by melanoma, glioblastoma, ovarian and lung carcinoma, and sarcoma cells [27, 105]. In the placenta, extravillous trophoblasts enter maternal spiral arteries to settle as endothelial-like cells; these cells create "flaccid conduits" with wide lumens for the influx of oxygenated maternal blood to the fetus (reviewed in reference [93]).

1.2.11. Th2-Type Immune Environment Induction

The mother's tolerance to the fetus and its placenta, and the host's tolerance to its tumor occur in a Th2-type immuno-logical environment (reviewed in reference [93]). Interleukins IL-4 and IL-10, TGFβ and various classes of immunoglobulins (not necessarily virus neutralizing, or complement-fixing, or ADCC-inducing antibodies) rule the Th2-type environment. A large number of infectious pathogens prevail in the host's Th2-type environment. In contrast, when the CD4$^+$ T cell disengaging from its immunological synapse formed with an antigen- presenting mature DC, secretes not IL-4, but IFNγ, in response, the host will create a Th1-type immunological environment. In the Th1-type immunological environment the host mobilizes immune CD8$^+$ T cells, which attack virally infected cells, cells infected by intracellular bacteria, unicellular parasites, and malignantly trans-formed cells. Cyto- and lymphokines (TNFα, IL-2, IL-12) promote these activities at the risk of parenchymal tissue destruction ("collateral damage"). T$_{REG}$ cell clones rise and terminate the immune reactions before their completion [64]; IL-10 production secures viral, bacterial and parasite persis-tence [8, 13], new clones of malignant cells arise that expropriate the host's cyto- and lymphokines for their own promotion (*vide supra*).

1.3. A New Armada of Young Oncologists Removes the Roadblocks

1.3.1. Elimination of T$_{REG}$ Cells. Neutralizing Hostile Chemokines

It is not easy to get rid of T$_{REG}$ cells; they use chemokines (SDF-1) and IL-2 for their locomotion and clonal expansion. Fludarabine and cyclophosphamide decimate their clones, but also kill immune CD4 and CD8 T cells exposing the host to fungal, mycobacterial, and protozoal infections. The CD25$^+$ T$_{REG}$ cells may be suppressed by the immuno-toxin denileukin diftitox. Pre-immunization of the host against the FoxP3$^+$ T$_{REG}$ cells may suppress their uprise [59]. Bicyclam derivatives, plerixafor (Mozobil) block the chemokines receptor CXCR, thus stem cells are released from the bone marrow into the circulation [30], whereas T$_{REG}$ cells (and suppressor macrophages or DCs) are deprived of their chemokines support.

1.3.2. Administering Chemotherapy After Tumor Vaccination

Cancer vaccines receive severe criticism because of lack of activity, not only in therapeutic, but also in preventive clinical trials. This author agrees that irradiated tumor cell and tumor lysate vaccines do not induce remissions of metastatic disease and seldom, if ever, prevent the recur-rence of surgically and incompletely removed cancers. The adverse criticism conspicu-ously left out viral oncolysates (VO), which were proven effective as a prophylactic vaccine against melanoma micrometastases at Emory University (Atlanta, GA), even though VO failed to induce remissions in estab-lished metastatic disease (reviewed in refer-ences [17, 94]). VO vaccination of patients with metastatic sarcomas was combined with chemotherapy and, in that clinical setting, it increased the response rates in comparison to that of patients receiving chemotherapy alone. In the cases of several other human tumor categories (pancreatic cancer; prostate cancer; small cell lung cancer), vaccinations against the metastatic cancer failed to score significant benefits, however, vaccinated patients experienced much improved response rates to chemotherapy (reviewed in reference [95]).

The newly designed cancer vaccines will refute the aspersions cast at them in general. A melanoma vaccine co-administered with IL-12 augmented immune reactivity of the high-risk recipients [41]. Indeed, documentation for generation of tumor antigen-specific T cells in vaccinated patients is very convincing [25, 49, 112]. Should not GM-CSF and IL-12 be a standard adjuvant for vaccination against cancer, as this combination may surpass IL-2 [63, 103]? In the case of multiple myeloma, the IL-12/GM-CSF combination was feasible with a most promising performance [40].

1.3.3. Collecting Immune Lymphocytes for Adoptive Therapy After Tumor Vaccination

The idea that post-vaccination immune lymphocytes will be either more immunoreactive or are produced in increased numbers was quite an obvious one [91]. It has now been documented that patients immunized with HER2-*neu* protein or peptide vaccines, yield immune CD4 and CD8 lymphocyte clones that could be expanded *in vitro* with IL-2. The immunoreactive clones were free of T_{REG} cell contamination, rendering them ready for adoptive immunotherapy [23, 49].

1.3.4. Combining Antibody Therapy with LAK Cell Adoptive Therapy

Monoclonal antibodies rituximab (anti-CD20) and trastuzumab (anti-HER2-*neu*) lyse their targeted B lineage lymphoma cells, or breast cancer cells, either by complement- or by ADCC-mediated reactions. It is the FcR-expressor NK cells, which potentiate the efficacy of these (and other) mcabs [2]. Joseph C. Horvath and this author proposed to combine these mcabs with autologous lymphokine-activated killer (LAK) cell infusions. However, the project was not financed; instead immunostimulatory lympho/cytokines (IL-2; IL-12) were co-administered at the Mayo Clinic (Rochester, NY) to patients receiving rituximab therapy with benefits claimed [2]. The Mount Sinai School of Medicine (New York, NY) proved that allogeneic NK cells potentiated the efficacy of trastuzumab [101].

1.3.5. Combining Cancer Vaccines and Adoptive Lymphocyte Therapy with Lymphokine Inducers of Th1-type Immune Reactions of the Host (IL-12)

Joseph C. Horvath and the author used the Emory University (Atlanta, GA) viral oncolysate (VO) melanoma vaccine [17, 94] with either IFNα, or IL-2, or GM-CSF added to it subcutaneously. Other cancer vaccines are being administered with low dose cyto/lymphokines combined with them. IL-12 is the latest addition. In non-randomized clinical trials, it is not possible to express statistically significant, evidence-based results. The consensus of opinion is that reduced dosage of cyclophosphamide diminishes the arousal of T_{REG} cells; and limited dosage of IFNα and/or IL-2 potentiate the efficacy of certain cancer vaccines [22, 41, 49, 63, 103, 112]. In the case of melanoma vaccines, caution is in order concerning the adjuvant administration of IL-2, inasmuch as an exceptional human melanoma subclone might have expropriated the IL-2-to-IL-2R circuit, as its growth loop (*vide supra*).

1.3.6. Repairing Damaged Lymphocytes and NK Cells. Activating Monocytes and Dendritic Cells

Kidney cancer cells not only secrete lympho-cytotoxic gangliosides (*vide supra*); the programmed death ligand-1 (PD-L1) of the B7 super family is paradoxically activated in kidney cancer and melanoma cells by IFNγ. An anti-PD-L1 mcab released immune helper CD4 lymphocytes to act in the direction of Th1-type anti-tumor immune reaction generation [10]. CD8$^+$ immune T cells proliferate and react to tumor antigens presented to them by heat shock protein 90 (HSP90)/tumor antigen-peptide complexes [51]. DCs expressing the NK(Vα24Vβ1)T cell ligand, when pulsed with a-galactosylceramide, regain their reactivity (that was suppressed by glycolipids of myeloma cell derivation) to kill CFD1d+ tumor (myeloma) cells [26]. The gangliosides squamous carcinoma cells release, downregulate MHC class I antigen-presenting molecules in DCs. Inhibition of glucosyl transferase in the tumor cells reduces the release of these gangliosides. Recombinant IL-15 restored the DCs ability to present antigens in MHC molecules to autologous T cells [106]. One of the earliest results with allogeneic lymphocyte therapy was reviewed well (including adoptive lymphocyte therapy for EBV-infected patients) [100]. Allogeneic lymphoid cells of healthy donors are exempt from the damages the T lymphocytes and NK cells of tumor-bearing patients are exposed to, and often fail to endure. Kidney carcinoma cells are highly vulnerable to allogeneic CD8$^+$ T lymphocytes taken from healthy donors, preferably matched siblings [28, 46].

1.3.7. Using Genetically Engineered Immune Lymphocytes for Adoptive Therapy

In the USA NIH, NCI, a complete remission was induced in a patient with metastatic melanoma with adoptive autologous T lymphocyte therapy; the lymphocyte were transfected with and expressed the TCR specific to a melanoma cell antigen [45]. The technology to raise immune T cell clones expressing TCR directed at specific tumor cell antigens for adoptive therapy, has now been readied from singled out individual patients to clinical trials [31]. Some limitations persist; one problem to deal with is the emergence of tolerogenic DCs, that suppress the reactive lymphocyte population [18, 33].

1.3.8. Converting the Stroma from Tumor-Friendly to a Tumor-Hostile Environment

Primary cancers developing in the hotbed of a chronic inflammatory environment are induced and supported by the stroma of the tumor bed (cited in references [88, 89]) (in which the opposite effect, the anti-sarcoma effects the Coley toxins were marveled about). Primary cancers induced by oncogenic viruses or by genetic mutations eventually and subsequently subvert their stroma to provide growth factors and blood vessels to the tumor. A large and established primary cancer switches its growth tactics after metastatic tumors are separated from it. At this point of its existence, the large established primary tumor will produce neo-angiogenesis inhibitors (endostatins; angiostatins) to suppress the establishment of its own metastases [32]. However, the counter-strategy of the metastases is to subvert their new niche for the induction of support. Surgical removal of the large established tumor relieves the metastases from the exposure to neo-angiogenesis inhibitors secreted by the established primary tumor. Post-amputation osteosarcoma patients experienced these tragic consequences quite conspicuously. This author believes that the pioneering Swedish natural IFN clinical trials preventing post-amputation lung metastases (cited in reference [81]) were due to the anti-angiogenic effects of the IFNs. The author's associates presented selected case histories of patients with silent micrometastases, which rapidly manifested and established themselves after the surgical removal of the primary tumor [43]. This is the clinical setting in which postoperatively anti-neoangiogenesis agents (endostatins, interferons), cancer vaccines, adjuvant chemo- or targeted therapy, and all other means of tumor-suppressive interventions should be applied. Endostatins were tried against established large and metastatic tumors (and failed); endostatins should be tested in neo-adjuvant trials against micrometastases.

There are no established treatment protocols that would convert a tumor-friendly stroma into a tumor-hostile environment. There are biologically active potentially effective compounds that may alter the activities of stromal cells in the tumor bed. The plant alkaloid halofuginone is a quinazolinone; it inhibits collagen synthesis; down-regulates the kinase p38MAPK, the apoptosis inhibitor NFκB, the immunosuppressor and Th2-type immunity inducer TGFβ, and the proto-oncogenes/oncogenes ErbB2 and Met; it is anti-neoangiogenic; it may activate the tumor suppressor gene WT. Its immunomodulatory effects are unpredictable: it inhibits IL-4, a pro-Th2 agent, but also may suppress IFNγ and TNFα, which are proTh1 agents (reviewed in reference [89]). The peri- or intratumoral injection of IL-2, IL-12, or GM-CSF offer the best chance to alter the circumstances in the tumor's microenvironment from a tumor-friendly to a tumor-hostile attitude [5, 34, 47].

1.3.9. Introducing Naturally Oncolytic or Genetically Engineered Oncolytic Virus Therapy in Combination with Other Means of Therapy

Naturally oncolytic viruses often limit their replicative cycles to tumor cells, that are deprived of endogenous IFN production [94].

In tumor cells, the H/KRas oncoproteins, the guaninetriphosphate (GTP)-Ras, dephosphorylate the enzyme of the dsRNA-activated protein kinase (PKR). Cells with the inactive enzyme can not initiate IFN production; thus the Ras oncogenes create an IFN-free intracellular environment within tumor cells. Most naturally oncolytic viruses (Newcastle disease virus, NDV; reovirus; vesicular stomatitis virus, VSV) are suppressed by INF-producer healthy cells; however, in tumor cells these viruses replicate uninhibitedly and actually kill the tumor cells when the new viral progeny burst out of the infected cells. The genetically engineered oncolytic viruses (adenoviruses, herpes viruses, measles virus, retrolentivirus) carry pro-apoptotic genes (p53), and cyto/lymphokine genes (INFγ, IL-2, IL-12, GM-CSF) into tumor cells. In expressing these genes, the tumor cell may die an apoptotic death or attract immune T cells or stimulate DCs to generate an anti-tumor immune reaction. In themselves, or in combination with other means of therapy (biologicals; targeted therapy; reduced dosage chemotherapy), viral therapy of human tumors will be incorporated into the armamentarium of strong antitumor agents in the very near future [109]. An ONYX oncolytic adenovirus-related agent is being licensed for cancer therapy in China [21, 114].

1.3.10. Discovering New Anti-Tumor Antibiotics

Building on the old tradition, emerging from Rutgers' Waksman Institute (New Brunswick, N.J.) of the 1960s and 1970s, that antibiotics can kill cancer cells (actinomycin), or alter the host reactions to the tumor, in favor of the host, several powerful antibiotics were developed elsewhere for cancer therapy (adriamycin and its derivatives, bleomycin, mithramycin, mitomycin, neocarzinostatin). Newer developments include rapamycin, geldanamycin (ansamycin) and tunicamycin.

Rapamycins suppress mTOR signaling, suppress the PI3K/Akt "cell survival pathway", downregulate the anti-apoptotic survivin, and upregulate the pro-apoptotic p53. Curcumin (diferuloylmethane) imitates rapamycin by inhibiting the phosphorylation of the mTOR/Akt complex. The ansamycin, 17-AAG inhibits HSP90 and arrests the cell cycle in G1. Leukemic cells arrested in G_1 undergo apoptosis. Gastrointestinal stromal cell tumors with mutated c-*kit* oncogene are killed by 17-AAG. This geldanamycin inhibits the unison between the ligand hepatocyte growth factor/scatter factor and its receptor, the oncogene Met. In bone marrow stromal cells (*vide supra*) supporting mutated hematopoietic cells of myelodysplasia, 17-AAG suppresses VEGF production. Combined with rapamycin, the two antibiotics switch off the constitutively activated PI3K/Akt pathway in myeloma cells. Tunicamycin inhibited the replication of the Rous sarcoma virus. It inhibited the locomotion and metastasis formation of rhabdomyosarcoma cells and prevented the activation of Ewing sarcoma cells by mevalonates (reviewed in reference [89]). The newest developments include 17-demethoxy-geldanamycin (to surpass 17-AAG); chrysomycins for topoisomerase II inhibition; leptomycin analogue kazusamycin for inhibition of nuclear translocation of proteins, rebeccamycin for topoisomerase I inhibition; reveromycin for EGF inhibition; and many others to follow.

1.4. An Addition: The Armamentarium of the United Innate/Adaptive Immune Systems

Opsonized phagocytes, Toll-like receptors and their ligands, chemokines and their receptors, complement precursors, intracellular Nod-receptors, lectin-like and other humoral antibacterial substances in the hemolymph and specialized cells in coeloma cavities and in the lymph constitute the innate immune system, that sustained unicellular and the first multicellular organisms for millennia. Inhibitory RNA (iRNA) was probably the first antiviral defense (in the literature, RNAi is used both for RNA interference and initiator RNA at the translation initiation from a codon). The original molecules recognized later as proto-oncogenes fulfilled essential biochemical tasks without inducing cancers. The ascidian protochordate, the *Botryllus*, is loaded with active retrotransposons, but it is not known to have cancers. The ancestors of NK cells circulate in its hemolymph. Dendritic cells and NK cells cooperated in the innate system, but the thymus and the mucosa-associated lymphatic systems did not exist before the Cambrian explosion. The lamprey and the hagfish possess "lymphoid cells" and these cells operate somatically rearranged variable (V), leucine-rich receptors with anticipatory diversification (D). An invariant stalk tethers the receptor to the cell surface but the receptor may be released (solubilized) to encounter and neutralize the antigen in tissue fluids outside the cell. The somatic hypermutations of B cell and T cell receptors evolved first in the ancestors of the sharks; it was in the mucosa-associated lymphatic tissues from the thymus down to the intestines, where the complete V(D)J and RAG/RSS (recombination activating genes and signal sequences) elements of the adaptive immune system first operated in unison. Transposons of probable prokaryotic origin inserted the genes of these systems into the genomes of ancestral sharks. In the united innate and adaptive immune systems, Toll-like receptors respond first and induce the production of inflammatory chemokines and cytokines, including various forms of interferons. Professional antigen presenting cells (dendritic cells) present MHC-restricted antigens to CD4, CD8 and NK cells. If the DC cell is fully mature and the CD4 cell responds with INFγ secretion, a Th1-type immunological environment will develop, in which TNFα, IL-2 and IL-12 rule and immune CD8 T lymphocyte clones expand to kill those host cells that express the target antigens. Either perforins will lyse the target cell, or a FasL-to-Fas receptor-induced caspase cascade will result in the fragmentation of nuclear DNA and the targeted cell dies apoptotic, or programmed cell death. If the DC is immature and the CD4 cell secretes IL-4, a Th2-type immunological environment will be created, in which IL-10 dominates and the B cell compartments produces antibodies to react with the target antigens, Of the receptors of NK cells, antigens presented by MHC molecules do not necessarily activate the killer receptors; the killer receptors are activated when the NK cell cannot find the MHC molecules loaded with self peptides or when the cell presents virally encoded antigens to the NK cell. Cells with MHC molecules loaded with self peptides activate the inhibitory NK cell receptors and the NK cells "let go" without launching an attack. The trophoblast of the fetus also activates inhibitory receptors of maternal NK cells. Tumor cells without clear identification of self are attacked and killed by NK cells. The fetal thymus generates regulatory CD4 T cells, which recognize self-reactive CD8 T cells; the regulatory T cells release TGFβ to antagonize clonal expansion of self-reactive CD8 T cells. Even when T_{REG} cells are removed from the patient's blood by immunomagnetic leukapheresis, these cells rapidly repopulate and continue to antagonize adoptively infused T_{REG} cell-depleted immune T cell populations; high-dose IL-2 failed to tilt the balance to the favor of immune T effector cells [3]. Could NK/LAK cells with their killer receptors activated perform better [1, 5]? The emergence of NK_{REG} cells for the protection of the fetus characterizes normal pregnancy, whereas this NK cell population is depleted in cases of miscarriage [4]. Do malignant tumors enroll the help of NK_{REG} cells? The chemokine, stromal-derived factor-1 is frequently produced by tumor cells and attracts into the tumor's microenvironment regulatory T cells, which express the receptor for this chemokine. Thus, the tumor with the help of an innate chemokine subverts the regulatory T cells for its own promotion. Even when TIL (tumor infiltrating lymphocytes), or NK/LAK (lymphokine-activated killer) cells are expanded by IL-2 *ex vivo* and then are re-infused into the tumor-bearing patient, the resident regulatory T cell clones rise to oppose this intervention of therapeutic intent. It is not known how many subclinical tumor cell colonies may be rejected in the lifetime of the human host by the united innate and adaptive immune systems; but it is clearly evident that malignant tumors have means to disconnect the two systems and to prevail in opposition to them. Even when a "cancer vaccine" fails to induce a remission, it renders the host more susceptible for chemotherapy [95]. In a vaccinated cancer-bearing patient, the balance of the effector immune T cell and the T/NK_{REG} cell populations may favor the former over the latter and adoptive immune lymphocyte-mediated immunotherapy may be more effective in the pre-vaccinated patient (Sinkovics, J.G: Cytotoxic Lymphocytes in the Armamentarium of the Human Host [5]). In this volume, citations are made of the Sendai virus, as it antagonizes T_{REG} cells when the virus is directly injected into tumors, thus releasing anti-tumor immune reactions without opposition [2].

This addition has been written in response to a special request from Professor Mikhail Kiselevsky, to whom the author expresses his gratitude for the invitation to contribute a chapter to this volume.

References

[1] Alileche A, Plaisance S, Han DS, Rubinstein E, Mingari C, Bellomo R, Jasmin C, Azzarone B (1993) Human melanoma cell line M14 secretes functional interleukin-2. Oncogene 8(7): 1791–1796

[2] Ansell SM (2003) Adding cytokines to monoclonal antibody therapy: does the concurrent administration of interleukin-12 add to the efficacy of rituximab in B cell non-Hodgkin lymphoma? Leuk Lymphoma 44(8):1309–1315

[3] Antoine M, Reimers OK, Dickson C, Kiefer P (1997) Fibroblast growth factor 3, a protein with dual subcellular localization, is targeted to the nucleus and nucleolus by the concerted action of two nuclear localization signals and a nucleolar retention signal. J Biol Chem 272(47):29475–29481

[4] Arnaud E, Touriol C, Boutonnet C, Gensac MC, Vagner S, Prats H, Prats AC (1999) A new 34-kilodalton isoform of human fibroblast growth factor 2 is cap dependently synthesized by using a non-AUG start codon and behaves as a survival factor. Mol Cell Biol 19(1):505–514

[5] Arora A, Su G, Mathiowitz E, Reineke J, Chang AE, Sable MS (2006) Neoadjuvant intratumoral cytokine-loaded microspheres are superior to postoperative autologous cellular vaccines in generating systemic anti-tumor immunity. J Surg Oncol 94(5):403–412

[6] Bachmann M, Möröy T (2005) The serine/threonine kinase Pim-1. Int J Biochem Cell Biol 37(4):726–730

[7] Basler M, Groettrup M (2007) Advances in prostate cancer immunotherapies. Drugs Aging 24(3):197–221

[8] Blackburn SD, Wherry EJ (20076) IL-10, T cell exhaustion and viral persistence. Trends Microbiol 15(4)P:143–146

[9] Blackwood EM, Lugo TG, Kretzner L, King MW, Street AJ, Witte ON, Eisenman RN (1994) Functional analysis of the AUG- and CUG-initiated forms of the c-Myc protein. Mol Cell Biol 5(5):597–609

[10] Blank C, Kuball J, Voelkl S, Wiendl H, Becker B, Walter B, Majdic O, Gajewski TF, Theobald M, Andreesen R, Mackensen A (2006) Blockade of PD-L1 (B7-H1) augments human tumor-specific T cell responses in vitro. Int J Cancer 119(2):317–327

[11] Bonavida B (2007) Rituximab-induced inhibition of antiapoptotic cell survival pathways: implications in chemo/immunoresistance, rituximab unresponsiveness, prognostic and novel therapeutic interventions. Oncogene 26(25):3629–3636

[12] Bontkes HJ, Kramer D, Ruizendaal JJ, Kueter EW, van Tendeloo VF, Meijer CJ, Hooijberg E (2007) Dendritic cells transfected with interleukin-12 and tumor-associated messenger RNA induce high avidity cytotoxic T cells. Gene Ther 14(4):366–375

[13] Brooks DG, Trifilo MJ, Edelmann KH, Teyton L, McGavern DB, Oldstone MB (2006) Interleukin-10 determines viral clearance or persistence *in vivo.* Nat Med 12(11): 1246–1248

[14] Burger JA, Tsukada N, Burger M, Zvaifler NJ, Del'Aquila M, Kipps TJ (2000) Blood-derived nurse-like cells protect chronic lymphocytic leukemia B cells from spontaneous apoptosis through stromal cell-derived factor-1. Blood 96(8):2655–2663

[15] Buschle M, Campana D, Carding SR, Richard C, Hoffbrand AV, Bernner MK (1993) Interferon gamma inhibits apoptotic cell death in B cell chronic lymphocytic leukemia. J Exp Med 177(1):213–218

[16] Bruening W, Pelletier J (1996) A non-AUG translational initiation event generates novel WT1 isoforms. J Biol Chem 271(15):8646–8654

[17] Cassel WA, Murray DR, Olkowski SZL (2005) Newcastle disease virus oncolysate in the management of stage III malignant melanoma. In: Reference 94, pp 677–689

[18] Coccoris M, de Witte MA, Schumacher TN (2005) Prospects and limitations of T cell receptor gene therapy. Curr Gene Ther 5(6):583–593

[19] Corcelette S, Massé T, Madjar JJ (2000) Initiation of transition by non-AUG codons in human T-cell lymphotropic virus type I mRNA encoding both Rex and Tax regulatory proteins. Nucleic Acid Res 28(7):1625–1634

[20] Coudrec B, Prats H, Bayard F, Amalric F (1991) Potential oncogenic effects of basic fibroblast growth factor requires cooperation between CUG and AUG-initiated forms. Cell Regul 2(9):709–718

[21] Crompton AM, Kirn DH (2007) From ONYX-015 to armed vaccinia viruses: the education and evolution of oncolytic virus development. Curr Cancer Drug Targets 7(2):133–139

[22] Czerniecki BJ, Koski GK, Koldovsky U, Xu S, Cohen PA, Mick R, Nisenbaum H, Pasha T, Xu M, Fox KR, Weinstein S, Orel SG, Vonderheidre R, Coukos G, DeMichele A, Araujo L, Spitz FR, Rosen M, Levine BL, June C, Zhang PJ (2007) Targeting HER-2/neu in early breast cancer development using dendritic cells with staged interleukin-12 burst secretion. Cancer Res 67(4):1842–1852

[23] Dang Y, Knutson KL, Goodell V, dela Rosa C, Salazar LG, Higgins D, Childs J, Disis ML (2007) Tumor antigen-specific T-cell expansion is greatly facilitated by *in vivo* priming. Clin Cancer Res 13(6):1883–1891

[24] Depeiges A, Degroote F, Espagnol MC, Picard G (2006) Translation initiation by non-AUG codons in Arabidopsis thaliana transgenic plants. Plant Cell Rep 25(1):55–61

[25] Dessureault S, Alsarraj M, McCarthy S, Hunter T, Noyes D, Lee D, Harkins J, Seigne J, Jennings R, Antonia SJ (2005) A GM-CSF/CD40L producing cell augments anti-tumor T cell responses. J Surg Res 125(2): 173–181

[26] Dhodapkar NV, Geller MD, Chang DH, Shimizu K, Fujii S, Dhodapkar KM, Krasovsky J (2003) A reversible defect in natural killer T cell function characterizes the progression of premalignant to malignant multiple myeloma. J Exp Med 197(12):1667–1676

[27] Döme B, Tímár J, Dobos J, Mészáros L, Raso E, Paku S, Kenessey I, Ostoros G, Magyar M, Ladányi A, Bogos K, Tóvári J (2006) Identification and clinical significance of circulating endothelial progenitor cells in human non-small cell lung cancer. Cancer Res 66(14):7341–7347

[28] Dörrschuck A, Schmidt A, Schnürner E, Glückmann M, Albrecht C, Wölfel C, Lennerz V, Lifke A, Di Natale C, Ranieri E, Gesualdo L, Huber C, Karas M, Wölfel T, Herr W (2004) CD8+ cytotoxic T lymphocytes isolated from allogeneic healthy donors recognize HLA classIa/Ib-associated renal carcinoma antigens with ubiquitous or restricted tissue expression. Blood 104(8):2591–2599

[29] Dupont PJ, Warrens AN (2007) Fas ligand exerts its pro-inflammatory effects via neutrophil recruitment but not activation. Immunology 120(1):133–139

[30] Editorial (2007) Plerixafor: AMD 3100, AMD3100, JM 3100, SDZ SID 791. Drugs R D 8(2):113–119

[31] Engels B, Noessner E, Frankenberger B, Blankenstein T, Schendel DJ, Uckert W (2005) Redirecting human T lymphocytes toward renal cell carcinoma specificity by retroviral transfer of T cell receptor genes. Human Gene Ther 16(&):799–810

[32] Folkman J (2002) Role of angiogenesis in tumor growth and metastasis. Semin Oncol 29(16): 15–18S

[33] Fujii S, Nishimura MI, Lotze MT (2005) Regulatory balance between the immune response of tumor antigen-specific T-cell receptor gene-transduced CD8 T cells and the suppressive effect of tolerogenic dendritic cells. Cancer Sci 96(12):897–902

[34] Galili U, Wigglesworth K, Abdel-Motal UM (2007) Intratumoral injection of alpha-gal glycolipids induces xenograft-like destruction and conversion of lesions into endogenous vaccines. J Immunol 178(7):4676–4687

[35] Gilboa E(2007) DC-based cancer vaccines. J Clin Invest 117(5):1195–1203

[36] Goillot E, Combaret V, Ladenstein R, Baubet D, Blay JY, Philip T, Favrot MC (1992) Tumor necrosis factor as an autocrine growth factor for neuroblastoma. Cancer Res 52(11):3194–3200

[37] Gomes AC, Costa T, Carreto L, Santos MA (2006) The molecular mechanism of changes in the genetic code. Mol Biol (Moskva) 40(4):634–639

[38] Gordon K, Fütterer J, Hohn T (1992) Efficient initiation of translation at non-AUG triplets in plant cells. Plant 2(5):809–813

[39] Han D, Pottin-Clemenceau C, Imro MA, Scudeletti M, Doucet C, Puppo F, Brouty-Boye D, Vedrenne J, Sahraoui Y, Brailly H, Poggi A, Jasmin C, Azzarone B, Indiveri F (1996) IL-2 triggers a tumor progression process in a melanoma cell line MELP derived from a patient whose metastasis increased in size during IL-2/IFN alpha biotherapy. Oncogene 12(5):1015–1023

[40] Hansson L Abdalla AO, Mosfegh A, Choudhury A, Rabbani H, Nilsson B, Osterborg A, Mellstedt H (2007) Long-term idiotype vaccination combined with interleukin-12 (IL-12), or IL-12 and granulocyte macrophage colony-stimulating factor, in early-stage multiple myeloma patients. Clin Cancer Res 13(5):1503–1510

[41] Hamid O, Solomon JC, Scotland R, Garcia M, Sian S, Ye W, Groshen SL, Weber JS (2007) Alum with interkeukin-12 augments immunity to a melanoma vaccine: correlation with time to relapse in patients with resected high-risk disease. Clin Cancer Res 13(1):215–222

[42] Höglund P, Klein E (2006) Natural killer cells and cancer. Semin Cancer Biol 16: 331–332

[43] Horak A, Horvath J, Sinkovics JG (1998) Cancer therapy by anti-angiogenesis. Arch Hung Med Assoc 6(2):9

[44] Huez I, Bornes S, Bresson D, Créancier L, Prats H (2001) New vascular endothelial growth factor isoform generates by internal ribosome

entry site-driven CUG translation initiation. Mol Endocrinol 15(12):2197–2210

[45] Johnson LA, Heemskerk B, Powell CJ, Cohen CJ, Morgan RA, Dudley ME, Robbins PF, Rosenberg SA (2006) Gene transfer of tumor-reactive TCR confers both high avidity and tumor reactivity to nonreactive peripheral blood mononuclear cells and tumor-infiltrating lymphocytes. J Immunol 177(9):6548–6559

[46] Kausche S, Wehler T, Schnürer E, Lennerz V, Brenner W, Melchior S, Gröne M, Nonn M, Strand S, Meyer R, Ranieri E, Huber C, Falk CS, Herr W (2006) Superior antitumor *in vitro* responses of allogeneic matched sibling compared with autologous patient CD8+ T cells. Cancer Res 66(23):11447–11454

[47] Kilinc MO, Aulakh KS, Nair RE, Jones SA, Alard P, Kosiewicz MM, Egilmez NK (2006) Reversing tumor immune suppression with intra-tumoral IL-12: activation of tumor-associated T effector/memory cells, induction of T suppressor apoptosis, and infiltration of CD8+ T effectors. J Immunol 177(10): 6962–6973

[48] Knuth A, Dippold W, Meyer zum Bueschenfelde KH (1984) Target level blocking of T-cell cytotoxicity for human malignant melanoma by monoclonal antibodies. Cell Immunol 83(2):398–403

[49] Knutson KL, Disis ML (2004) IL-12 enhances the generation of tumor antigen-specific Th11 CD4 T cells during *ex vivo* expansion. Clin Exp Immunol 135(2):322–329

[50] Köpke AK, Leggatt PA (1991) Initiation of translation at an AUA codon for an archaebacterial protein gene expressed in E. coli. Nucleic Acid Res 19(19):5169–5172

[51] Li ZL, Chang JW, Zhang SM, Ma FL, Zhang HS, Ma TX (2004) Generation of specific cytotoxic T lymphocytes induced by tumor-derived heat shock protein 90-peptide complexes *in vitro*. Zhonghua Yi Xue Za Zhi (Beijing) 84(20):1701–1704

[52] Liang H, Hittelman W, Nagarajan L (1996) Ubiquitous expression and cell cycle regulation of the protein kinase PIM-1. Arch Biochem Biophys 330(2):259–265

[53] Marth C, Egle D, Auer D, Rössler J, Zeimet AG, Vergote I, Daxenbichler G (2007) Modulation of CA-125 tumor market shedding in ovarian cancer cells by erlotinib or cetuximab. Gynecol Oncol 105(3):716–721

[54] McKallip R, Li R, Ladisch S (1999) Tumor gangliosides inhibit the tumor-specific immune response. J Immunol 163(7):3718–3726

[55] Mehdi H, Ono E, Gupta KC (1990) Initiation of translation at CUG, GUG, and ACG codons in mammalian cells. Gene 91(2):173–178

[56] Miranda I, Silva, Santos MA (2006) Evolution of the genetic code in yeasts. Yeast 23(3): 203–213

[57] Mosca PJ, Lyerly HK, Clay TM, Morse MA, Lyerly HK (2007) Dendritic cell vaccines. Front Biosci 12:4050–4060

[58] Muralidhar S, Veytsmann G, Chandran B, Ablashi D, Doniger J, Rosenthal LJ (2000) Characterization of the human herpesvirus 8 (Kaposi's sarcoma-associated herpesvirus) oncogene, kaposin (ORF K12). J Clin Virol 16(3):203–213

[59] Nair S, Boczkowski D, Fassnacht M, Pisetsky D, Gilboa E (2007) Vaccination against the forkhead family transcription factor Foxp3 enhances tumor immunity. Cancer Res 67(1):371–380

[60] Németh AL, Medveczky P, Tóth J, Siklódi E, Schlett K, Patthy A, Palkovits M, Ovádi J, Tokési N, Németh P, Szilágyi L, Gráf L (2007) Unconventional translation initiation of human trypsinogen 4 at a CUG codon with an N-terminal leucine. A possible means to regulate gene expression. FEBS J 274(6):1610–1620

[61] Noiman S, Yaniv A, Tsach T, Miki T, Tronick SR, Gazit A (1991) The Tat protein of equine infectious anemia virus is encoded by at least three types of transcripts. Virology 184(2): 521–530

[62] Ogino T, Moriai S, Ishida Y, Ishii H, Katayama A, Miyokawa N, Harabuchi Y, Ferrone S (2007) Association of immunoescape mechanisms with Epstein-Barr virus infection in nasopharyngeal carcinoma. Int J Cancer 120(11):2401–2410

[63] Oosterwijk-Wakka JC, Tiemessen DM, Bleumer I, de Vries IJ, Jongmans W, Adema GJ, Debruyne FM, de Mulder PH, Oosterwijk E, Mulder PF (1997) Vaccination of patients with metastatic renal cell carcinoma with autologous dendritic cells pulsed with autologous tumor antigens in combination with interleukin-2: a phase I study. J Immunother 25(6):500–508

[64] Orentas RJ, Kohler ME, Johnson BD (2006) Suppression of anticancer immunity by regulatory T cells: back to the future. Semin Cancer Biol 16:137–149

[65] Peabody DS (1989) Translation initiation at non-AUG triplets in mammalian cells. J Biol Chem 264(9):5031–503

[66] Podack ER (1988) Cytolytic Lymphocytes and Complement: Effectors of the Immune System. Volume II. CRC Press, Boca Raton 1–235

[67] Prats AC, De Billy G, Wang P, Darlix JL (1989) CUG initiation codon used for the synthesis of a cell surface antigen coded by the murine leukemia virus. J Mol Biol 205(2):363–372

[68] Qin JZ, Kamarashev J, Zhang CL, Dummer R, Burg G, Döbbeling U (2001) Constitutive and interleukin-7- and interleukin-15-stimulated DNA binding of STAT and novel factors in cutaneous T cell lymphoma cells. J Invest Dermatol 117(3):583–589

[69] Raval G, Biswas S, Rayman P, Biswas K, SA G, Ghosh S, Thornton M, Hilston C, Das T, Bukowski R, Finke J, Tannenbaum CS (2007) TNF-alpha induction of GM2 expression on renal cell carcinomas promotes T cell dysfunction. J Immunol 178(10):6642–6652

[70] Reeves ME, Royal RE, Lam JS, Rosenberg SA, Hwu P (1996) Retroviral transduction of human denditic cells with a tumor-associated antigen gene. Cancer Res 56(24):5672–5677

[71] Rosenberg SA, Dudley ME (2004) Cancer regression in patients with metastatic melanoma after the transfer of autologous anti-tumor lymphocytes. Proc Natl Acad Sci USA 101(S2):14639–14645

[72] Sadler R, Wu L, Forghani B, Renne R, Zhong W, Herndier B, Ganem D (1999) A complex translational program generates multiple novel proteins from the latently expressed kaposin (K12) locus of Kaposi's sarcoma-associated herpesvirus. J Virol 73(7):5722–5730

[73] Santos MA, Tuite MF (1995) The CUG codon is decoded *in vivo* as serine and not lucine in Candida albicans. Nucleic Acid Res 23(9):1481–1486

[74] Saris CJ, Domen J, Berns A (1991) The pim-1 oncogene encodes two related protein-serine/threonine kinases by alternative initiation at AUG and CUG. EMBO J 10(3):655–664

[75] Schlitz RL, Shih DS, Rasty S, Montelaro RC, Rushlow KE (1992) Equine infectious anemia virus gene expression: characterization of the RNA splicing pattern and the protein products encoded by open reading frames S1 and S2. J Virol 66(6):3455–3465

[76] Schmitt A, Hus I, Schmitt M (2007) Dendritic cell vaccines for leukemia patients. Expert Rev Anticancer Ther 7(3):275–283

[77] Schwab SR, Shugart JA, Horng T, Malarkannan S, Shastri N (2004) Unanticipated antigens: translation initiation at CUG with leucine. PLoS Biol 2(11):366 (19 pages)

[78] Shevach EM (2004) Fatal attraction: tumors beckon regulatory T cells. Nat Med 10(9):900–901

[79] Shinohara H, Yagita H, Ikawa Y, Oyaizu N (2000) Fas drives cell cycle progression in glioma cells via extracellular signal-regulated kinase activation. Cancer Res 60(6): 1766–1772

[80] Shirako Y (1998) Non-AUG translation initiation in a plant RNA virus: a forty-amino-acid extension is added to the N terminus of the soil-borne wheat mosaic virus capsid protein. J Virol 72(2):1677–2682

[81] Sinkovics JG (1986) The Swedish adjuvant leukocyte IFN trials. In: Medical Oncology an Advanced Course. Sinkovics JG, single author. Marcel Dekker, New York, volume II 1455

[82] Sinkovics JG (1986) A reappraisal of cytotoxic lymphocytes in human tumor immunology. In: Cancer Biology and Therapeutics. Cory JG, Szentivanyi A, editors. Plenum Press, New York London 225–253

[83] Sinkovics JG (1988) Oncogenes and growth factors. CRC Crit Rev Immunol 8(4):217–298

[84] Sinkovics JG (1995) The graft-versus-leukemia GvL reaction: its early history, value in human bone marrow transplantation and recent developments concerning its mechanism and induction. In: Autologous Marrow and Blood Transplantation. Proc 7th Internat Symposium 1994, Arlington, Texas. Dicke KS. Keating A, editors. Cancer Treatment Research & Educational Institute, Arlington 305–318

[85] Sinkovics JG (1997) Malignant lymphoma arising from natural killer cells: report of the first case in 1970 and newer developments in the FasL → FasR system. Acta Microbiol Immunol Hung 44(3):295–306 (Erratum: the Fas receptor is CD95)

[86] Sinkovics JG (2005) A notable phenomenon recapitulated. A fusion product of a murine lymphoma cell and a leukemia-virus-neutralizing antibody-producer host plasma cell formed spontaneously and secreting the specific antibody continuously. Acta Microbiol Immunol Hung (Budapest) 52(1):1–40

[87] Sinkovics JG (2005) The first observation (in the late 1960s) of fused lymphoid cells continuously secreting a specific antibody. Bull Mol Med (Cluj Napoca/Kolozsvár) 26(W):61–80

[88] Sinkovics JG (2007) Adult human sarcomas. I. Basic science. Expert Rev Anticancer Ther 7(1):31–56

[89] Sinkovics JG (2007) Adult human sarcomas. II. Medical oncology. Expert Rev Anticancer Ther 7(2):183–210

[90] Sinkovics JG, Cabiness JR, Shullenberger CC (1972) Monitoring *in vitro* immune reactions to solid tumors. Front Rad Ther Oncol 7:99–119

[91] Sinkovics JG, Horvath JC (2000) Vaccination against human cancers. Int J Oncol 16:81–96

[92] Sinkovics JG, Horvath JC (2001) Virological and immunological connotations of apoptotic and anti-apoptotic forces in neoplasia. Int J Oncol 19:473–488

[93] Sinkovics JG, Horvath JC (2005) Human natural killer cells: a comprehensive review. Int J Oncol 27:5–47

[94] Sinkovics JG, Horvath JC, authors, editors (2005) Viral Therapy of Human Cancers. Marcel Dekker, New York iii-xiii 1–829

[95] Sinkovics JG, Horvath JC (2006) Evidence accumulating in support of cancer vaccines combined with chemotherapy: a pragmatic review of past and present efforts. Int J Oncol 29:765–777

[96] Sinkovics JG, Horvath JC (2006) The molecular biology and immunology of glioblastoma multiforme (GMF) with the presentation of an immunotherapy protocol for a clinical trial. Acta Microbiol Immunol Hung 53(4): 367–429

[97] Sinkovics JG, Shirato E, Gyorkey F, Cabiness JR, Howe CD (1970) Relationship between lymphoid neoplasms and immunologic functions. In: Leukemia-Lymphoma. A Collection of Papers Presented at the Fourteenth Annual Clinical Conference on Cancer, 1969 at The University of Texas M. D. Anderson Hospital and Tumor Institute at Houston, Texas. Year Book Medical Publishers, Chicago 53–92

[98] Sinkovics JG, Shirato E, Martin FG, Cabiness JR, White ED (1971) Chondrosarcoma. Immune reactions of a patient to autologous tumor. Cancer 27:782–793

[99] Sinkovics J, Szakács J, Horváth J, Györkey F, Györkey P, Gergely AS (2006) Kaposi-sarcoma. Orvosi Hetilap (Budapest) 147(13):617–621

[100] Slavin S, Naparstek E, Nagler A, Ackerstein A, Weiss L, Or R (1995) Allogeneic cell-mediated immunotherapy (allo-CMI) using matched peripheral blood lymphocytes for prevention and treatment of relapse following bone marrow transplantation. In: Autologous Marrow and Blood Transplantation. Proc 7th Int Symposium, 1994. Dicke KA, Keating A, editors. The Cancer Treatment Research and Educational Institute, Arlington, Texas 271–280

[101] Stein MN, Shin J, Gudzowaty O, Bernstein AM, Liu LM (2006) Antibody-dependent cytotoxicity to breast cancer targets despite inhibitory KIR signaling. Anticancer Res 26(3A): 1759–1763

[102] Straube C, Wehner R, Wendisch M, Bornhäuser M, Bachmann M, Rieber EP, Schmitz M (2007) Bortezomib significantly impairs the immunostimulatory capacity of human myeloid blood dendritic cells. Leukemia 21(7):1454–1471

[103] Stritzke J, Zunkel T, Steinmann J, Schmitz N, Uharek L, Zeis M (2003) Therapeutic effects of idiotype vaccination can be enhanced by the combination of granulocyte-macrophage colony-stimulating factor and interleukin-1 in a myeloma model. Br J Haematol 120(1): 27–35

[104] Takahashi T, Tanaka M, Ogasawara J, Suda T, Murakami H, Nagata S (1996) Swapping between Fas and granulocyte colony-stimulating factor receptor. J Biol Chem 271(29):17555–17560

[105] Tímár J, Tóth J (2000) Tumor sinuses – vascular channels. Pathol Oncol Res 6(2):83–86

[106] Tourkova IL, Shurin GV, Chatta GS, Perez L, Finke J, Whiteside TL, Ferrone S, Shurin MR (2005) Restoration by IL-15 of MHC class I antigen-processing machinery in human dendritic cells inhibited by tumor-derived gangliosides. J Immunol 175(5): 3045–3052

[107] Uzzo RG, Rayman P, Kolenko V, Clark PE, Cathcart MK, Bloom T, Novick AC, Bukowski RM, Hamilton T, Finke JH (1999) Renal cell carcinoma-derived gangliosides suppress nuclear factor-kappaB activation in T cells. J Clin Invest 104(6):769–776

[108] Vagner S, Touriol C, Galy B, Audigier S, Gensac MC, Amalridc F, Bayard F, Prats H, Prats AC (1996) Translation of CUG- but not AUG-initiated forms of human fibroblast growth factor 2 is activated in transformed and stressed cells. J Cell Biol 135(5): 1391–1402

[109] Vähä-Koskela MJ, Heikkilä JE, Hinkkanen AE (2007) Oncolytic viruses in cancer therapy Cancer Lett 254(2):178–216

[110] Vile FG (2006) Viral mediated cell fusion: viral fusion – the making or breaking of a tumor? Gene Ther 13(15):1127–1130

[111] Wada A, Tada Y, Kawamura K, Takiguchi K, Tatsumi K, Kuriyama T, Takenouchi T, O-Wang J, Takawa M (2007) The effects of FasL on inflammation and tumor survival are

dependent on its expression levels. Cancer Gene Ther 14(3):262–267

[112] Weber J, Sondak VK, Scotland R, Philips R, Wang F, Rubio V, Stuge TB, Groshen SG, Gee C, Jeffery GG, Sian S, Lee PP (2003) Granulocyte-macrophage-colony-stimulating factor added to a multipeptide vaccine for resected stage II melanoma. Cancer 97(1):186–200

[113] Xia X (2005) Mutation and selection on the anticodon of tRNA genes in vertebrate mitochondrial genomes. Gene 345(1):13–20

[114] Yu W, Fang H (2007) Clinical trials with oncolytic adenovirus in China. Curr Cancer Drug Targets 7(2):141–148

References to Addendum

[1] Farag SS, Fehniger TA, Beckner B, Blaser BW, Caliguri MA (2003) New directions in natural killer cell-based immunotherapy of human cancer. Expert Opin Biol Ther (32):237–250

[2] Kurooka M, Kaneda Y (2007) Inactivated Sendai virus particles eradicate tumors by inducing immune responses through blocking regulartory T cells. Cancer Res 67(1):227–236

[3] Powell DJ, de Vries CR, Allen T, Ahmadzadeh M, Rosenberg SA (1997) Inability to mediate prolonged reduction of regulatory T cells after transfer of autologous CD25-depleted PBMC and interleukin-2 after lymphodepleting chemotherapy. J Immunother 30(4):438–4

[4] Shigeru S, Akitoshi N, Subaru MH, Shiozaki A (2007) The balance between cytotoxic NK cells and regulatory NK cells in human pregnancy. J Reprod Immunol June 8 EPUB

[5] Sinkovics JG: 2007 Cytotoxic Lymphocytes in the Armamentarium of the Human Host. Manuscript of the monograph with over 1800 references, 12 Tables and 12 Figures submitted to Publisher.

[6] Woan K, Reddy V (2007) Potential therapeutic role of natural killer cells in cancer. Expert Opin Biol Ther 7(1):17–29

2. Tumor microenvironment genesis and implications on cancer immune response

GIANFRANCO BARONZIO

Family Medicine Area ASL1 Legnano
(Mi) and Radiotherapy
Hyperthermia Service
Policlinico di Monza
Monza
Italy

ISABEL FREITAS

Department of Animal Biology and IGM-CNR
Center for Histochemistry and Cytometry
University of Pavia
Pavia
Italy

Keywords: Cancer cells, tumor microenvironment, hypoxia, fibroblasts, macrophages, lymphocytes, myeloid cells, T regulatory cells (T_{reg}), tumor interstitial fluid (TIF), chronic inflammation, immune activity suppression

Abstract

A tumor mass is an association of normal cells and epigenetically modified cells in continuous evolution. Different normal cells are forced to survive in a hostile environment produced in contact with cancer cells. In fact, fibroblasts and a complex infiltrate of neutrophils, macrophages, lymphocytes and mast cells work in concert with neoplastic cells to create a distinctive microenvironment that allows tumor progression. Fibroblasts can be considered orchestra conductors that contribute to the production of inflammatory reaction and neovasculature at the tumor periphery. This reaction is initially an attempt to restrain tumor growth but this capacity is progressively lost in the environment that ensues. In this review we will describe the various pathophysiological interactions among the different cell populations carrying to the tumor stroma generation. Special emphasis will be attributed to the interstitial fluid, neoangiogenesis and the hypoxic areas present in the tumor area that determine failure and the evasion from the immune system *in situ*.

M.V. Kiselevsky (ed.), Atlas Effectors of Anti-tumor Immunity, 25–43.

2.1. Pathophysiologic Mechanisms Generating Tumor Hypoxia, Angiogenesis and Tumor Interstitial Fluid (TIF)

The majority of human neoplasias are of epithelial origin and cancer cells are the result of the accumulation of somatic mutations in these epithelial cells [41]. Neoplastic cells however do not live alone. To survive inside the tumor area they need to create contact and interaction with a network of cell types that make up the normal context of the original tissue. The normal cell types that make up the non-tumor components include transformed fibroblasts (or cancer-associated fibroblasts, *CAFs*), lymphocytes, neutrophils, endothelial cells inflammatory cells, adipocytes, tumor-associated macrophages (*TAMs*), eosinophils and mast cells [77].

Neoplastic and non-neoplastic cells are in turn embedded in a supporting structure, the extra cellular matrix (*ECM*), which is composed of a variable proportion of proteins and polysaccharides (glycosaminoglicans, proteoglycans and glycoproteins) organized in a 3D network. The complex of cellular components and *ECM* represent the tumor stroma. Furthermore, ECM can act as a reservoir of growth factors permitting both normal and neoplastic cells to exchange information and nutritive substances [34, 111]. Intermingled between the *ECM* and the cellular context, a liquid phase is also present. Liquid-rich areas are particularly abundant in the tumor mass, forming liquid pouches defined by Gullino as the tumor interstitial fluid (*TIF*) [39, 40] (Figures 2.1 and 2.2).

A tumor is a continuously evolving structure which, according to current models, shows two main phases: an avascular and a vascular phase [10, 79]. The growth of tumors beyond a critical mass >1–2 mm^3 (10^6 cells) is dependent on an adequate blood supply [26, 103]. Up to a distance from host vessel of 100–200 μm the initial foci of neoplastic cells (*avascular phase*) receive their nutrients and oxygen by diffusion (Figure 2.3). Beyond

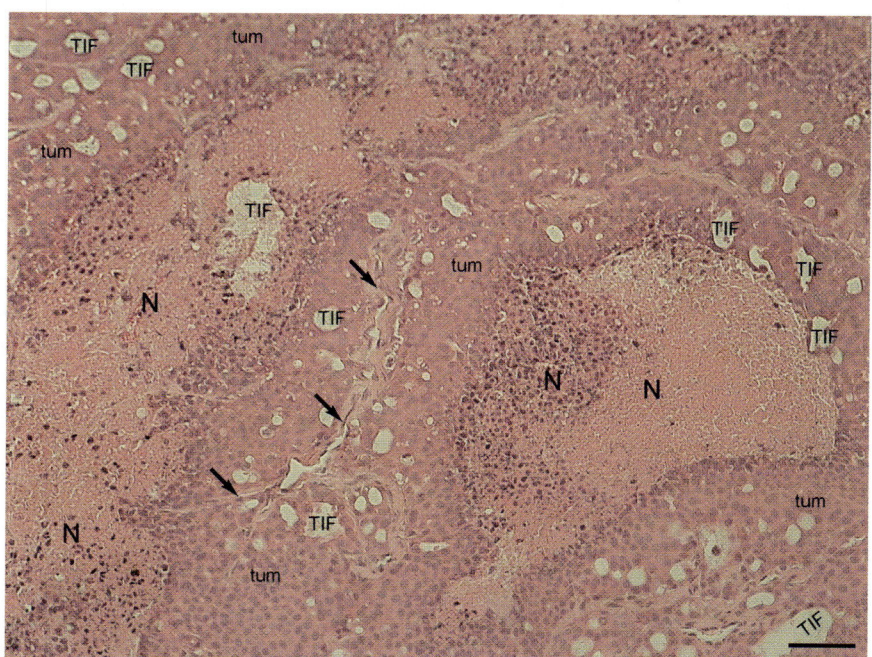

Figure 2.1. Tumor cuffs around blood vessels (arrows). H&E. N: necrosis; tum: tumor cells; TIF: tumor interstitial fluid. Scale bar: 50 μm

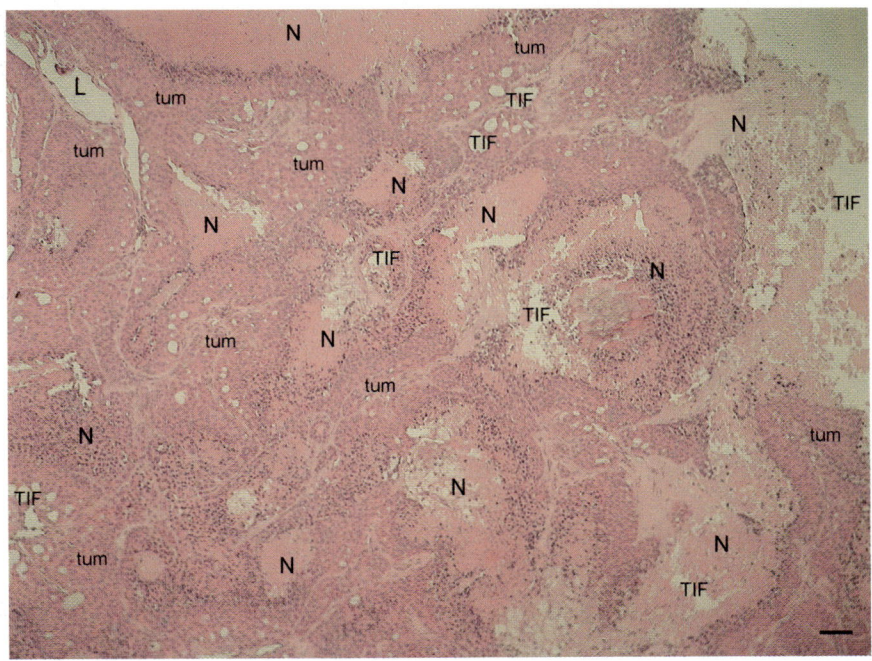

Figure 2.2. Tumor microenvironments under low magnification. H&E. N: necrosis; tum: tumor cells; TIF: tumor interstitial fluid; L: lymph vessels. Scale bar: 50 μm

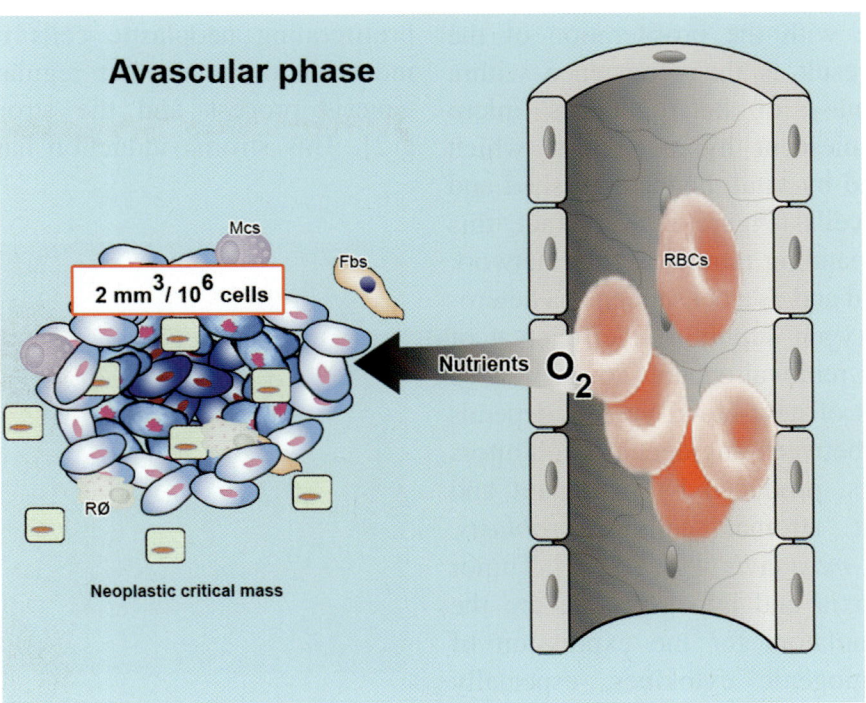

Figure 2.3. Tumor mass surrounded by normal cells and recruited macrophages and fibroblasts. Until a mass of 2 mm³, cancer cells obtain nutritive substances and oxygen by diffusion

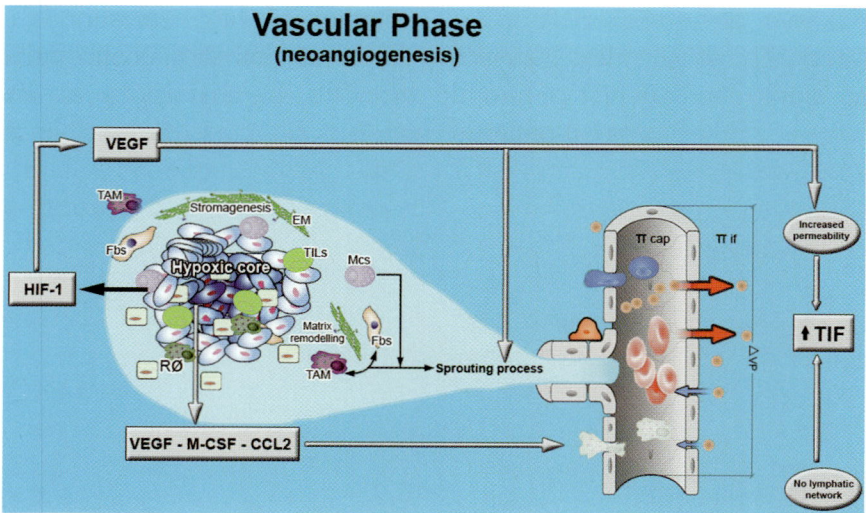

Figure 2.4. The principal steps which carry to the tumor neoangiogenesis are illustrated

this distance and beyond a critical mass of $2\,mm^3$, hypoxia occurs and the need for an adequate blood supply is crucial (*vascular phase*) (Figure 2.4) [26, 103].

However, the establishment of a neovascular supply in the attempt to overcome hypoxia is inefficient, irregular and may not keep in pace with the proliferation of the tumor. The result is the persistence within the tumor mass of heterogeneous micro regions of quiescent hypoxic cells, which are surrounded by vital, better nourished and proliferating cells (Figure 2.5). In fact, this constantly expanding tumor vascular network is disorganized and as a consequence a heterogeneity of oxygen supply and efficiency of waste product removal occurs [26, 103].

The genesis of new blood vessels depends on a balance between angiogenesis inhibitors and promoters, produced by malignant and non-malignant stromal cells (*fibroblasts, macrophages, mast cells*) [10, 25, 77]. Tumor regional hypoxia and hypoglycemia are the principal stimulators for the expression of local pro-angiogenic cytokines, especially vascular endothelial growth factor (VEGF) (Figure 2.4) [10, 25, 26, 79, 104]. The early response gene that encodes hypoxia inducible factor-1 (HIF-1) and in particular

its subunits (HIF-1a and -1b) regulate VEGF expression. HIF-1 is a protein of 120 kDa, a member of the basic helix-loop-helix superfamily transcription factors, and its expression is very sensitive to oxygen concentration (1% O_2) [87].

The adaptation to hypoxia by formerly proliferating neoplastic cells results in the induction of genes that regulate the angiogenesis process and the stroma induction [12]. This stroma induction has been called

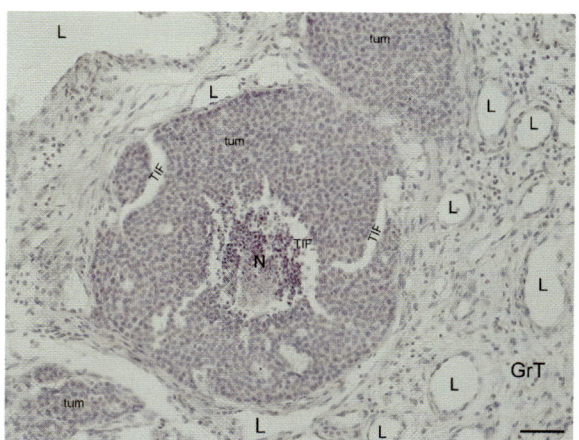

Figure 2.5. A tumor cord with inner necrosis (N) apparently nourished by lymph vessels (L) and the tumor interstitial fluid (TIF): Hematoxylin. GT: granulation tissue. Scale bar: 50 μm

by some authors the tumor stromagenesis process [7]. Recent studies have shown that HIF-1 and VEGF transcripts are over-expressed by several human neoplastic cells including breast, prostate, gastric, colon, lung, bladder and endometrium cells and they are more active in hypoxic and necrotic areas. VEGF is correlated to vascular density, especially in brain tumors and it is associated with bad prognoses [43, 58]. VEGF, which also acts as a vascular permeability factor (VPF) is a 32–44-KDa protein exerting different effects on endothelial cells (EC), going from EC motility to increased perme-ability [43]. It becomes active by binding to three high-affinity tyrosine kinase receptors [VEGFR-1(flt-1), VEGFR-2(KDR/Flk-1) and VEGFR-3(Flt-4)] which are highly expressed on endothelial tumor vessels but not on mature vessels [68]. They exert different effects on endothelial cells (ECs). In particular, VEGFR-1 mediates EC motility, VEGFR-2 regulates vascular permeability and VEGFR-3 lymphoangiogenesis [49]. The increased permeability induced by VEGF associated to an altered Starling's equation of capillary forces working in the tumor context leads to TIF formation [22, 30, 64]. TIF is a fluid mixture intermingled among the various cells that compose the stroma and is characteristic of most solid tumors [30, 39, 40]. This fluid is derived from plasma leaked from venules rendered hyper-permeable due to VPF/VEGF expression by hypoxic tumor cells after clotting with the tumor mass [22]. Therefore, at the moment of its genesis, the TIF is made up of serum, rich in nutrients and platelet-derived growth factors. It is important to recall that in the wound healing process, tumor stromatoge-nesis mimics [22]. A key role of the exudate is that of nourishing the cells of the granu-lation tissue and carrying away their waste products. The TIF has therefore a trophic role for tumor and stromal cells. However, whereas in wound healing lymphatic vessels the TIF

progressively accumulates in areas opposing low mechanical resistance, in particular at the necrosis edge and along the connective tissue that sheathes muscle and nerve fibers; furthermore, its overproduction at the tumor edge facilitates the process of invasion. The accumulation of TIF in confined spaces causes a progressive increase of the tumor inter-stitial fluid pressure (TIFP). In addition, the TIF generates shear stress and/or mechanical stretch that can influence the proliferation, apoptosis and/or differentiation of malignant and stromal cells via an integrin-mediated mechanotransduction process [74, 94].

Starling's law is the simplest mathematical description of liquid compartmentalization between the circulation and the interstitial fluid [13, 95]. Water flux across the capillary membrane is determined by a difference of hydrostatic pressure existing between the arterial and the venous end of capillary [a − v Δp], which normally drives filtration from the plasma into the interstitium, and the osmotic pressure of proteins, Π, which acts to absorb fluid into the plasma. The expression of the rate at which water moves across the capillary wall can be expressed in quantitative terms by the following equation:

$$\mathbf{J_v} = \mathbf{K_f}[(\mathbf{a} - \mathbf{v\Delta p} - \mathbf{p_{if}}) - (\Pi_{cap} - \Pi_{if})] - \mathbf{L} \qquad (2.1)$$

where $\mathbf{J_v}$ is the flux of water from capillary to interstitium, $\mathbf{K_f}$ is the hydraulic conduc-tance, Π_{cap} is the osmotic pressure in the capillary and Π_{if} is the osmotic pressure in the interstitium. Associated with these factors, a lymphatic drainage ($\mathbf{L}$) factor must be considered. All these parameters are altered in the tumor. In fact, in the tumor capillary the arterial venous pressure difference (a − vΔp) component does not exist, since the venous pressure is near to that at the arterial end of the capillary, due to the increased arteri-ovenous anastomosis present in the neovas-culature. Since albumin leaks abundantly due to the increased permeability induced by

VPF/VEGF in the endothelium of venules and capillaries, the increased venous reabsorption that normally happens at the venous end of the capillary in cancer is lost. Lymphatics are present at the tumor periphery but not inside the tumor mass [5, 6, 11]. Altogether, these factors cooperate to create a progressive increase of *TIFP* from the periphery to the center of the tumor [93].

In conclusion, from the pathophysiological point of view, the process of tumor expansion is characterized by rapid growth and alteration of tumor microenvironment due to the inability of tumor neovasculature to supply oxygen nutrients at an adequate rate. The ensuing hypoxic microenvironments are characterized by low oxygen tension, increased extracellular lactate concentration leading to low extracellular pH (pH$_e$), high interstitial fluid pressure, glucose deficiency, multidrug resistance and tendency to metastatization [26, 103].

2.2. Examples of Carcinomas Microanatomy

Our group has studied two experimental models of a solid tumor: first an Ehrlich carcinoma induced by inoculation of Ehrlich ascites tumor cells in the skeletal muscle of the hind leg of a normal mouse and currently the mammary tumors spontaneously developed by MMTV-*neu (erbB-2)* transgenic mice. Both these tumor models share the presence of hypoxic/necrotic regions, a hypercellular, granulation-like tissue at the tumor periphery, chaotic neoangiogenesis and TIF infiltrations (Figures 2.5 and 2.6). Cuff-like formations around blood vessels with outer necrosis were seen in both tumor types; in the transgenic model tumor cords with outer capillaries and inner necrosis were also present.

Figures 2.5 and 2.6 show representative tumor sections displaying malignant cell masses with perinecrotic/hypoxic regions [29], necrotic cells, a vascular stroma and peripheral, granulation-like tissue.

In both models we noticed that the width of the viable cords (peripheral blood vessels, inner necrotic regions) or cuffs (central blood vessel, external necrosis) of tumor cells were in general lower than 150 μm, compatibly with the oxygenation capacity of the vessel and the oxygen and nutrients demand of the tumor cells [29]. Cells distant from the blood vessels, which receive lower concentrations of oxygen and blood-borne nutrients, were seen to be quiescent and metabolically poorly active. Generally cells in the perinecrotic region were very small, rounded up and intertwined, forming strand-like structures. Cells closer to the blood vessels were larger, polygonal and formed a pluristratified-like epithelium. It is worth recalling that although they eventually die as indicated by the large necrotic areas, tumor hypoxic cells have a remarkable high capacity to cope and adapt to oxygen deprivation, low pH and nutrient starvation [29].

As already mentioned, tumor stroma induction has been shown to closely resemble a wound repair process [22] in which an initial phase of hyper- permeability of blood vessels leads to diffuse liquid accumulation (*TIF*).

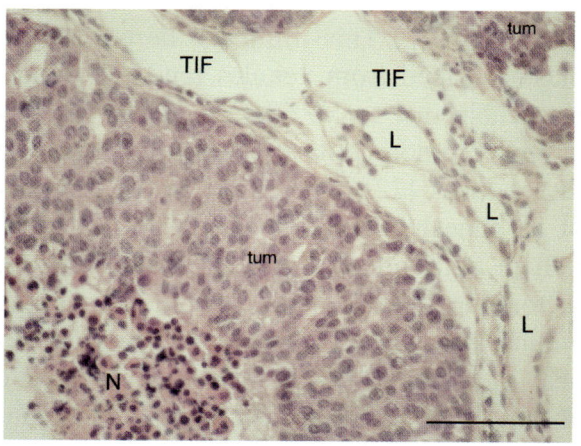

Figure 2.6. Detail under higher magnification of a tumor cord. H&E. N: necrosis; L: lymph vessels; TIF: tumor interstitial fluid. Scale bar: 50 μm

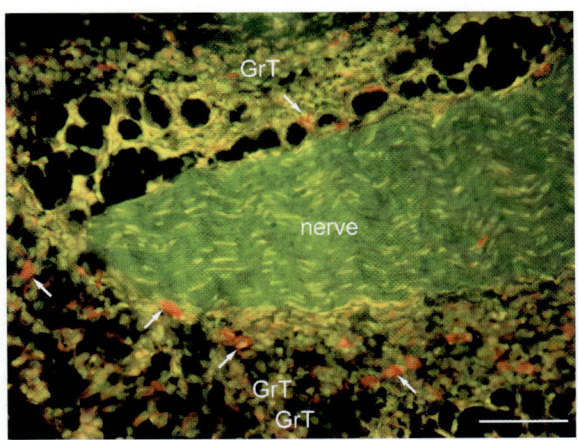

Figure 2.7. Abundance of mast cells (arrows) in the granulation tissue (GrT) at the tumor periphery. A nerve can be seen. Acridine Orange. Scale bar: 50 μm

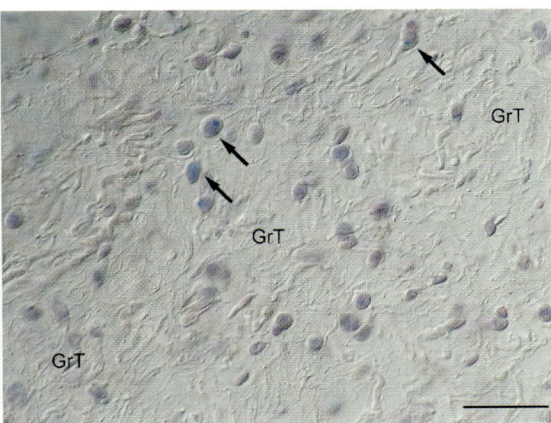

Figure 2.8. Iron (III)-containing mononucleated cells in the granulation tissue (GrT). Perls' reaction. Scale bar: 20 μm

We have previously reported that light and electron microscopical analyses of the Ehrlich tumor revealed non-random distribution of stromal cells (*fibroblasts, macrophages, mast cells and adipocytes in regions involved in angiogenesis and tumor invasion*)[28].

Mast cells in particular were present in high numbers at the tumor periphery (Figure 2.7) [22]. This region was supported by a fibrin-rich provisional stroma. Generally, fibrin is formed after wounding or whenever plasma leaks out from blood vessels forming a fibrinous exudate that provides a scaffolding into which new microvessels migrate [16, 22]. Besides mast cells, fibroblasts and leukocytes were abundant in the granulation-like tissue at the tumor invasion edge. Similar findings were reported in colorectal cancer by Menon et al. [60]; these AA have demonstrated that leukocyte infiltration in the tumor epithelium compartment was correlated with a better prognosis, whereas leukocyte located in the tumor stroma or at the advancing margin of the tumor did not affect prognosis. Similar findings have been seen by other authors for ductal breast carcinoma [44].

We have furthermore reported that stromal cell location within the tumor mass suggested an involvement with the preliminary phases of angiogenesis. As a matter of fact, TIF infiltrations with a morphology similar to that of the irregular blood vessels, were surrounded by mast cells, macrophages, adipocytes and proliferating endothelial-like cells (Figures 2.7–2.10) [27].

An enzyme histochemical study of Ehrlich carcinoma revealed that perinecrotic (hypoxic cells) can be characterized by intense lactate dehydrogenase (LDH), acid phosphatase and purine nucleoside phosphorylase (PNP) but low xanthine oxidoreductase activity, compatible with the use of glycolysis, (auto)

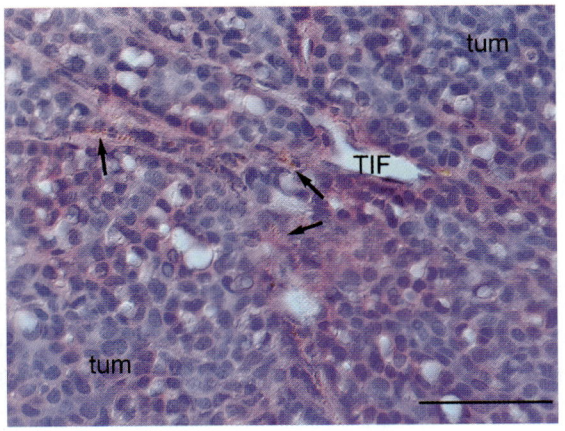

Figure 2.9. Hemosiderin-containing macrophages (arrows) within the tumor parenchyma. H&E. TIF: tumor interstitial fluid. Scale bar: 50 μm

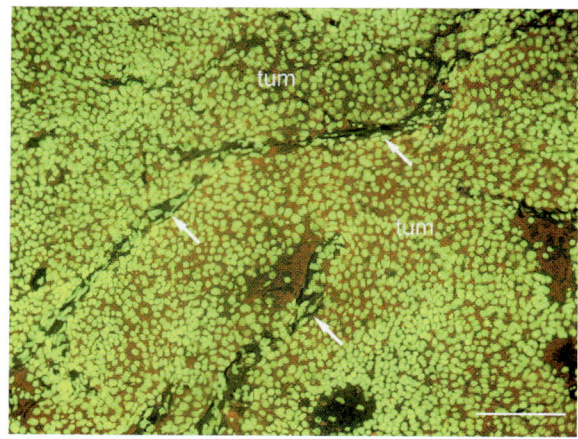

Figure 2.10. Blood vessels (arrows) in the tumor parenchyma. Acridine Orange. Scale bar: $50\,\mu$m

phagocytosis and purine salvage strategies to survive in such hostile microenvironments [29]. The poor eosinophilia of most necrotic areas and the relative absence of macrophages in the necrosis suggest that materials released from dead tumor cells are utilized as nutrition surrogates by the cells distant from the vasculature.

The TIF infiltration patterns in the two models of carcinomas were dissimilar to the infiltrations seen in a poorly-vascularized but fast growing MS2 fibrosarcoma. In this last case, the mesenchyma-derived tumor cells apparently opposed little mechanical resistance to the infiltration of the serum-derived fluid; we speculated that the oxygen-dissolved in the TIF, its platelet-derived growth factors and the plasma-bound nutrients supported tumor growth without need for angiogenesis [29, 30].

2.3. Role Played by Stromal Cells in Cancer Microenvironments

The neoplastic tissue can be described as a triad formed by tumor tissue, endothelium and cellular components of the stroma. Several cell types constituting the stroma have been recognized to play a critical role in this triad, namely: fibroblasts, macrophages, mast cells, eosinophils, tumor infiltrating lymphocytes (*TILs*), regulatory T cells (*CD4$^+$ CD25$^+$ Foxp3*), IDO cells and myeloid cells.

2.3.1. Fibroblasts

Fibroblasts are a cell type that synthesizes and maintains the extracellular matrix of many animal tissues. Fibroblasts provide a structural framework (stroma) for many tissues, and play a critical role in wound healing. They are morphologically heterogeneous, with diverse appearances depending on their location and activity (for a complete review see Eiden [24]). Recent evidence suggests that fibroblasts play a critical role not only in tumor support but they may even help tumor progression and metastatization [4]. Both resident and recruited fibroblasts are involved in tumor progression. Once recruited fibroblasts become activated they proliferate and differentiate into myofibroblasts, assuming specific characteristics. These phenotypically evidenced fibroblasts are generally called CAFs (Cancer Associated Fibroblasts). CAFs are perpetually activated cells that neither revert to normal phenotype nor undergo apoptosis, expressing filaments like α-smooth muscle actin [48]. Cross-talk through different cytokines, chemokines and growth factors takes part between cancer cells and CAFs. Cancer cells recruit fibroblasts from circulating CD34-positive hematopoietic progenitors cells in presence of TGF-β, PDGF and GM-CSF. As these progenitor cells reach the tumor area they secrete elevated levels of stromal-derived factor 1 (SDF-1) (also called CXCL12) which play a central role in the promotion of tumor growth and angiogenesis. CAF derived SDF-1 stimulates cancer cell growth directly through the CXCR4 receptor displayed on tumor cells and also recruits endothelial progenitor cells (EPCs), which play a crucial role in induced neoangiogenesis [60, 69]. Furthermore, Silzle et al. [91] have also emphasized the role of

CAFs in the peritumor inflammatory reaction (leukocyte infiltration) and in the immune modulation.

2.3.2. Macrophages

Macrophages are defined as a population of cells derived from progenitors cells (CD34$^+$) in the bone marrow, which differentiate to form blood monocytes, circulate in blood and, after entering tissues, become tissue macrophages [45, 101]. The blood monocytes are young cells that already possess migratory, chemotactic, pinocytic and phagocytic activities as well as receptors for IgG Fc-domains and iC3b complement. Under migration into tissues, monocytes undergo further differentiation, becoming multifunctional tissue macrophages. The principal role of macrophages is to phagocytose foreign invaders and to remodel the tissue.

Macrophages are attracted to a damaged site by chemical substances through chemotaxis, triggered by a range of different stimuli including damaged cells, pathogens, histamine released by mast cells and basophils and cytokines released by resident macrophages already present at the damaged tissue. In the case of tumors the hypoxic core, through the upregulation the HIFs 1 and 2, induces a series of cytokines and chemokines (VEGF, M-CSF, CCL2), which recruit circulating monocytes across the tumor vasculature. After recruitment they become the prominent part of the stromal compartment and exhibit a distinctive phenotype and are termed *tumor-associated macrophages* (TAMs) [76] (Figures 2.9–2.11). TAMs are characterized by low expression of the differentiation-associated macrophage antigens, carboxypeptidase M and CD51. This shift indicates a high constitutive expression of inflammatory cytokines IL-1 and IL-6 associated to a low expression of TNF-α, they are classified according to cluster differentiation as

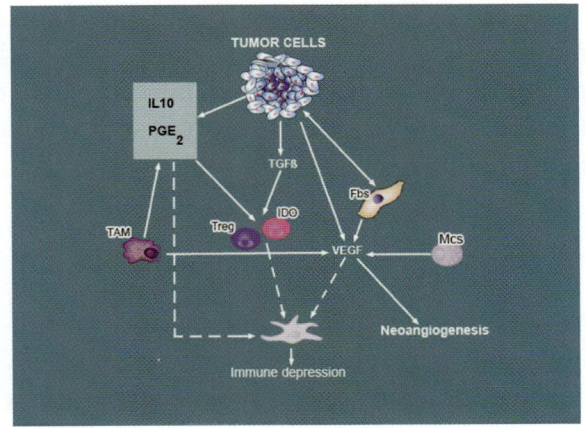

Figure 2.11. Simplified diagram of tumor evasion. Cellular and factors interested

CD45$^+$CD14$^+$ [45, 101]. Distinctive phenotypes have been recognized as associated to tumor mass and have been classified as M1 and M2 phenotypes. The two phenotypes can be distinguished by their different production of cytokines and chemokines, L-citrulline and iNOS, polarizing signals (IL-4, IL-13, IL-10), lipid metabolism and tissue remodeling [90, 102]. Inside the tumor mass the M2 type represents the prominent component of solid tumor, which has been associated and in some cases with poor prognosis. This kind of polarized macrophage have many protumoral functions and produce angiogenic factors and immune-suppressive cytokines such as IL-10 (Figure 2.11). We can distinguish further among M2 macrophages three other subforms denominated M$_2$a, M$_2$b and M$_2$c. These subforms under the presence of various polarizing signals show specific functional properties. M$_2$a. for example. in the presence of IL-4 and IL-13 express a type II immune response, M$_2$b in the presence of IC and agonists of TLRs or IL-1R activate Th2 response, whereas M$_2$c cells under the pressure of IL-10 can acquire a prominent immuno-suppressive activity [90, 102].

Phagocytosis is induced when the phospatidylserine receptors of macrophages come in contact with phospatidylserine externalized on the membranes of damaged or dying cells. Afterwards, a down regulation message, constituted by IL-10, TGF-β and prostaglandin 2 (PGE-2) is induced, which tries to block the inflammatory response and the remodeling activity.

2.3.3. Mast Cells

Mast cells derive from bone marrow progenitors that migrate into tissue, where they become resident cells. They contain many granules rich in histamine, heparin and serine proteases such as tryptase and chymase. Although best known for their role in allergy and anaphylaxis mast cells play an important protective role in wound healing, angiogenesis and inflammation [19, 97]. Mast cells under physiological conditions are localized close to capillaries, lymphatic channels and nerves (Figure 2.7) and their localization can explain their involvement in tumor angiogenesis [19]. In many solid and hematologic tumors (e.g. lung carcinoma, gastric cancer, melanoma, and chronic lymphocytic leukemia) an increased number of mast cells has been reported and in some cases their elevated count has been associated with tumor invasion [57, 80]. Among mast cells two identifiable types can be recognized (MC_T and MC_{TC} cells in humans) according to the content of their granules and their responsiveness to stimuli. The phenotypic expression of mast cells is not fixed and can vary according to the environmental conditions [19]. In addition, they are versatile and can share many growth factors and cytokines with TAMs, such as (Il-8, VEGF, PDGF, histamine, PGE_2). As TAMs they have a dual role as they can either inhibit or promote tumor growth, according to the stromal conditions. Mast cell recruitment to tumors is induced by various factors, including hypoxia, cellular damage, tissue ischemia and tumor-derived chemoattractants, including stem cell factor (SCF), interleukins-3 (IL-3) and IL-4 [57]. These in turn produce various cytokines,

such as tumor necrosis factor-α (TNF-α), IL-1, IL-4 and IL-6, which can induce apoptosis of tumor cells. Mast cells are also known to stimulate anti-tumor lymphocytes through IL-8 and RANTES [15]. Furthermore, as demonstrated by Samoszuk et al., degranulating mast cells are restricted to tumor fibrous tissue, and in this area they abundantly secrete heparin, which has been shown to inhibit the growth of primary and metastatic tumors [80]. In particular, the inhibition was observed when colonies of UACC-812 human breast cancer were co-cultured with fibroblasts [80]. In conclusion, the majority of experimental studies show a correlation between mast-cell infiltration and tumor progression. Recent research supports this conclusion, as co-injection of mast cells with an inoculum of rat sarcoma tumors resulted in enhanced tumor growth, whereas pharmacologically decreasing the quantity of mast cells slowed tumor growth [46, 81].

2.3.4. TILs

TILs can have prognostic significance and are recognized as the main effector of antitumor immune response [110]. Yu and Fu however, outline that among the various subset of CD4+ T cells that accumulate in the tumor environment, a special subset of CD4 + CD25+ regulatory T cells (*T reg*) is also accumulated. These T reg are able to suppress tumor specific T-cell response thereby hindering tumor rejection. Furthermore, the authors conclude that their presence decrease the prognostic significance of TILs [110]. The morphology of TILs and T reg is described elsewhere in this book.

2.3.5. Eosinophils

Tumor associated eosinophilia seems a favorable prognostic marker for many tumors except in Hodgkin's disease [18]. Their antitumor activity relies on their tight contact with tumor cells and their interaction with mast cells, endothelial cells and fibroblasts/myofibroblasts [62]. Their interaction with and influence on fibroblasts suggests the importance of eosinophils for tissue remodeling and fpr their importance as immune effector cells towards tumors [18, 62]. Recent studies outlined that the principal stimuli for eosinophil cell recruitment occur in part through signals released from areas of necrosis and that their presence is correlated with the persistence of inflammation in the tumor area [17, 110]. Furthermore, eosinophils can synergize with reactive oxygen species (ROS) produced by macrophages to kill tumor cells [65], but as for other cells in the tumor microenvironment, they are regulated by surface molecules, extracellular components and cell–cell interaction. Improved methods to evaluate their activity and contribution to tumor state are required.

2.4. Immune Competent Cells Dysfunction Created by Tumor Microenvironment

Although tumors are frequently infiltrated by dendritic cells (DCs) and tumor infiltrating lymphocytes (TILs), these immune cells are functionally compromised. The abnormalities are more evident for TILs than for circulating lymphocytes and suggest that such abnormalities are caused or induced by suppressive mechanisms or environmental conditions present inside the tumor mass. Explanations for this failure include: insufficient activation of tumor – specific T cells, tolerance to tumor antigens, regulatory T cells and hostile tumor microenvironment. As already mentioned, the hostile microenvironment is characterized by low oxygen tension, low extracellular pH_e, high interstitial fluid pressure, glucose deficiency, multidrug resistance, increased extracellular lactate concentration and tendency to metastatization. Emerging evidence points out that not only tumor cells but also lymphocytes within the tumor mass are subjected to a stressful hypoxic and acidic environment that can modify their response to mitogen and their cytokine production. Several factors have been identified: 1) **Metabolites** (pO_2, pH_e, *PGE$_2$*, *histamine*, *ROS*); 2) **Cytokines – growth factors** (*VEGF, TGF-β, IL-10*); 3) **Failure of lymphocyte homing** (decreased expression of adhesion molecules); 4) **presence of Suppressor T cell subsets (T reg, Myeloid cells, IDO cells)**.

2.4.1. Metabolites

2.4.1.1. pO_2

Oxygen concentration decreases from the tumor periphery towards the tumor inner areas and depends on the distance from the nutritive vessel. The partial decrease in oxygen tension can affect IL-2 activity and TNF treatment, as demonstrated by Sampson and Chaplin [82]. These authors have shown that the response to TNF was dependent on oxygen concentration. In fact, the resistance to TNF treatment of cells incubated at various oxygen tensions increased with the decrease of oxygen concentration in the incubation medium. Some authors have postulated that this TNF treatment resistance was correlated to the decreased induction of ROS and to the up-regulation of endogenous soluble receptors in the hypoxic tumor microenvironment [73, 84].

2.4.1.2. pH_e

The low extracellular pH_e is due to the accumulation of H^+ ions in the tumor interstitium. As reported by Jain there are at least two sources of H^+ ions: lactic acid and carbonic acid. The former results from anaerobic glycolysis and the latter from conversion of CO_2 and H_2O via carbonic anhydrase [32]. Acidic extracellular pH_e can inhibit the proliferation of lymphocytes, can affect the release of perforins and can lower the cytotoxic activity of LAK cells against tumor cells [51]. Dendritic cell's activity (differentiation and antigen expression) can also be affected by tumor micromilieu, as demonstrated by Gottfried in a 3-dimensional model [37]. These authors conclude that lactic acid accumulation can contribute to tumor escape mechanisms.

2.4.1.3. Arachidonic Acid Metabolites (PGE_2)

The role of prostaglandins in immunoregulation is complex. Prostaglandins affect cell differentiation as well as target cell interaction. In humans the cells responsible for prostaglandin production are the macrophages and the tumor cells themselves. Prostaglandin synthesis is regulated by cycloxigenase (COX) gene expression. Two separate gene products, COX-1 and COX-2, are expressed at high levels by tumors interacting with effector lymphocytes. *In vitro*, prostaglandins have been shown to inhibit lymphocyte mitogenesis, cytolysis and antibody production. Clinical studies have demonstrated that macrophages from patients with Hodgkin's disease produces excess amounts of prostaglandins E_2. Furthermore, administration of prostaglandin inhibitors (COX2 inhibitors) to patients with breast and lung cancers, permitted macrophages *in vitro* to acquire enhanced cytotoxicity for tumor target cells. Thus prostaglandin production by tumor cells has been suggested as a mechanism by which tumor cells can escape the host's immune surveillance [75]. Four PG receptors have been demonstrated in mice and humans: EP1, EP2, EP3 and EP4. The suppression of T cells by PGE2 is mediated via EP2 and EP4 receptors. Both receptors share similar intracellular signaling pathways that involve binding to G proteins, stimulation of adenylate cyclase and generation of increased intracellular levels of cyclic AMP [106]. Furthermore, PGE2 exerts an inhibitory action on Dendritic cells reducing their differentiation, maturation and their ability to present antigens [75, 106].

2.4.1.4. Histamine

Mast cells are the major source of histamine (HA) and its production is under the control of various cytokines such as IL-1, IL-3, IL-12, IL-18, TNF-α, and macrophage colony stimulating factor (MCSF) [2]. HA has been demonstrated to polarize naïve CD4$^+$ T cells toward a Th2 phenotype acting upon a H2 receptor of Dendritic cells increasing Il-10 and decreasing Il-12 secretion [59]. In certain kinds of tumors such as melanoma, renal cell carcinoma and acute leukemia. HA has, however, shown an immune boosting effect in association with IL-2 therapy [1]. *In vitro*, studies indicate that HA exerts its effect through the inhibition of ROS generated by macrophages and on the abrogation of their inhibitory activity on Natural Killers [1]. Studies by Outila indicate that HA and PGE2 together exert mainly an inhibitory effect on the mediated cellular immunity impairing T cell and macrophage antitumor activity [99, 100].

In conclusion, new studies indicate that histamine deregulates the balance between TH1 and TH2 cells, enhancing secretion of TH2 cytokines such as IL-4, IL-5, IL-10 and IL-13, whist inhibiting production of TH1 cytokines IL-2 and IFN-γ and monokine IL-12 [23, 71, 98]. Furthermore, HA endogenous synthesis in tumor tissues suppresses local tumor immunity and promotes colon tumor growth in mice [98].

2.4.1.5. ROS, Myeloid Cells

Myeloid cells are immature cells found in the bone marrow and not normally in the peripheral blood; they are the most primitive precursors in the granulocytic series, that matures to develop into the promyelocyte and eventually in granular leukocytes; they accumulate in tumor-bearing hosts and suppress antigen-specific T cell response. In cancer patients, myeloid cells express the myeloid marker CD33 but lack expression of the MHC class II molecule. According to Gabrilovich, myeloid cells might represent a source of TAMs and of endothelial cells [50, 76]. In any case, they are regulated by ROS, which are produced in abundance in cancer patients. ROS may affect the differentiation of myeloid cells acting on several transcription factors (e.g. NF-kB, AP-1) [83]. In animal models their presence has been associated with tumor progression and with a state of immune suppression. They explicate their immune suppression through the production of TGF-β, ROS, L-arginine metabolism and peroxinitrite [83].

2.4.2. Cytokines and Growth Factors

2.4.2.1. VEGF

Vascular endothelial factor has been demonstrated not only to promote angiogenesis but to suppress anti-tumor immune response, principally by hampering leukocyte recruitment [21] and by inhibiting CD34$^+$ cell differentiation into dendritic cells [38]. An indirect confirmation to the inhibitory effect of VEGF on DCs comes from the studies by Gabrilovich et al. These authors have shown that the combined treatment of peptide-pulsed DCs and anti-VEGF antibody results in a prolonged and much more pronounced antitumor effect [33, 70].

2.4.2.2. TGF-β

In mammals, there are three isoforms of TGF-ß, TGF-ß1, 2, and 3 which are each the product of a separate gene. All these isoforms bind to the same receptors and exert similar pleiotropic effects on cell behavior. The most studied is TGF-ß1 which is secreted by fibroblasts and the tumor itself and has a dual effect depending on tumor stage. In fact, it can restrain tumor growth at an early stage but can be a promoter of invasiveness in an advanced stage [72]. TGF-β exert its effects on almost

all the cells of the immune system such as lymphocytes, natural killers (NKs), DCs, mast cells, neutrophils and macrophages, regulating their proliferation and differentiation [56]. The inhibitory effects of TGF-ß are the following: inhibition of T-cell growth, of Cytotoxic cells differentiation, of cytokine production (IL-2; INF−γ) with the shift toward Th2 pattern. Furthermore, it induces T-Cell anergy and down-regulates cytotoxic activity and the adhesion/co-stimulatory molecules [8].

2.4.2.3. IL-10

IL-10 is produced by tumor cells or TILs and can down-regulate antigen-presenting activity, cytokine expression and anti-tumor activities of monocytes by inhibiting the production of anti-tumor effector molecules (e.g. IL-12). It blocks, furthermore, cell-mediated effector cell functions by inhibiting cytokine secretion (e.g. IFN-gamma, TNF-alpha) in Th1 cells, and protects tumor cells from CTL-mediated lysis. Its elevated expression in various human tumors indicates its important regulatory role in the regulation of the anti-tumor immune response [61]. IL-10 cooperates with other tumor/stroma secreted cytokines, PGE2 and TGF-β, to increase the local production of T regulatory cells inducing tumor tolerance [96]. The crucial role of their association and the immunosuppressive effect on dendritic cell function has been highlighted and confirmed by other authors [52, 78, 105].

2.5. STAT3

The Janus family of tyrosine kinase (Jack) and STAT family of transcription factors are critically important in cellular differentiation, proliferation and apoptosis [78]. These signaling proteins have been demonstrated to be critical for DCs differentiation as well. The excessive production of VEGF, IL-10 and gangliosides in the tumor medium can induce the activation of Jack 2 and STAT3 in myeloid cells, thus inhibiting their differentiation and maturation. The excessive accumulation of immature DCs and myeloid cells, as previously reported, is responsible for the generation of tolerance and tumor immune suppression [66, 67].

2.5.1. Presence of Suppressor T Cell Subsets (T_{reg}, Myeloid Cells, IDO Cells)

2.5.1.1. T_{reg} (CD4$^+$CD25$^+$) Cells

CD4$^+$Cd25$^+$ or regulatory T cells (T_{reg} cells) represent a stable proportion of 5–12% of circulating T cells in mice and humans. They are quiescent cells with a long lifespan, identified by expression of 1) high levels of Cd25 (CD25^{hi}), 2) the forkhead/winged helix transcription factor (Foxp3), 3) high levels of intracytoplasmatic T-lymphocyte-associated antigen 4) (CTLA-4), 5) the glucocorticoid-induced tumor necrosis factor receptor (GITR) surface marker [36, 89, 107]. Their function is to maintain self-tolerance and an increased pool of these cells compared to healthy controls has been found in the peripheral blood of patients suffering from different epithelial malignancies. (lung, breast, colorectal, gastric, pancreatic and esophageal cancers) [108]. Another interesting aspect is the over-expression of galectin-1 binding proteins on the surface of naturally occurring regulatory cells and the fact that their inhibition significantly reduces their regulatory effect [35]. The over-expression of galectin-1 binding proteins can be induced by hypoxia, as happens for certain cancer lines and seems associated with a modulation of immune privilege and overall survival [53]. In fact galectin-1 has many effects on T-cell homeostasis, survival and function ranging from Il-2 decreased secretion to the favoring of IL-10 secretion. Furthermore, its over-expression in tumor stroma has been reported to be involved in tumor progression [20].

Confirmation of the involvement of tumor microenvironment on T_{reg} activity comes from the work of Curiel et al., who have clearly demonstrated the fatal attraction of T_{reg} towards tumor hypoxic areas [20]. The increased infiltration in malignant epithelial cancers is obtained under the influence of the chemokine CCL22, a chemokine able to also recruit macrophages that are specifically produced by tumor and stroma cells in the hypoxic areas [3].

2.5.1.2. Myeloid Cells (See Above "Myeloid Cells, ROS")

IDO cells. Indoleamine 2,3-dioxygenase (IDO) is a rate limiting enzyme in the catabolism of tryptophan, induced in various pathologic states including neoplasia. Different *in vitro* studies have shown that this induction is consequent to the activation of antigen-presenting cells (APCs), such as macrophages and DCs. The production of IDO cells by specific subsets of DCs, probably induced by the hostile tumor microenvironment [63], can influence the killing activity of lymphocytes against cancer cells and T-cell proliferation. IDO seems to be important for NK cells activity as demonstrated by Kai et al. [47], and as counter regulation of immune activation and inflammation [47], however the presence of these IDO cells in the tumor draining lymph nodes can induce tumor-tolerance and immune-evasion.

Dendritic cells. DCs are essential for the initiation of immune responses by capturing, processing and presenting antigens to T cells. In addition to their important role as professional APCs, inside the tumor area they show a reduced activity (immaturity) due to the over-expression of immunosuppressive and pro-inflammatory prostanoids from arachidonic acid (AA) by the action of cyclooxygenase (COX) enzymes [9, 106, 109]. Associated with PGE$_2$ histamine, IL10 stimulate DCs to differentiate into Th2 cell-promoting effector DCs and to tumor immunity paralysis [31, 42, 109]. Other molecules over-expressed in the tumor microenvironment, such as VEGF and Jak2/STAT3, have been implicated in the block of dendritic cell maturation and in a decrease in its activity of antigen presenting cells [31, 89].

2.6.   Failure of Lymphocyte Homing

Adhesion molecules. Tumor immunotherapy success or failure is strongly dependent on leukocyte migration into the tumor area [14]. In fact, leukocytes and macrophages, before reaching the target tissue (tumor site), undergo a series of sequential steps during extravasation from blood into tissues: tethering, rolling, adhesion and diapedesis. Among these steps, the leukocytes' adhesion to tumor endothelium is critical and occurs through the expression of specific adhesion molecules, such as: L-selectin ligands, alpha-4beta-7 integrin adhesion receptors (a4b7) and mucosal addressing cell adhesion molecule-1 (CAM-1). Several animal experiments have shown that in the presence of VEGF a significantly decreased expression of these adhesion molecules occurs, determining a decline in leukocyte arrival into the tumor mass [14, 38, 70].

Effects of tumor environment on cytokines production and treatment. Besides the impaired tumor infiltration by immune competent cells, tumor environment (hypoxia, acidic pH) itself unfavorably modifies T lymphocytes, NK cells and macrophage activity [55, 88]. In fact, this kind of tumor environment alters the pattern of secreted cytokines towards an immunosuppressive T_H2 pattern, permitting tumor escape from immune surveillance [51, 54, 55, 86, 92].

2.7.   Conclusions

In the majority of cases, cancer cells are recognized as foreign by specific cytotoxic lympho-

cytes $CD8^+$, however, they are not spontaneously eliminated by the immune system. This failure to recognize cancer cells as foreign bodies is initially found inside the tumor mass and then becomes a peripheral effect [86, 92]. The hostile microenvironment that neoplastic cells create in concert with the recruited macrophages and fibroblasts is responsible for this failure [Figures 2.4 and 2.11]. The recruited cells lose their anti-tumor capacity and their activity becomes able to facilitate tumor progression [92]. Probably hypoxia is the principal factor responsible for all these effects. More observations on other pathological states, such as inflammation, can lead to a better understanding of this factor in the near future [85].

Abbreviations. TAMs: Tumor Associated Macrophages; VEGF: Vascular Endothelial Growth Factor; HIF: Hypoxia-inducible Factor; IL: interleukin; TNF-a: tumor necrosis factor alpha; M-CSF: macrophage colony stimulating factor; TILs: tumor infiltrating Lymphocytes; ROS: reactive oxygen species; TGF-β: transforming growth factor Beta; NKs: natural killer cells; IDO: Indoleamine 2,3-dioxygenase; APCs: Antigen presenting cells; DCs: dendritic cells; iNOS: inducible nitric oxide synthase, IC: immune complexes; TLRs: toll-like receptors; IL-1R: Interleukin one receptor; T_{reg} cells: regulatory T cells

References

[1] Agarwala S S, Sabbagh M H (2001) Histamine dihydrochloride: inhibiting oxidants and synergism IL-2 mediated immune activation in the tumor microenvironment. Expert Opin Biol Ther 1: 869–879

[2] Akdis C A, Blaser K (2003) Histamine in the immune regulation of allergic inflammation. J Allergy Clin Immunol 112: 15–22

[3] Allavena P, Marchesi F, Mantovani A (2005) The role of chemochines and their receptors in tumor progression and invasion: potential new target of biological therapy. Curr Cancer Ther Rev 1: 81–92

[4] Ariztia E V, Lee C J, Gogoi R et al. (2006) The tumor microenvironment: key to early detection. Crit Rev Clin Lab Sci 43: 393–425

[5] Baronzio G, Freitas I, Kwaan H C (2003) Tumor microenvironment and hemorheological abnormalities. Semin Thromb Hemost Oct 29(5): 489–497

[6] Bates D O, Hillman N J, Williams B et al. (2002) Regulation of microvascular permeability by vascular endothelial growth factors. J Anat 200: 581–97

[7] Beacham D A, Cukierman E (2005) Stromagenesis: the changing face of fibroblastic microenvironments during tumor progression. Semin Cancer Biol 15: 329–341

[8] Beck C, Schreiber H, Bowley D A (2001) Role of TGF-β in immune-evasion of cancer. Microsc Res Tech 52: 387–395

[9] Bell D, Chomarat P, Broyles D et al. (1999) In breast carcinoma tissue, immature dendritic cells reside within the tumor area, whereas mature dendritic cells are located in the peritumor areas. J E M 190: 1417–1425

[10] Berges G, Benjamin L (2002) Tumorigenesis and the angiogenic switch. Nat Rev Cancer 3: 401–410

[11] Boucher Y, Leunig M, Jain R K, Jain R K (1996) Tumor angiogenesis and interstitial hypertension. Cancer Res 56(18): 4264–4266

[12] Boudreau N, Myers C (2003) Breast cancer-induced angiogenesis: multiple mechanisms and the role of the microenvironment. Breast Cancer Res 5: 140–146

[13] Brace R A, Guyton A C (1979) Interstitial fluid pressure: capsule, free fluid, gel fluid, and gel absorption pressure in subcutaneous tissue. Microvasc Res 18: 217–228

[14] Carlos T M (2001) Leukocyte recruitment at sites of tumor: dissonant orchestration. J Leukoc Bio l70: 171–184

[15] Ch'ng S, Sullivan M, Yuan L et al. (2006) Mast cells dysregulate apoptotic and cell cycle genes in mucosal squamous cell carcinoma. Cancer Cell Int 6:1–7

[16] Collen A, Koolwijk P, Kroon M et al. (1998) Influence of fibrin structure on the formation and maintenance of capillary-like tubules by human microvascular endothelial cells. Angiogenesis 2(2):153–165

[17] Cormier S A, Taranova A, Bedient C et al. (2006) Pivotal advance: eosinophil infiltration of solid tumors is an early and persistent inflammatory host response. J Leukoc Bio l79: 1131–1139

[18] Costello R, O' Callaghan T, Sebahoun G (2005) Eosinophiles et response antitumorale. La revue de medicine interne 26: 479–484

[19] Crivellato E, Ribatti D (2005) Involvement of mast cells in angiogenesis and chronic inflammation. Curr Drug targets 4: 9–11

[20] Curiel T J, Coukos G, Zou L et al. (2004) Specific recruitment of regulatory T cells in ovarian carcinoma fosters immune privilege and predicts reduced survival. Nature Med 10: 942–949

[21] Dirkx A E, Oude Egbrink M G, Kuijpers M J et al. (2003) Tumor angiogenesis modulates leukocyte-vessel wall interactions in vivo by reducing endothelial adhesion molecule expression. Cancer Res 63: 2322–2329

[22] Dvorak H F (1986) Tumors: wound that not heal. Similarities between tumor stroma generation and wound healing. N Engl J Med 315: 1650–1659

[23] Elenkov I J, Webster E, Papanicolaou D A, Fleisher T A, Chrousos G P, Wilder R L (1998) Histamine potently suppresses human IL-12 and stimulates IL-10 production via H2 receptors. J Immunol 161: 2586–2593

[24] Eyden B (2005) The myofibroblast: a study of normal, reactive and neoplastic tissue, with emphasis on ultrastructure. Part1-Normal and reactive cells. J Submicrosc Cytol Pathol 37: 1–96

[25] Folkman J (1971) Tumor Angiogenesis: therapeutic implications. N Engl J Med 285: 1182–1186

[26] Freitas I, Baronzio G F (1991) Tumor hypoxia, reoxygenation and oxygenation strategies: possible role in photodynamic therapy. J Photochem Photobiol B Biol 11: 3–30

[27] Freitas I, Baronzio G F, Barni S et al. (1992) Tumor angiogenesis: evidence of new blood channels from plasma infiltrations. EXS 61: 81–84

[28] Freitas I, Baronzio G F, Bertone V et al. (1991) Stroma formation in Ehrlich carcinoma. I. Oedema phase. A mitosis burst as an index of physiological reoxygenation? Anticancer Res 11(2): 569–578

[29] Freitas I, Bono B, Bertone V et al. (1996) Characterization of the metabolism of perinecrotic cells in solid tumors by enzyme histochemistry. Anticancer Res 16: 1491–1502

[30] Freitas I, Baronzio G F, Bono B et al. (1997) Tumor interstitial fluid: misconsidered component of the internal milieu of a solid tumor. Anticancer Res 17(1A): 165–172

[31] Fricke I, Gabrilovich D I (2006) Dendritic cells and tumor microenvironment: a dangerous liaison. Immunol Invest 35(3–4): 459–483

[32] Fukumura D, Jain R (2006) Tumor microenvironment abnormalities: Causes, consequences, and strategies to normalize. J Cell Biochem 14: [Epub ahead of print]

[33] Gabrilovich D I, Ishida T, Nadaf S et al. (1999) Antibodies to vascular endothelial growth factor enhance the efficacy of cancer immunotherapy by improving endogenous dendritic cell function. Clin Cancer Res 5(10): 2963–2970

[34] Gadea B B, Joyce J (2006) Tumor-host interactions: implications for developing anti-cancer therapies. Expert Rev Mol Med 8: 1–32

[35] Garin M I, Chu C C, Golshayan D et al. (2007) Galectin-1: a key effector of regulation mediated by CD4+CD25+ T cells. Blood 109: 2058–2065

[36] Gavin M, Rudensky A (2003) Control of immune homeostasis by naturally arising regulatory CD4+ T cells. Current Opinion in Immunology 15: 690–696

[37] Gottfried E, Kunz-Schughart L, Ebner S et al. (2006) Tumor-derived lactic acid modulates dendritic cell activation and antigen expression. Blood 107: 2013–2021

[38] Griffioen A W, Tromp S C, Hillen H F (1998) Angiogenesis modulates the tumor immune response. Int J Exp Pathol 79: 363–368

[39] Gullino P M (1966) The internal milieu of tumors. Prog Exp Tum Res 8: 1–25

[40] Gullino P M (1975) Extracellular compartments of solid tumors. In Beckert FB (ed.), Cancer, a comprehensive treatise. Vol. 3, Biology of tumors: Cellular biology and growth, Plenum, New York: 327–354

[41] Hanahan D, Weinberg R (2000) The hallmarks of cancer. Cell 100: 57–70

[42] Harizi H, Gualde N (2006) Pivotal role pf PGE2 and IL-10 in the cross–regulation of Dendritic cell-derived inflammatory mediators. Cell Mol Immunol 3: 271–277

[43] Hoeben A, Landuyt B, Highley M S et al. (2004) Vascular endothelial growth factor and angiogenesis. Pharmacol Rev 56(4): 549–580

[44] Horny H P and Horst H A (1986) Lymphoreticular infiltrates in invasive ductal breast cancer: a histological and immunohistological study. Virchows Arch A Pathol Anat Histopathol. 409: 275–286

[45] Hume D A, Ross L, Himes S R et al. (2002) The mononuclear phagocyte system revisited. J Leukoc Biol 72: 621–627

[46] Ichim C V (2005) Revisiting immunosurveillance and immunostimulation: implications for cancer immunotherapy. J Transl Med 3: 1–13

[47] Kai S, Goto S, Tahara K et al. (2004) Indoleamine 2,3-dioxygenase is necessary for cytolytic activity of natural killer cells. Scand J Immunol 59(2): 177–182

[48] Kalluri R, Zeisberg M (2006) Fibroblasts in cancer. Nat Rev Cancer. 6: 392–401

[49] Karkkainen M J, Petrova T V (2000) Vascular endothelial growth factor receptors in the regulation of angiogenesis and lymphangiogenesis. Oncogene 19(49): 5598–5605

[50] Kusmartev S, Gabrilovich D I (2006) Role of immature myeloid cells in mechanisms of immune evasion in cancer. Cancer Immunol Immunother 55: 237–245

[51] Lardner A (2001) The effects of extracellular pH on immune function. J Leukoc Biol 69: 522–530

[52] Larmomier N, Marron M, Zeng Y et al. (2007) Tumor-derived CD4 + Cd25* regulatory T cell suppression of dendritic cell function involves TGF-β and IL-10. Cancer Immuniol. Immunother 56: 48–59

[53] Le Q-T, Shi G, Cao H et al. (2005) Galectin-1: A link between tumor hypoxia and tumor immune privilege. J Clin Oncol 23: 8932–8941

[54] Lewis C E, Pollard J W (2006) Distinct role of Macrophages in different tumor microenvironments. Cancer Res 66: 605–612

[55] Lewis J S, Lee J A, Underwood J C E et al. (1999) Macrophage response to hypoxia: relevance to disease mechanisms. J Leukoc Biol 66: 889–900

[56] Li M O, Wan Y Y, Sajabi S et al. (2006) Transforming growth factor -.-β regulation of immune responses. Annu Rev Immunol 24: 99–146

[57] Lowe D, Jorizzo J, Hutt M S (1981) Tumor associated eosinophilia: a review. J Clin Pathol 34: 1343–1348

[58] Mabjeesh N J, Amir S (2007) Hypoxia–inducible factor (HIF) in human tumorigenesis. Histol Histopathol 22: 559–572

[59] Mazzoni A, Young H A, Spitzer J H et al. (2001) Histamine regulates cytokine production in maturing dendritic cells, resulting in altered T cell polarization. J Clin Invest 108: 1865–1873

[60] Menon A G, Fleuren G J, Alphenaar E A et al. (2003) A basal membrane-like structure surrounding tumor nodules may prevent intraepithelial leukocyte infiltration in colorectal cancer. Cancer Immunol Immunother 52: 121–126

[61] Mocellin S, Marincola F M, Young H A (2005) Interleukin-10 and the immune response against cancer: a counterpoint. J Leukoc Biol 78: 1043–1051

[62] Munitz A, Levi-Shaffer F (2004) Eosinophils: new role for old cells. Allergy 59: 268–275

[63] Munn D H (2006) Indoleamine 2,3-dioxygenase, tumor induced tolerance and counter regulation. Curr Opin Immunol 1: 220–225

[64] Nagy J A, Feng D, Vasile E, Wong W H et al. (2006) Permeability properties of tumor surrogate blood vessels induced by VEGF-A. Lab Invest 86(8): 767–780

[65] Nathan C F, KLebanoff S J (1982) Augmentation of spontaneous macrophage-mediated cytolysis by eosinophils peroxidase. J Exp Med 155: 1291–1308

[66] Nefedova Y, Gabrilovich D I (2007) Targeting of Jak/STAT pathway in antigen presenting cells in cancer. Curr Cancer Drug Targets 7(1):71–77

[67] Nefedova Y, Huang M, Kusmartsev S et al. (2004) Hyperactivation of STAT3 is involved in abnormal differentiation of dendritic cells in cancer. J Immunol 172: 464–474

[68] Neufeld G, Cohen T, Gengrinovitch S, Poltorak Z (1999) Vascular endothelial growth factor (VEGF) and its receptors. FASEB J 13: 9–22

[69] Orino A, Weinberg R A (2006) Stromal fibroblasts in cancer: A novel tumor promoting cell type. Cell Cycle 5: 1597–1601

[70] Oyama T, Ran S, Ishida T, Nadaf S et al. (1998) Vascular endothelial growth factor affects dendritic cell maturation through the inhibition of nuclear factor-kappa B activation in hemopoietic progenitor cells. J Immunol 160: 1224–1232

[71] Packard K A, Khan M M (2003) Effects of histamine on Th1/Th2 cytokine balance. Int Immunopharmacol 3: 909–920

[72] Pardali K, Moustakas A (2007) Actions of TGF-β as tumor suppressor and pro-metastatic factor in human cancer. Biochimica et Biophisica acta 1775: 21–62

[73] Park Y M K, Anderson R L, Spitz D R et al. (1992) Hypoxia and resistance to hydrogen peroxide confer resistance to tumor necrosis factor in murine L929 cells. Radiat Res 131: 162–168

[74] Ping C N, Hinz B, Swartz M A (2005) Interstitial fluid flow induces myofibroblast differentiation and collagen alignment in vitro. J Cell Sci 118: 4731–4739

[75] Pockaj B A, Basu G D, Pathangey L B et al. (2004) Reduced T-Cell and dendritic Cell function is related to cycloxigenase-2 overexepression and prostaglandin E 2 secretion in patients with breast cancer. Ann of Surg Oncol 11: 328–339

[76] Pollard J (2004) Tumor-educated Macrophages promote tumor progression and metastasis. Nat Rev Cancer 4: 71–78

[77] Polverini P J (1995) The pathophysiology of angiogenesis. Crit Rev Oral Biol Med 6: 230–247

[78] Rane G S, Reddy E S (2000) Janus kinases: components of multiple signalling pathways. Oncogene 19: 5662–5679

[79] Ribatti D, Vacca A, Danmacco F (1999) The role of vascular phase in solid tumor growth: a historical review. Neoplasia 1: 293–302

[80] Said M, Wiseman S, Yang J et al. (2005) Tissue eosinophilia: a morphologic marker for assessing stromal invasion in laryngeal squamous neoplasms. BMC Clin Pathol 5: 1–8

[81] Samoszuk M, Kanakubo E, Chan J K (2005) Degranulating mast cells in fibrotic regions of human tumors and evidence that mast cell heparin interferes with the growth of tumor cells through a mechanism involving fibroblasts. BMC Cancer 5: 1–10

[82] Sampson L E, Chaplin D J (1994) The influence of microenvironment on the cytotoxicity of TNFa in vitro. Int J Radiat Oncol Biol Phys 29: 467–471

[83] Sauer H, Wartenberg M, Hesheler J (2001) Reactive oxygen species as intracellular messengers during cell growth and differentiation. Cell Physiol Biochem 11: 173–186

[84] Scannel G, Waxman K, Kaelm G J et al. (1993) Hypoxia induces a human macrophage cell line to release tumor necrosis factor a and its soluble receptors in vitro. J Surg Res 54: 281–285

[85] Schwartz L (2004) Cancer. Between glycolysis and physical constraint. Springer. Berlin, Heidelberg, New York

[86] Seliger B (2006) Strategies of tumor immune evasion. Biodrugs 19: 347–354

[87] Semenza G L (2000) HIF-1: mediator of physiological and pathophysiological responses to hypoxia. J Appl Physiol 88: 1474–1480

[88] Severin T, Muller B, Giese G et al. (1994) pH–Dependent LAK cell Cytotoxicity. Tumor Biol 15: 304–310

[89] Shevach E M (2001) Certified professionals: CD4(+)CD25(+) suppressor T cells. J Exp Med 193(11): F41–46

[90] Sica A, Schioppa T, Mantovani A et al. (2006) Tumor-associated Macrophages are a distinct M2 polarized population promoting tumor progression: potential targets of anti-cancer therapy. EJC 42: 717–727

[91] Silzle T, Randolph G J, Kreutz M et al. (2004) The fibroblast: sentinel cell and local immune modulator in tumor tissue. Int. J. Cancer 108: 173–180

[92] Stewart T J, Greeneltch K M, Lutsiak M E C et al. (2007) Immunologic response can have both pro- and antitumor effects: implications for immunotherapy. Expert Rev Mol Med 9: 1–20

[93] Stohrer M, Boucher Y, Stangassinger M, Jain R K (2000) Oncotic pressure in solid tumors is elevated. Cancer Res 60(15): 4251–4255

[94] Swartz M A, Boardman K, Jr C (2002) The role of interstitial stress in lymphatic function and lymphangiogenesis. Annals of the New York academy of sciences 979:197–210

[95] Tamsma J T, Keizer H J, Meinders A E (2001) Pathogenesis of malignant ascites: Starling's law of capillary hemodynamics revisited. Ann Oncol 12: 1353–1357

[96] Taylor A, Verhagen J, Blaser K et al. (2006) Mechanisms of immune suppression by interleukin-10 and transforming growth factor-β: the role of T regulatory cells. Immunology 117: 433–442

[97] Theoharides T C, Conti P (2004) Mast cells: the Jekyll and Hyde of tumor growth. Trends Immunol 25: 235–241

[98] Tomita K, Okabe S (2005) Exogenous histamine stimulates colorectal cancer implant growth via immunosuppression in mice. J Pharmacol Sci 97: 116–123

[99] Uotila P (1993) Inhibition of prostaglandin E_2 formation and histamine action in cancer immunity. Cancer Immunol Immunother. 37: 251–254

[100] Uotila P (1996) The role of cyclic AMP and oxygen intermediates in the inhibition of cellular immunity in cancer. Cancer Immunol Immunother 43: 1–9

[101] Van Furth (1992) Production and migration of monocytes and kinetics of Macrophages. In van Furth R. (ed.), Mononuclear phagocytes Dordrecht, Kluwer Academic Publishers: 3–12

[102] Van Ginderachter J A, Movahedi K, Ghassabeh G H et al. (2006) Classical and alternative activation of mononuclear phagocytes: picking the best of both words for tumor promotion. Immunobiology 211: 487–501

[103] Vaupel P, Kallinowski F, Okunieff P (1989) Blood flow, oxygen and nutrient supply and metabolic microenvironment of human tumors, a review. Cancer Res 49: 6449–6465

[104] Vaupel P (2004) The role of hypoxia-induced factors in tumor progression. Oncologist 9 (5): 10–17

[105] Wahl S A, Swisher J, Mc Cartney-Francis N et al. (2004) TGF-β: the perpetrator of immune suppression by regulatory T cells and suicidal T cells. J Leukoc Biol 76: 15–24

[106] Wang D, Du Bois R N (2006) Prostaglandins and cancer. Gut 55: 115–122

[107] Wing K, Ekmark A, Karlsson H et al. (2002) Characterization of human CD25+ CD4+ T cells in thymus, cord and adult blood. Immunology 106: 190–199

[108] Wolf A M, Wolf D, Steurer M et al. (2003) Increase of regulatory T-cells in the peripheral blood of cancer patients. Clinical Cancer Res 9: 606–612

[109] Yang A S, Lattime E C (2003) Tumor-induced Interleukin 10 Suppresses the Ability of Splenic Dendritic Cells to Stimulate CD4 and CD8 T-Cell Responses. Cancer Res 63(9): 2150–2157

[110] Yu P, Fu Y-X (2006) Tumor-infiltrating Lymphocytes friends or foes? Lab Invest 86: 231–245

[111] Zalatnai A (2006) Molecular aspects of stromal-parenchymal interactions in malignant neoplasms. Curr Mol Med 6: 685–693

3. Natural killer cells. Lymphokine-activated killers

IRINA ZH. SHUBINA
NN Blokhin Russian Cancer Research Center RAMS
Laboratory of Cell Immunity
Moscow
Russia

OLGA V. LEBEDINSKAYA
EA Vagner Perm Medical Academy
Department of Histology
Embryology and Cytology Perm
Russia

EVGENIA O. KHALTURINA
IM Setchenov Medical Academy
Department of Microbiology
Virology and Immunology
Moscow
Russia

IRINA O. CHIKILEVA
NN Blokhin Russian Cancer Research Center RAMS
Laboratory of Cell Immunity
Moscow
Russia

MIKHAIL V. KISELEVSKY
NN Blokhin Russian Cancer Research Center RAMS
Laboratory of Cell Immunity
Moscow
Russia

Keywords: NK, Interleukin-2, lymphokine-activated killer cells, cytotoxic activity

Abstract

Tumors can escape from adaptive immune reactions mediated by cytotoxic T-lymphocytes via down-regulation or complete loss of major histocompatibility class I molecules. Some, and perhaps most, of tumors also seem to lack tumor-specific antigens that may be recognized by adaptive immunity. However, transformed cells with deficiencies in surface expression of major histocompatibility class I molecules are targets of natural killer cells – effectors of the innate immune system. Their function does not depend on recognition of complexes of specific antigens with major histocompatibility class I molecules. Interleukin-2 induces proliferation and activation of natural killer cells. Lymphocytes incubated in the presence of interleukin-2 are termed as lymphokine-activated killer cells. Lymphokine-activated killer cells have high proliferative activity and effectively lyse different types of tumor cells.

M.V. Kiselevsky (ed.), Atlas Effectors of Anti-tumor Immunity, 45–63.

Natural killer (NK) cells are lymphocytes of the innate immunity. They are different from effectors of the adaptive immunity, such as T- and B-lymphocytes and do not have their specific cell surface markers (CD3, CD19, CD20 etc.). Their morphology is typical for large granular lymphocytes. Numerous secretory granules in the cytoplasm indicate their intensified activity. NK cells comprise about 5–15% of all the lymphocytes. Generally lymphocytes, which express CD16 and CD56 antigens but do not have component of T-cell receptor CD3, are considered to be NK cells. NK cells also have receptors for interleukin-2 (IL-2) and therefore may be activated by endogenous or exogenous cytokine. In contrast to T-cells, NK cells do not require antigen presentation for recognition of their targets. NK cells as well as neutrophils may be considered an "early line of defense" of the immune system, which includes activation of neutrophils, tissue macrophages, monocytes, because they can lyse transformed cells by contact without prior activation [5, 7, 17, 20, 39, 40, 49, 51, 61, 66]. NK cells can kill tumor cells in antigen-independent manner. That is their major difference from T-cells. The main mechanism of NK-cell function, called natural cytotoxicity, is involved in the destruction of various targets such as tumor cells and virus-infected cells, which generally have certain deficiencies (down-regulation or lack) in expression of major histocompatibility class I (MHC-I) surface molecules. NK cells were also found to recognize specific molecules that are up-regulated in cellular stress. NK function is inhibited by MHC-I molecules expressed on normal cells. Tumor cells can have decreased MHC-I expression and lose tissue-specific markers during their malignant trans-formation. They thus escape from adaptive immunity but become targets of NK cells that are activated as a result of lacking "self" – MHC molecules, while T-cells recognize foreign peptides in the context of a "self" – set of MHC molecules expressed in a individual. The majority of the NK cells in human blood ($\geq 95\%$) belong to $CD56^{dim}CD16^+$ cytolytic subset. These cells carry homing receptors for inflamed peripheral sites and contain perforin to rapidly mediate cytotox-icity. The minor NK subset in blood ($\leq 5\%$) is $CD56^{bright}CD16^-$ cells. These NK cells have no perforin, but increasingly secrete interferon-γ (IFN-γ) and tumor necrosis factor β (TNF-β) as a result of activation and are superior to the $CD56^{dim}CD16^+$ NK subset in these functions. In addition, they display homing markers for secondary lymphoid organs, namely CC-receptor 7 (CCR7) and CD62L (ligand). The main activating receptors constitutively found on all NK cells in peripheral blood are NKG2D and natural cytotoxicity receptors (NCRs) NKp30 and NKp46. Activating receptors bind stress-induced ligands. For example, NKG2D recognizes MHC-I chain-related proteins A and B as well as UL16 binding proteins (ULBPs) that are up-regulated on epithelial tumors, leukemia, some melanoma and T-cell lymphoma cell lines. Besides that, NKG2D ligands can be induced by viral and bacterial infections [2, 3, 9, 13, 16, 22, 25, 29, 33, 37, 38, 54, 57, 59].

Most inhibitory NK receptors recognize MHC-I molecules on target cells. They can be divided into two groups, detecting either common allelic determinants of MHC-I, or MHC-I expression in general. Killer inhibitory receptors (KIRs) presenting the first group recognize polymorphic HLA-B and -C molecules. Inhibitory receptors detecting MHC-I expression in general are more heterogeneous. They include the leukocyte Ig-like receptor 1/Ig-like transcript 2 molecule with a broad speci-ficity for different MHC-I molecules and CD94/NKG2A heterodimer, specific for HLA-E. MHC-I allele specific KIRs are expressed on subsets of $CD56^{dim}CD16^+$

cytolytic NKs, whereas immunoregulatory CD56^{bright}CD16$^-$ NK subset expresses uniformly CD94/NKG2A and lacks KIRs. CD56^{dim}CD16$^+$ cytolytic NKs are probably terminally differentiated effectors that have the entire panel of special activating and inhibitory receptors to detect even allelic HLA loss and thus can readily lyse malignant cells. On the contrary, CD56^{bright}CD16$^-$ NK cells might perform an immunoregulatory function in secondary lymphoid tissues. Data from recent studies show that NK cells play a major role in anti-tumor immunity. For example, immunologically deficient athymic-nude mice that lack all T-cells have a similar rate of tumor development to that of syngenic immunocompetent mice [10, 23, 24, 28, 32, 36, 44, 45, 58, 64]. Certain cytokines, such as IL-2, increase NK-cell cytotoxicity. Activated NK cells are able to lyse a wide range of tumor cells including tumor cells expressing autologous MHC-I molecules. Such cells were termed lymphokine-activated killers (LAKs) [21, 25, 27, 36, 47, 48].

As defined by S. Rosenberg et al. [19] LAKs are activated killer cells, which display LAK activity and are generated from a lymphoid population by *in vitro* activation in the presence of IL-2. The phenomenon of lysis of isolated or cultured tumor cells by lymphocytes activated with IL-2 *in vitro* was termed LAK phenomenon or LAK activity. Although there are no inter-individual or interspecies histocompatibility barriers for cell lysis, normal fresh tissues are resistant to LAK's lytic effect. LAK activity does not require prior effector sensitization with antigens of target cells. IL-2 is sufficient for lymphocyte activation [3, 21, 25, 30, 43].

Primarily, the LAK phenomenon was observed in the result of the activation of the total lymphoid cell populations obtained from different mouse and human tissues. Such populations contained different cell types, including T-, B- and NK cells. A more detailed study of the phenomenon by Yang et al. determined that most LAK precursors are NK cells. A lot of the following studies of LAK phenomenon applying human lymphocytes confirmed that most LAK precursors are found in a small subset of peripheral blood mononuclear cells (PBMCs) with phenotypic features of NK cells (CD11b$^+$, CD16$^+$, CD56$^+$, CD57$^+$). The most active were the cells derived from CD3$^-$/CD16$^+$/CD56$^+$ precursors. CD3$^+$/CD16$^-$/CD56$^-$ T-cells displayed moderate activity when activated with IL-2. Cell phenotypes did not change after activation. LAK activity was due mainly to a small subpopulation of PBMC, including CD3$^-$/CD56$^+$ cells. Although another subset of CD3$^+$/CD56$^+$ lymphocytes with minor LAK activity was also described [6, 41, 42, 55]. The LAK phenomenon is mainly determined by lymphocytes, which demonstrate NK-cell phenotype and functions.

3.1. NK and LAK-Cell Mechanisms of Action

The process of cell lysis resulting from the interaction of LAK or NK cells with tumor cells may be subdivided into five phases (Figure 3.1):

- NK or LAKs recognize target tumor cells;
- effector cells bind to target cells;
- lymphocytes release cytotoxic substances;
- target tumor cells die.

CD16$^+$-LAKs kill antibody-coated cells via a mechanism called antibody-dependent cytotoxicity [32, 38]. This is mediated by low-affinity Fcγ receptor, CD16. Cytolitic effect of LAK and NK cells on target cells is achieved by secretion of cytotoxic substances such as perforin and granzyme, accumulated in cytoplasmic granules. One of the granzymes (granzyme B) is a serine protease activating caspase-8, with subsequent induction of apoptotic proteolytic cascade.

Activated lymphocytes express Fas ligand (FasL) and induce apoptosis of transformed cells by interaction of FasL with Fas receptor (FasR) on target cells. Studies on mice deficient in perforin, granzyme or FasL showed that these are the main effector molecules of cytotoxicity. FasL expression is characteristic for many immune cells and different tissues. IFN-γ or IL-2 up-regulate FasL expression in mononuclear leukocytes (MNLs). FasL belongs to the TNF family, including TNF-α, lymphotoxin, CD30L, CD40L, CD27L, as well as TRAIL (TNF-related apoptosis-inducing ligand). Membrane bound FasL induces apoptosis as a result of direct cell contact, whereas soluble form of FasL acts as an autocrine or paracrine factor of cell "suicide" or "murder" neighbor cells [11, 14, 15, 26, 51, 52, 53, 56]. Thus, perforin/granzyme or Fas/FasL mechanisms may act simultaneously or independently to induce apoptosis of target cells (Figure 3.2).

3.2. Generation of LAKs. Their Anti-Tumor Effects

Activation of MNLs *in vitro* in the presence of IL-2 generates LAK cells, which effectively lyse tumor cells. NK cells, a major population of LAKs, express the p75β chain of IL-2R and LFA-1 (lymphocyte function associated antigen-1) when stimulated by IL-2. Therefore, MNLs incubation with IL-2 induces selective activation of NK cells and a rapid increase of NK-activity in LAKs. Cytotoxic activity of MNLs or NK cells alone similarly increased during a short incubation in the presence of IL-12. The studies showed that the IL-12 activating rate was lower than that of IL-2 and similar to IFN-γ. The maximal increase of NK-cell activity was registered with a combination of IL-2 and IL-12 as stimulating factors with additive effect. IL-2 and IL-12 induce mRNAs

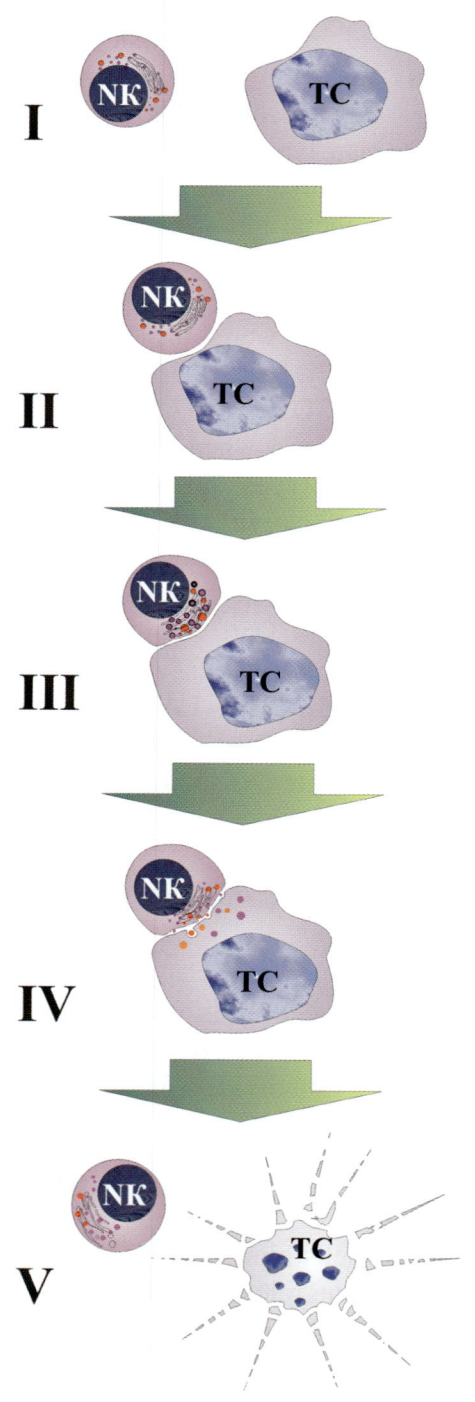

Figure 3.1. Schematic presentation of interactions between LAKs and tumor cells. I – NK or LAKs recognize target tumor cells; II – effector cells bind to target cells; III – accumulation of granules containing cytotoxic substances; IV – lymphocytes release cytotoxic substances; V – target tumor cells die (Refs. [3, 21, 25, 30, 43])

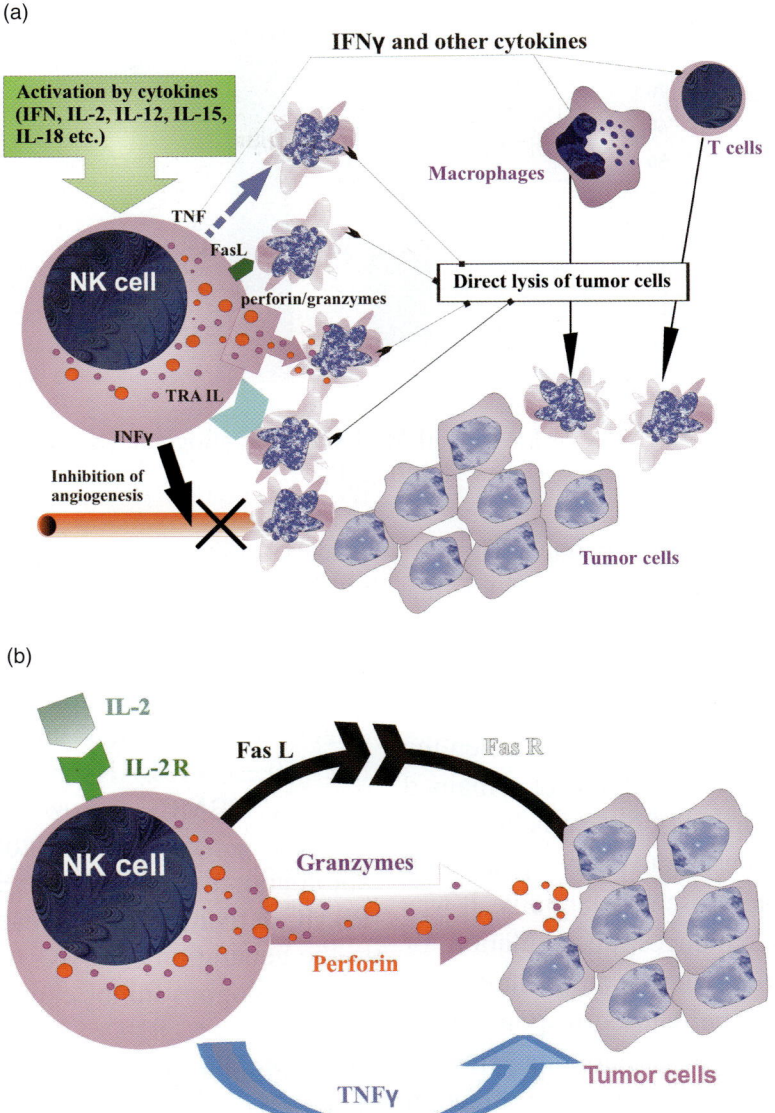

Figure 3.2. Mechanism of antitumor activity of NK. **a** – Interaction of effectors of anti-tumor immunity; **b** – Perforin/granzyme and Fas/FasL mechanisms (Refs. [11, 14, 15, 26, 51, 52, 56])

coding perforin and granzymes A and B [4, 12, 31, 60, 62, 63, 67]. Earlier, cytotoxic activity of LAKs was considered to depend on two major populations: NK-cells and cytotoxic T-lymphocytes. However, further studies showed that the LAK phenomenon was due primarily to the activity of typical NK cells [42]. Studies with electron microscopy and antibodies to CD16 marker conjugated with colloid gold proved directly that NK cells are the main mediators of LAK activity. The results revealed that CD16[+]-cells of the LAK population penetrated deep into target tumor cells with their pseudopodia, while their cytoplasmic granules and vacuoles accumulated in the sites of cell contact [18].

IL-2 or/and IL-12 induced a gradual increase in the proportion of NK cells in cultured MNLs. The proportion of NK cells in the total population of LAKs reached 70% by day 9 of incubation in the presence of cytokines. Even low concentrations of IL-2

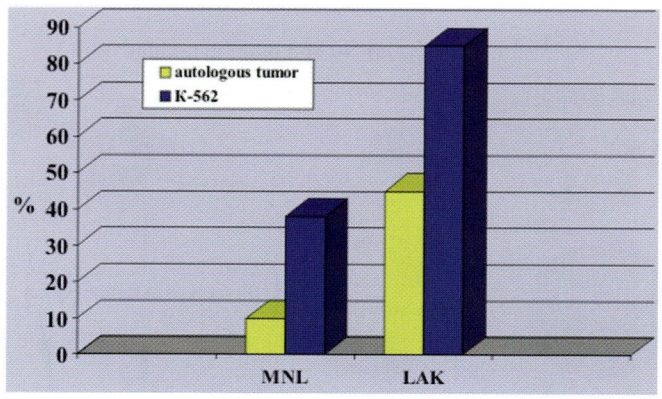

Figure 3.3. Cytotoxic activity of LAKs and MNLs against allogenic (K-562) and autologous tumor cells

combined with IL-12 led to enhanced proliferation of NK cells. The number of CD56$^+$ T-cells had increased several-fold by the second day of PBMC incubation with IL-2, though their cytotoxic activity was low. However, during further cultivation, when the percentage of CD56$^+$ T-cell subset remained the same, the proportion of NK cells increased significantly and the cytotoxicity of the total LAK-cell population rose substantially. It was shown that IL-12 induces up-regulation of NK-cell proliferation without augmentation of their cytotoxicity. The data corresponds well to the concept of the pre-stimulating effect of IL-12 but it has minimal stimulating effect on latent lymphocytes [1, 8, 34, 35, 68].

PBMCs from healthy donors have physiological (spontaneous) anti-tumor activity towards allogeneic tumor cells. A population of PBMCs can be generated into LAKs during cultivation in the presence of IL-2. Generally, LAKs are considered as NK-like cells, which cytotoxic effect does not require antigen presentation in the context of MHC-I molecules. Determination of their cyotoxic function involves a test on NK-sensitive immortalized cell lines such as human leukemia K-562. LAKs of healthy donors present higher NK activity, than PBMCs of the same donors. They reach the peak of their activity by the third day of cultivation.

PBMCs of cancer patients also have high spontaneous NK activity and lyse about 45 ± 6% of K-562 cells. However, their cytolytic effect on autologous tumor cells is very low (10 ± 6%). LAKs generated from cancer patients' PBMC in vitro have a higher rate of NK activity and cytotoxicity towards autologous tumor cells (35 ± 6%). Therefore PBMC activation in the presence of IL-2 leads to the generation of LAKs that can efficiently lyse autologous tumor cells (Figure 3.3) [25].

3.3. Phenotype, Morphology and Cytotoxic Activity of LAK Cells

Our research group thoroughly investigated morphological and phenotypical changes in LAKs during the process of their generation. LAKs may be derived from different sources of precursor cells. The most commonly used initial cells for activation are mononuclear leukocytes (MNLs). Spleens surgically removed during gastrectomy in gastric cancer patients can be also used as an appropriate source of lymphocytes for subsequent LAK generation. We also generated LAKs from mouse (CBA line) spleens for experimental purposes. Lymphocytes may be isolated from malignant effusions and tumor-infiltrating leukocytes as well.

LAKs derived from MNLs from different donors have variable donor-specific phenotypic features [65]. However, the highest cytotoxic activity was registered in NK-LAKs with phenotypic features of NK cells. This finding shows that the most important phenotypic feature of LAKs is a high expression rate of NK markers (CD16, CD56) and a lower subset of T-cells characterized by the expression of CD3, CD4 and CD8, compared with initial MNLs. LAKs have an enhanced expression rate of activation antigens (CD25, CD38) and adhesion molecules (CD57, CD58) (Figures 3.4, 3.5).

The percentage of cells expressing CD16 and CD56 (NK markers), CD58, CD25 (IL-2R subunit) and HLA-DR significantly increased within 24 hours after the start of cultivation with IL-2 ($p \leq 0.001$). This tendency continued on the third day of incubation (Figure 3.6). The number of $CD16^+$, $CD56^+$, $CD58^+$ and HLA-DR$^+$ cells

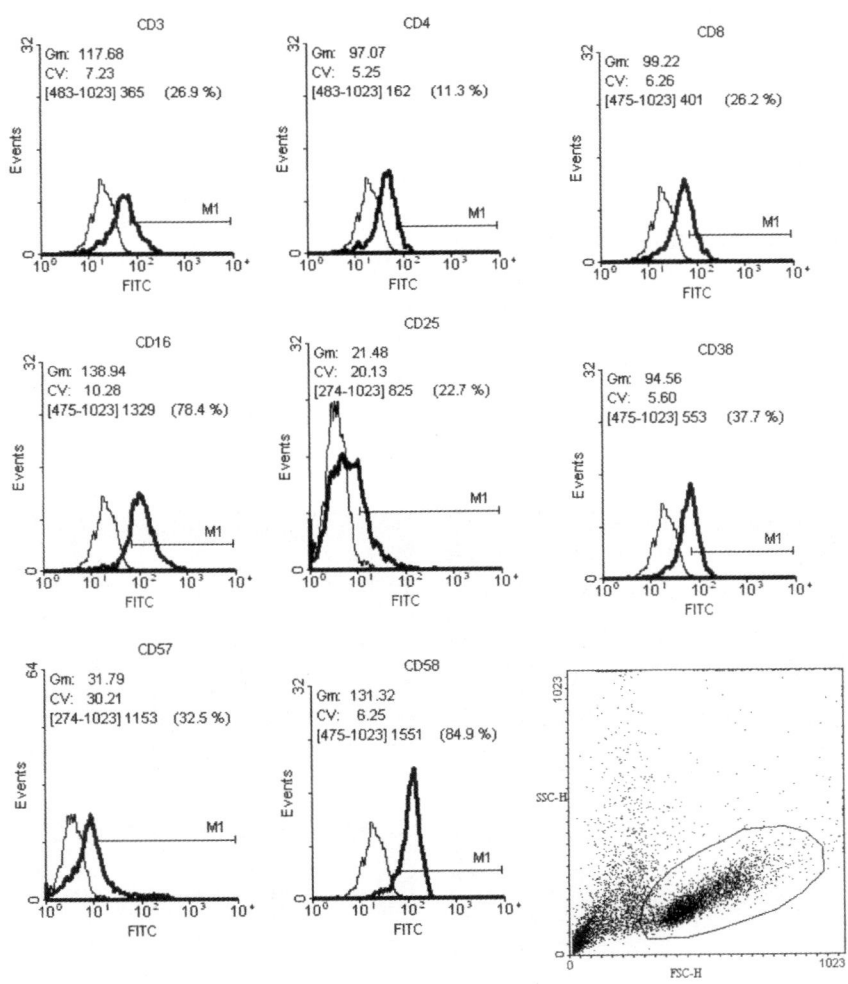

Figure 3.4. Expression of cell surface antigens by LAKs generated from human donor PBMCs (72 hours of incubation with IL-2). Histograms: left – isotypic control; right – samples labeled with fluorescent dye-conjugated antibodies to cell surface antigens (CD3, CD4, CD8, CD14, CD25, CD38, CD56, CD57, CD58, HLA-DR). Dot-plot presents forward and side light scattering. Events - number of cells, FITC, PE – logarithms of fluorescence intensity corresponding to fluorescent dyes FITC (fluorescein isothiocyanate) and PE (phycoerythrin)

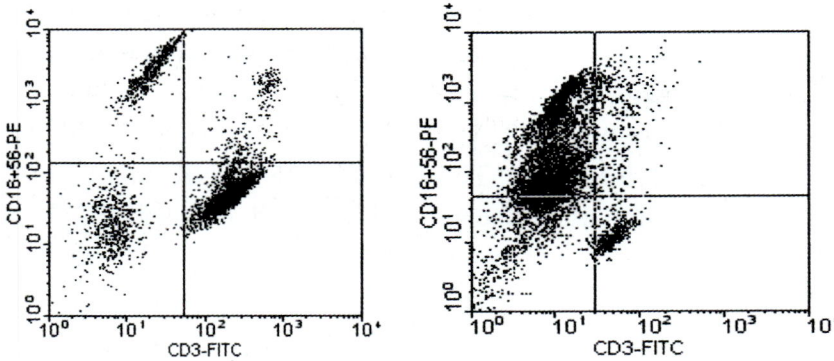

Figure 3.5. Expression of T-cell and NK markers by PBMC-derived LAKs (72 hours of incubation with IL-2). Left – PBMCs; right – LAKs labeled with fluorescent dye-conjugated antibodies to cell surface antigens (CD3/ CD16,CD56). FITC (fluorescein isothiocyanate) and PE (phycoerythrin)

was still much higher in comparison to initial MNLs until days 5 and 7 of incubation.

Typical LAKs are large lymphoid cells. Most of them look like prolymphocytes or immunoblasts with basophilic and pyroninophilic cytoplasm (Figures 3.7–3.9). The Pyroninophilic character of LAK cytoplasm may be explained by RNA-accumulation. Mitotic cells are often observed in LAK samples (Figure 3.10).

On incubation day, two groups of large lymphoid cells with wide rims of cytoplasm were detected in cell cultures that were much larger than latent lymphocytes (Figure 3.11). They proliferated intensively and formed huge colonies of large cells and adhered firmly to plastic (Figures 3.12, 3.13). On day 3, a lot of blast cells with eccentrically located nuclei, multiple nucleoli, and a wide rim of

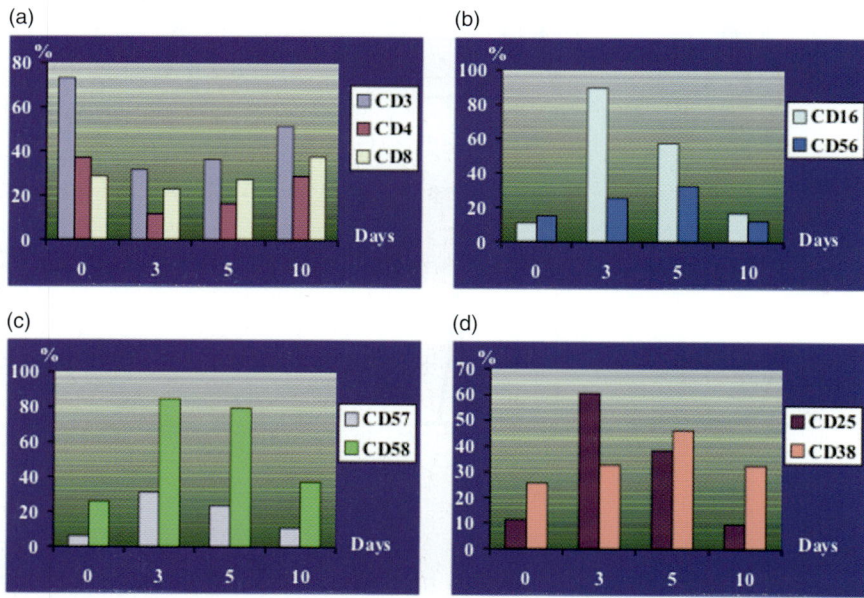

Figure 3.6. IL-2 effect on the expression of molecular markers on human PBMC cell surface (expression rate, $p \pm s_p$,%). **a** – Expression of T-cell markers (CD3, CD4, CD8); **b** – Expression of NK-cell markers (CD16, CD56); **c** – Expression of adhesion molecules (CD57, CD58); **d** – Expression of activation molecules (CD25, CD38)

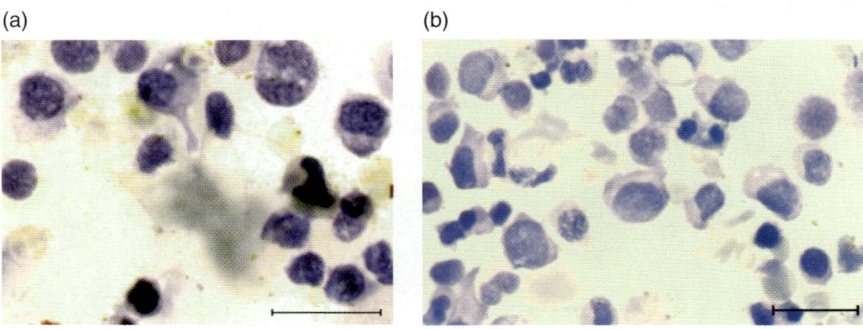

Figure 3.7. PBMC-derived LAKs Micrographs of samples of cell suspensions: **a** – day 3 of incubation with IL-2; Scale bar: 20 μm; **b** – day 5 of incubation with IL-2; Romanovsky-Giemsa azure II-eosin staining; Scale
bar: 20 μm

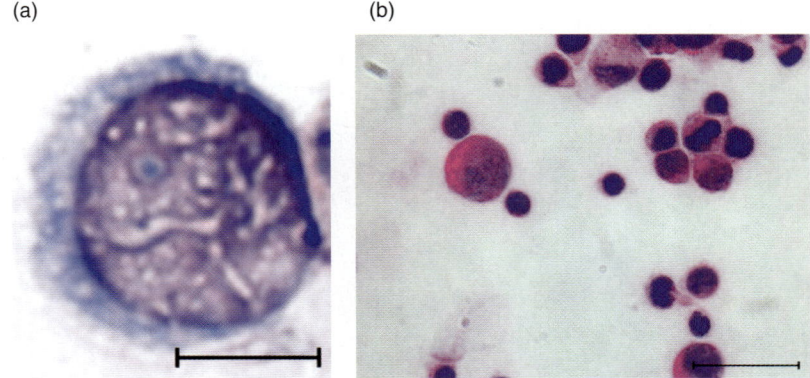

Figure 3.8. Immunoblast in LAK population Micrographs of samples of cell suspensions: **a, b** – day 5 of incubation with IL-2; Scale bar: 5 μm; **a** – Romanovsky-Giemsa azure-eosin staining; **b** – Brachet methyl green – pyronine staining; Scale bar: 20 μm

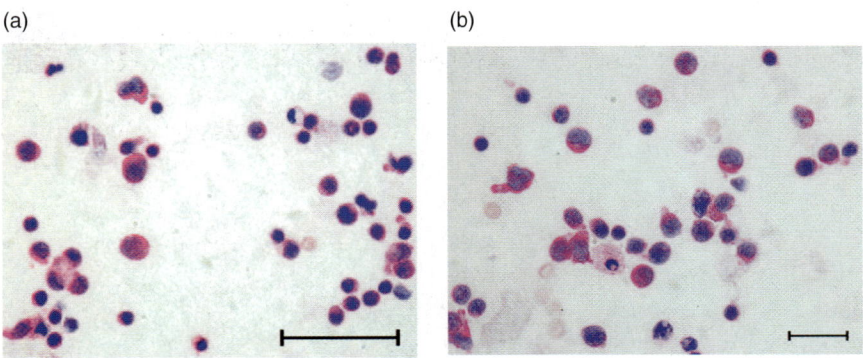

Figure 3.9. Pyroninophilic PBMC-derived LAKs Micrographs of samples of cell suspensions: **a** – day 3 of incubation with IL-2; Scale bar: 50 μm; **b** – day 5 of incubation with IL-2; Brachet methyl green – pyronine staining; Scale
bar: 20 μm

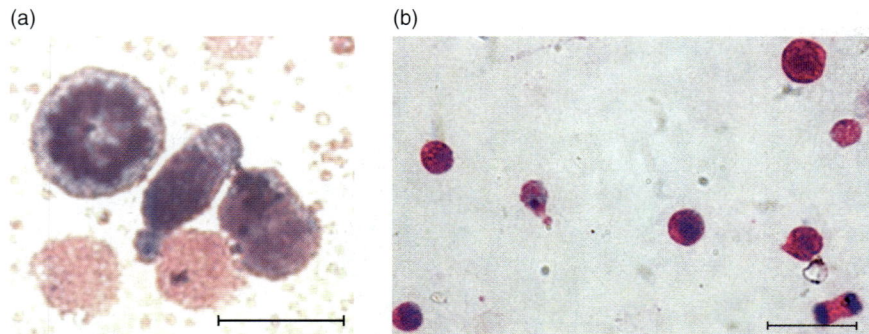

Figure 3.10. Mitotic cells in LAK samples Micrographs of samples of cell suspensions: **a** – day 3 of incubation with IL-2; Romanovsky-Giemsa azure-eosin staining; Scale bar: 10 μm; **b** – day 5 of incubation with IL-2; Brachet methyl green – pyronine staining; Scale bar: 20 μm

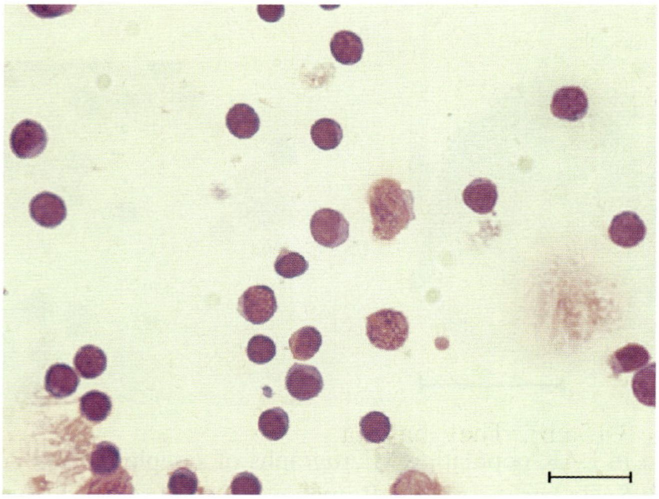

Figure 3.11. PBMC-derived LAKs on day 2 of incubation with IL-2. Micrographs of samples of cell suspensions: Romanovsky-Giemsa azure II-eosin staining; Scale bar: 20 μm

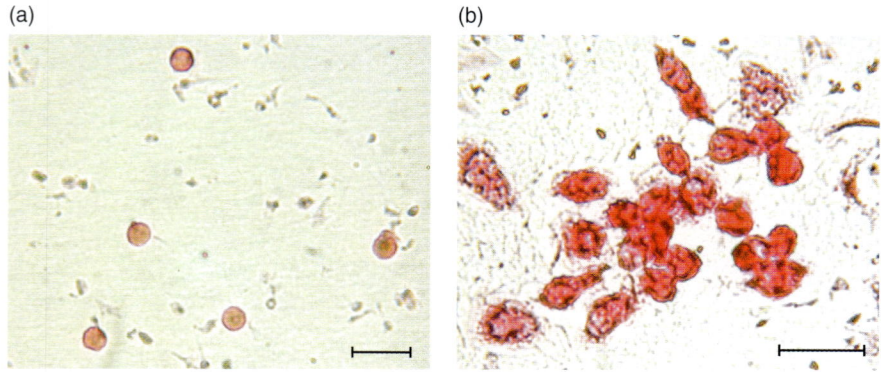

Figure 3.12. PBMCs and LAKs Micrographs of adherent cells. Ziehl fuchsin staining, **a** – Before incubation with IL-2, Scale bar: 20 μm; **b** – After 48 hours of incubation with IL-2; Scale bar: 10 μm

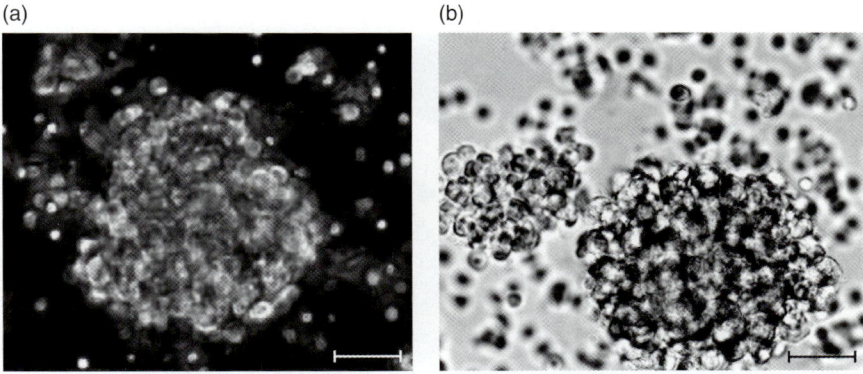

Figure 3.13. Phase-contrast micrographs of PBMC-derived LAK suspensions (48 hours of incubation with IL-2): **a** – In dark field Scale bar: 20 μm; **b** – In bright field; Scale bar: 20 μm

basophilic cytoplasm were observed in the cell culture. By day 5, most mononuclear cells were presented by blasts, prolymphocytes and pyroninophilic lymphocytes. An increased number of blasts and activated lymphocytes was registered for 7–10 days (Figure 3.14). The dynamics of cell surface antigen expression correlated with the changes in the percentage of activated cell forms during PBMC incubation in the presence of IL-2. Electron micrographs of LAKs show their typical morphology of large granular lymphocytes (Figures 3.15a,b). They have a lot of mitochondria and polyribosomes in a

wide rim of cytoplasm. Active RNA biosynthesis is revealed by Bernard electron histochemical cell treatment (Figure 3.15c). LAKs contact with dendritic cells and macrophage-like cells using their cytoplasmic protrusions (Figure 3.16).

Starting from incubation day 10, large macrophage-like cells were seen in the LAK population. They had eccentrically located nuclei (the feature typical for dendritic cells) and vacuolated basophilic cytoplasm (Figure 3.17a), which contained a bright pyroninophilic component (Figure 3.17b). They displayed some other

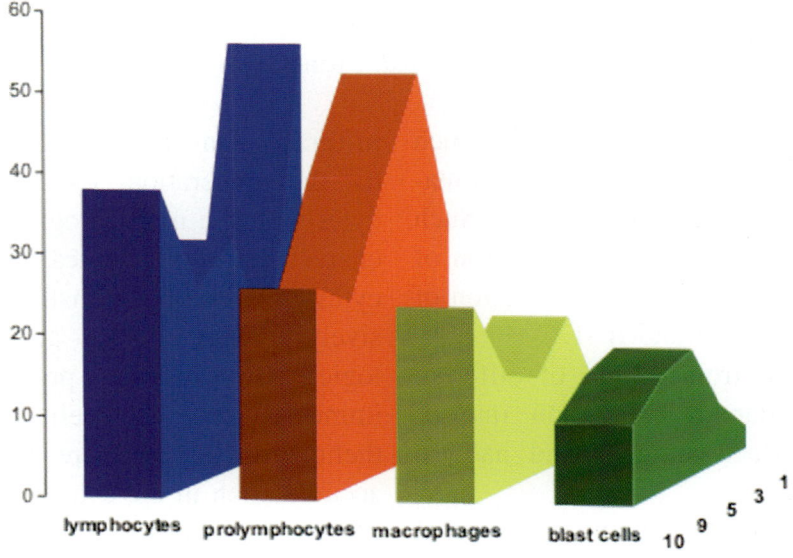

Figure 3.14. Dynamics of cell composition in LAKs (days 1–10)

(a)

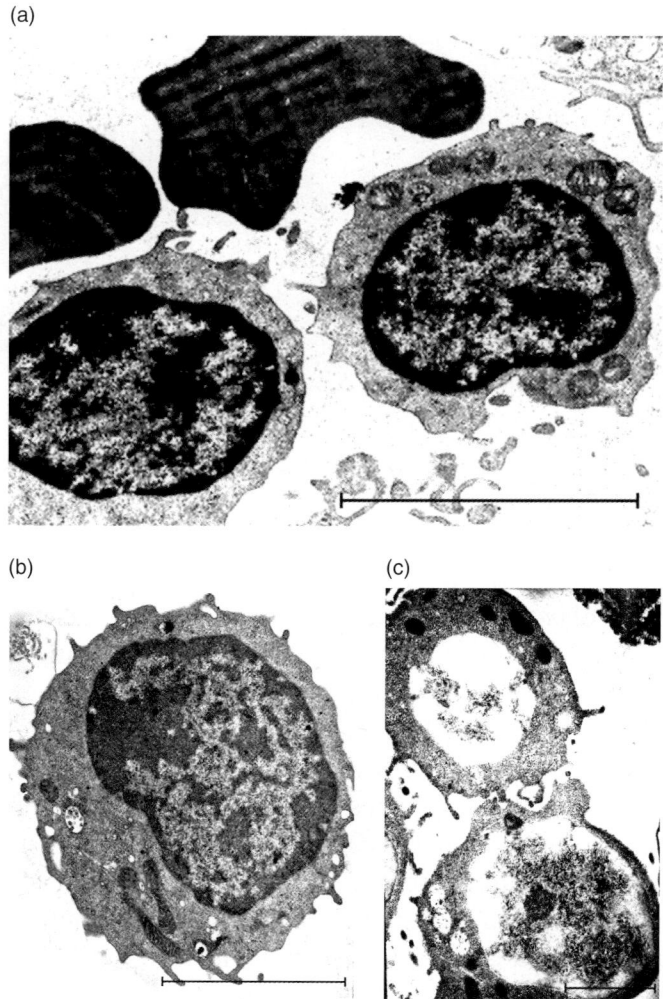

Figure 3.15. PBMC-derived LAKs day 5 of incubation with IL-2 Electron micrographs of samples of
cell suspensions: **a** – Lymphocytes; Scale bar: 10 μm; **b** – Blastic form; Scale bar: 5 μm;
c – Bernard electron histochemical cell treatment;
Scale bar: 5 μm

characteristic features of dendritic cells, such as long membrane protrusions and spontaneous clustering with lymphocytes. Such cells might provide additional stimulation of LAK cells, by cell interaction or secretion of cytokines such as IL-12 and IL-1.

LAKs generated from MNLs of different origin were similar in expression rate of different cell surface antigens and had no significant variations.

The results have demonstrated that incubation of MNLs obtained from different sources (peripheral blood, spleen and tumor infiltrates) in the presence of IL-2 leads to the generation of activated lymphocytes with the morphological and phenotypic characteristics of typical LAKs. Lymphocytes undergo blast-transformation and intensively proliferate. They acquire the morphological features of prolymphocytes and immunoblasts. The cells activate biosynthetic processes that are revealed by RNA-accumulation in the cytoplasm and numerous cellular organelles necessary for biosynthesis. The process of cell activation is also reflected by up-regulated expression of activation

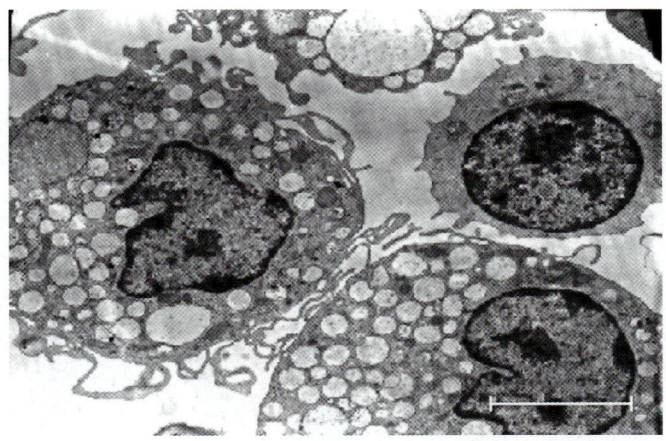

Figure 3.16. Macrophage-like cells in PBMC-derived LAK populations. Day 14 of incubation with IL-2. Electron micrographs of samples of cell suspensions: contacts of LAKs and macrophage-like cells; Scale bar: 5 μm

markers (CD38, CD25 and HLA-DR) as well as adhesion molecules (CD58). During prolonged incubation (more than 10 days) the lymphoid population is gradually replaced by macrophage-like cells.

We compared cytotoxic NK-activity to the K-562 leukemia cell line of LAKs derived from MNLs of different origin (blood, spleen, liver metastases and malignant effusions). All LAK groups showed high NK-activity related to ratios of target and effector cells. The maximal lysis of tumor cells was observed at the ratios of 1:2 and 1:5. However, LAKs obtained from MNLs infiltrating metastatic regions of livers effectively lysed tumor cells,

even at the ratio of target cells and LAKs 1:0.5 (47% of cell lysis) (Figure 3.18).

NK cells and LAKs can lyse tumor cells of different origin [46, 47, 50]. Different ability, of various lymphocyte populations to respond to IL-2 stimulation and subsequently lyse tumors, may be explained by a different expression rate of inhibitory NK receptors on their surfaces (KIR and CD94/NKG2A) [25].

Freshly isolated MNLs and the MNL-derived LAKs displayed cytotoxic activity towards tumor cells of different origin (Tables 3.1, 3.2 and Figures 3.19–3.21). The maximal cytotoxic activity was observed at

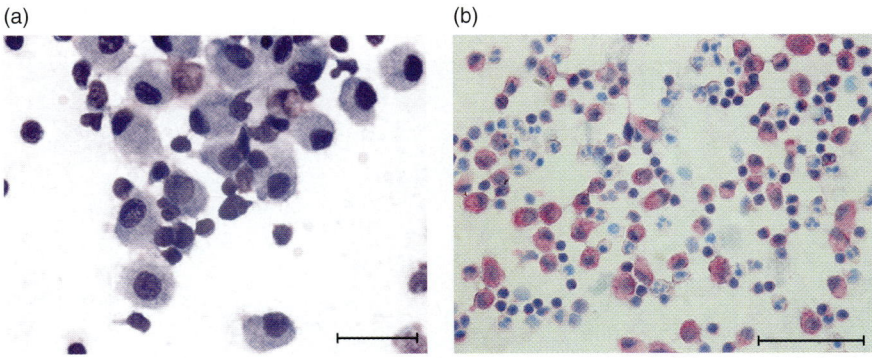

Figure 3.17. Macrophage-like cells in PBMC-derived LAK populations. Day 14 of incubation with IL-2 Micrographs of samples of cell suspensions: **a** – Romanovsky-Giemsa azure-eosin staining; Scale bar: 20 μm; **b** – Brachet methyl green – pyronine staining; Scale bar: 50 μm

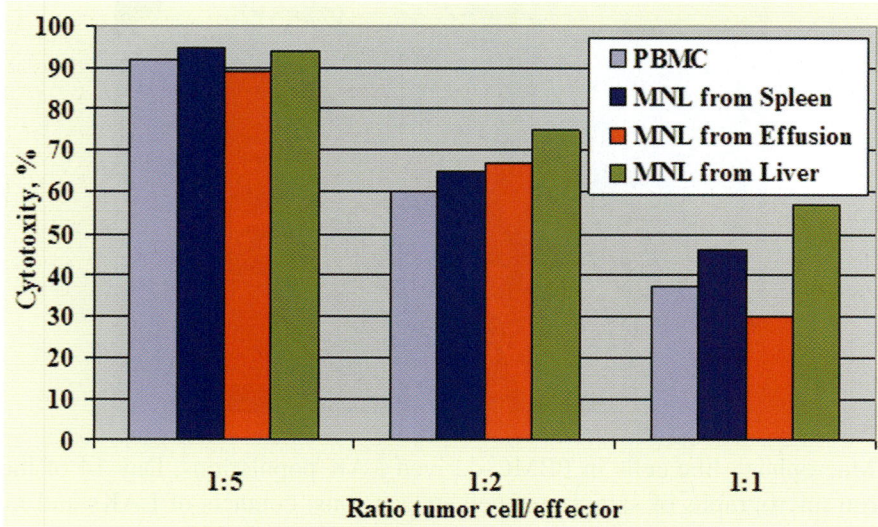

Figure 3.18. NK-activity towards K-562 leukemia cell line of LAKs derived from MNLs of different origin. PBMC – LAK generated from PBMC. MNL from spleen – LAK generated from spleen MNLs. MNL from malignant effusion – LAK generated from malignant effusion MNLs. MNL from liver – LAK generated from liver TIL

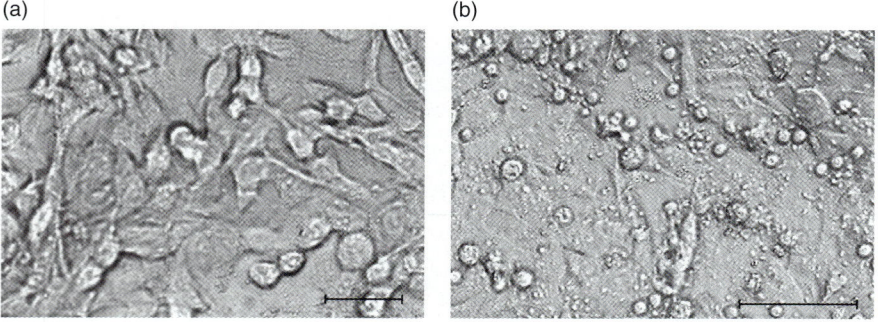

Figure 3.19. Non-small cell lung cancer A-549 cells before **a** and after addition of LAKs **b**. Ratio of targets/effectors 1:5. Micrographs of cell suspensions; Scale bar: **a** – 20 μm; **b** – 50 μm

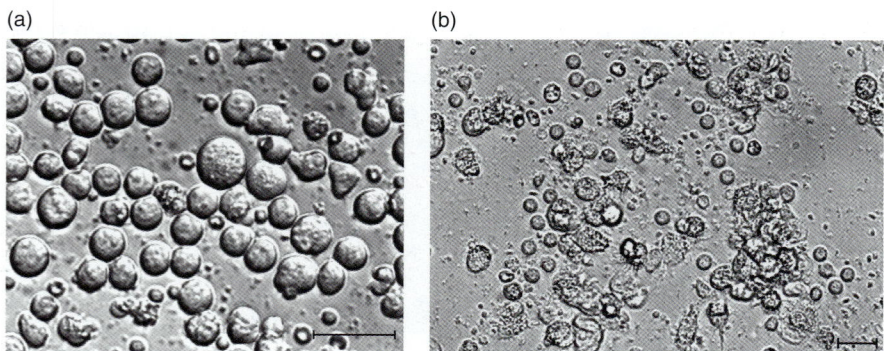

Figure 3.20. Erythroblastic leukemia K-562 cells before **a** and after **b** addition of LAKs. Ratio of targets/effectors 1:5. Micrographs of cell suspensions; Scale bar: 20 μm

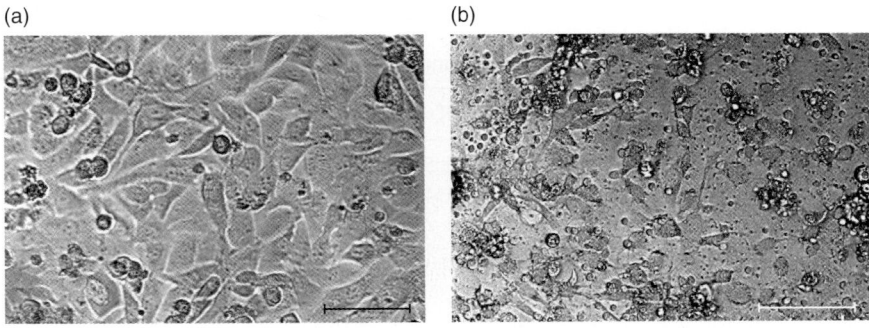

Figure 3.21. Ovarian cancer SKOV-3 cells before **a** and after **b** addition of LAKs. Ratio of targets/effectors 1:5. Micrographs of cell suspensions; Scale bar: 20 μm

Table 3.1. Cytotoxic activity of PBMCs and LAKs against solid tumor cell lines (%)

Ratio Targets/Effectors	Non-small Cell Lung Cancer A-549		Colon Cancer Colo		Ovarian Cancer SKOV-3		Breast Cancer MCF7	
	PBMCs	LAKs	PBMCs	LAKs	PBMCs	LAKs	PBMCs	LAKs
1:5	58 ± 5	77 ± 6*	68 ± 10	86 ± 5*	28 ± 9	52 ± 10*	10 ± 5	63 ± 6*
1:2	53 ± 5	60 ± 6	41 ± 5	69 ± 6*	25 ± 9	40 ± 9*	8 ± 2	36 ± 5*
1:1	42 ± 3	58 ± 6	33 ± 3	57 ± 3*	20 ± 5	30 ± 8	6 ± 3	27 ± 7*

* Statistically significant differences compared to PBMCs, $p \leq 0.05$.

Table 3.2. Cytotoxic activity of PBMCs and LAKs against hematoblastic tumor cell lines (%)

Ratio Targets/Effectors	B-cell Lymphoma Raji		Erythroblastic Leukemia K 562	
	PBMCs	LAKs	PBMCs	LAKs
1:5	48 ± 3	59 ± 4*	68 ± 10	86 ± 5*
1:2	33 ± 5	40 ± 3	41 ± 5	69 ± 6*

* Statistically significant differences compared to PBMCs $p \leq 0.05$.

the ratio of tumor target cells/effectors 1:5 in all tested cell lines.

LAKs showed significantly higher activity compared to that of freshly isolated MNLs in killing tumor cells at all ratios of targets and effectors. The highest cytotoxic activity of both MNLs and LAKs was registered towards leukemia cell lines K-562 and Raji as well as towards non-small cell lung cancer line A-549. Other cell lines such as SCOV3, Colo and MCF7 were less susceptible to the lytic function of MNLs and LAKs.

Both MNLs and LAKs had no significant cytotoxic effect towards normal human fibroblasts and embryonic cells of the calf LEC (lung embryonic cells) line (Table 3.3 and Figures 3.22, 3.23).

Both MNLs and LAKs have selective cytotoxic activity towards tumor cells of different origin. The IL-2 effect leads to up-regulation of NK-activity (cytolysis of NK-sensitive cell lines such as K-562) as well as cytotoxic activity towards other, different tumor cell lines. Altogether LAKs do not significantly influence the viability of normal cells.

The maximal LAKs number was obtained by day 3–5 of PBMC incubation with IL-2, but high proliferation rates and cytotoxicity were registered until day 10. Therefore,

Table 3.3. Cytotoxic activity of PBMCs and LAKs against normal cells (%)

Ratio Targets/Effectors	Calf Embryo Lung Cells LEC		Skin Fibroblasts	
	PBMCs	LAKs	PBMCs	LAKs
1:5	20 ± 3	24 ± 5	18 ± 3	32 ± 5
1:2	12 ± 5	15 ± 4	22 ± 4	23 ± 5
1:1	20 ± 3	20 ± 2	15 ± 4	17 ± 2

* Statistically significant difference, $p \leq 0.05$.

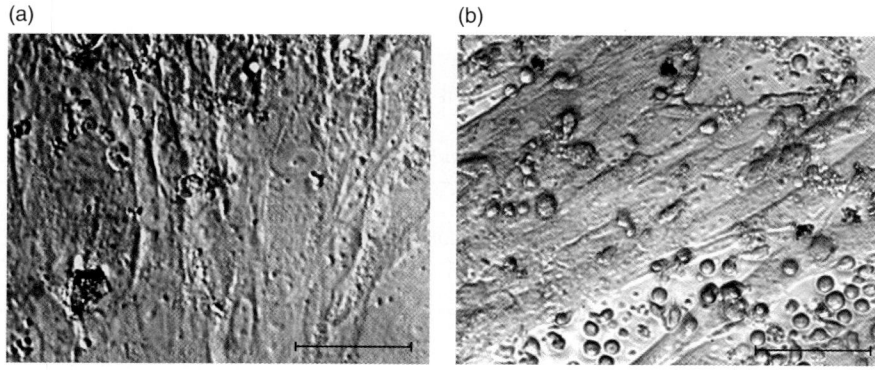

Figure 3.22. Human fibroblasts derived from donor skin before **a** and after **b** addition of LAKs. Ratio of targets/effectors 1:5. Micrographs of cell suspensions; Scale bar: **a** – 30 μm; **b** – 50 μm

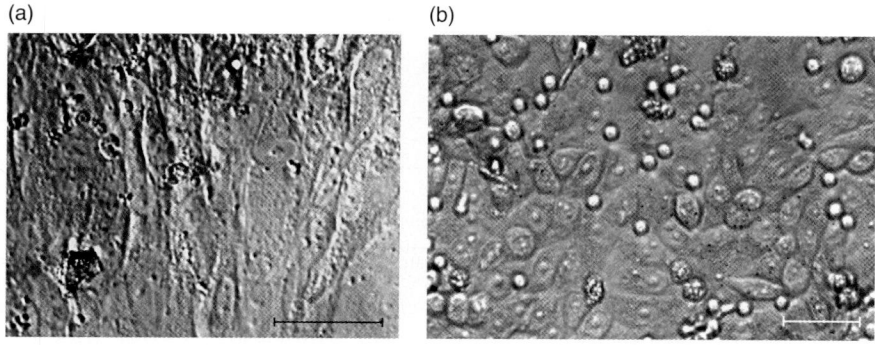

Figure 3.23. Calf LEC (lung embryonic cells) line before **a** and after **b** addition of LAKs. Ratio of targets/effectors 1:5. Micrographs of cell suspensions; Scale bar: 20 μm

better terms for including LAKs in adoptive anti-cancer immunotherapy are days 3–5 of their incubation with IL-2, when they present the optimal rate of proliferation and cytotoxic activity.

LAKs comprise mixed populations of mononuclear cells activated by IL-2. Their cytotoxic activity is apparently due to their major constituents – activated NK cells.

Selective cytotoxic effects of LAKs toward tumor cells of different origin makes them attractive for anti-cancer immunotherapy.

References

[1] Allavena P, Paganin C, Zhou D et al. (1994) Interleukin-12 is chemotactic for natural killer cells and stimulates their interaction with vascular endothelium. Blood 84:2261–2268.

[2] Aptsiauri N, Cabrera T, Mendez R et al. (2007) Role of altered expression of HLA class I molecules in cancer progression. Adv Exp Med Biol. 601:123–1231.

[3] Barlozzari T, Reynolds CW, Herberman RB (1983) *In vivo* role of natural killer cells: involvement of large granular lymphocytes in the clearance of tumor cells in anti-asialo GM1-treated rats. J Immunology 131(2): 1024–1027.

[4] Bendall LJ, Kortlepel K, Gottlieb DJ (1995) GM-CSF enhances IL-2-activated natural killer cell lysis of clonogenic AML cells by upregulating target cell expression of ICAM-1. Leukemia 9(4):677–684.

[5] Campbell J, Qin S, Unutmaz D et al. (2001) Unique subpopulations of CD56$^+$ NK and NK-T peripheral blood lymphocytes identified by chemokine receptor expression repertoire. J Immunol 166(11):6477–6482.

[6] Cao JP, Jiang ZM, Zhang XC et al. (2005) The proliferation, phenotype change and anti-tumor activity of cytokine induced killer cells. Xi Bao Yu Fen Zi Mian Yi Xue Za Zhi 21(5):583–586.

[7] Chan WC, Gu LB, Masih A et al. (1992) Large granular lymphocyte proliferation with the natural killer-cell phenotype. Am J Clin Pathol 97(3):353–358.

[8] Chehimi J, Starr SE, Rengaraju M et al. (1992) Natural killer cell (NK) stimulatory factor increases the cytotoxic activity of NK cells from both healthy donors and human immunodeficiency virus-infected patients. J Exp Med 75(3):789–796.

[9] Cooper MA, Fehniger TA, Turner SC et al. (2001) Human natural killer cells: a unique innate immunoregulatory role for the CD56^{bright} subset. Blood 97(10):3146–3151.

[10] Costello RT, Fauriat C, Sivori S et al. (2004) NK cells: innate immunity against hematological malignancies? Trends Immunol 25(6):328–333.

[11] Derby E, Reddy V, Kopp W et al. (2001) Three-color flow cytometric assay for the study of the mechanisms of cell-mediated cytotoxicity. Immunol Lett 78(1):353–359.

[12] Donskov F, Basse PH, Hokland M (1997) Expression and function of LFA-1 on A-NK and T-LAK cells: role in tumor target killing and migration into tumor tissue. Nat Immunol 15 (2–3):134–146.

[13] Dunn C, Chalupny NJ, Sutherland CL, Dosch S, Sivakumar PV, Johnson DC, Cosman D (2003) Human cytomegalovirus glycoprotein UL16 causes intracellular sequestration of NKG2D ligands, protecting against natural killer cell cytotoxicity. J Exp Med 197(11):1427–1439.

[14] Ebert EC (2004) Interleukin-12 up-regulates perforin- and Fas-mediated lymphokine-activated killer activity by intestinal intraepithelial lymphocytes. Clin Exp Immunol 138(2):259–265.

[15] Facchetti P, Tacchetti C, Prigione I et al. (1999) Ultrastructural and functional studies of the interaction between IL-12 and IL-2 for the generation of lymphokine-activated killer cells. Exp Cell Res 253(2):440–453.

[16] Falk CS, Noessner E, Weiss EH, Schendel DJ (2002) Retaliation against tumor cells showing aberrant HLA expression using lymphokine activated killer-derived T cells. Cancer Res 62(2):480–487.

[17] Ferlazzo G, Münz C (2004) NK cell compartments and their activation by dendritic cells. J Immunol 172(3):1333–1339.

[18] Gong YH, Guo X, Zhang XQ (1994) Immuno-electron microscopic studies on the process of tumor cytolysis mediated by lymphokine activated NK cell. Zhonghua Bing Li Xue Za Zhi 23(1):17–19.

[19] Grimm EA, Mazumder A, Zhang HZ, Rosenberg SA (1982) Lymphokine-activated killer cell phenomenon. Lysis of natural killer-resistant fresh solid tumor cells by interleukin 2-activated autologous human peripheral blood lymphocytes. J Exp Med 155(6):1823–1841.

[20] Herberman RB, Nunn ME, Lavrin DH (1975) Natural cytotoxic reactivity of mouse lymphoid cells against syngeneic and allogeneic tumors. I. Distribution of reactivity and specificity. Int J Cancer 2:216–229.

[21] Herberman RB, Hiserodt J, Vujanovic N et al. (1987) Lymphokine-activated killer cell activity. Immunol Today 8:178–181.

[22] Ikeda H, Chamoto K, Tsuji T et al. (2004) The critical role of type-1 innate and acquired immunity in tumor immunotherapy. Cancer Sci 95(9):697–703.

[23] Jacobs R, Hintzen G, Kemper A et al. (2001) CD56^{bright} cells differ in their KIR repertoire and cytotoxic features from CD56^{dim} NK cells. Eur J Immunol 31(10):3121–3137.

[24] Kärre K, Ljunggren HG, Piontek G, Kiessling R (1986) Selective rejection of H-2-deficient lymphoma variant suggests alternative immune defense strategy. Nature 319(6055):675–678.

[25] Kiselevsky MV (2003) Adoptive immunotherapy of malignances. Vestnik RAMS 3:40–44.

[26] Komatsu F, Kajiwara M (2000) CD18/CD54(+CD102), CD2/CD58 pathway-independent killing of lymphokine-activated killer (LAK) cells against glioblastoma cell lines T98G and U373MG. Oncol Res 12(1):17–24.

[27] Konjević G, Spuzić I (2002). The possibilities of modulation of NK cell activity. Glas Srp Akad Nauka 47:89–101.

[28] Lanier LL (1998) NK cell receptors. Annu Rev Immunol 16(1):359–393.

[29] Lee SJ, Son YO, Kim H et al. (2007) Suppressive effect of a standardized mistletoe extract on the expression of activatory NK receptors and function of human NK cells. J Clin Immunol 27(5):477–485.

[30] Lefor AT, Rosenberg SA (1991) The specificity of lymphokine-activated killer (LAK) cells in vitro: fresh normal murine tissues are resistant to LAK-mediated lysis. J Surg Res 50(1):15–23.

[31] Licato LL, Grimm EA (1999) Multiple interleukin-2 signaling pathways differentially regulated by microgravity. Immunopharmacol 44(3):273–279.

[32] Long EO (1999) Regulation of immune responses through inhibitory receptors. Annu Rev Immunol 17:875–904.

[33] Maeurer MJ, Gollin SM, Martin D et al. (1996) Tumor escape from immune recognition. J Clin Invest 98(7):1633–1641.

[34] Masztalerz A, Everse LA, Otter WD (1997) Presence of cytotoxic B220 + CD3 + CD4 − CD8− cells correlates with the therapeutic efficacy of lymphoma treatment with IL-2 and/or IL-12. J Immunother 27(2):107–115.

[35] Melder RJ, Rosenfeld CS, Herberman RB, Whiteside TL (1989) Large-scale preparation of adherent lymphokine-activated killer (A-LAK) cells for adoptive immunotherapy in man. Cancer Immunol Immunother 29(1):67–73.

[36] Mestas J, Hughe CCW (2004) Of mice and not men: differences between mouse and human immunology. J Immunol 172:2731–2738.

[37] Moretta A, Bottino C, Vitale M et al. (2001) Activating receptors and coreceptors involved in human natural killer. Annu Rev Immunol 19:197–223.

[38] Nirmala R, Narayanan PR (2002) Flow cytometry – a rapid tool to correlate functional activities of human peripheral blood lymphocytes with their corresponding phenotypes after in vitro stimulation. BMC Immunol 3:9.

[39] Ortaldo JR, Winkler-Pickett R, Kopp W et al. (1992) Relationship of large and small CD3–CD56[+] lymphocytes mediating NK-associated activities. J Leukoc Biol 52:287–295.

[40] Papazahariadou M, Athanasiadis GI, Papadopoulos E et al. (2007) Involvement of NK cells against tumors and parasites. Int J Biol Markers 22(2):144–153.

[41] Phillips JH, Lanier LL (1986) Dissection of the LAK phenomenon. J Exp Med 164(3):814–825.

[42] Phillips JH, Gemlo BT, Myers WW et al. (1987) In vivo and in vitro activation of natural killer cells in advanced cancer patients undergoing combined recombinant interleukin-2 and LAK cell therapy. J Clin Oncol 5(12):1933–1941.

[43] Potapnev MP, Garbuzenco TS, Goncharova NV et al. (1994) Discrepancy between direct and antibody-dependent cytotoxic activities of human LAK cells. Immunol Lett 41(1):13–17.

[44] Raulet DH, Vance RE, McMahon CW (2001) Regulation of the natural killer cell receptor repertoire. Annu Rev Immunol 19:291–330.

[45] Raulet DH (2003) Roles of the NKG2D immunoreceptor and its ligands. Nat Rev Immunol 3(10):781–790.

[46] Rayner AA, Grimm EA, Lotze MT et al. (1985) Lymphokine-activated killer (LAK) cell phenomenon. IV. Lysis by LAK cell clones of fresh human tumor cells from autologous and multiple allogeneic tumors. J Natl Cancer Inst 75(1):67–75.

[47] Rivoltini L, Cattoretti G, Arienti F et al. (1991) The high lysability by LAK cells of colon-carcinoma cells resistant to doxorubicin is associated with a high expression of ICAM-1, LFA-3, NCA and a less-differentiated phenotype. Int J Cancer 47(5):746–754.

[48] Romagnani C, Juelke K, Falco M et al. (2007) CD56brightCD16-killer Ig-like receptor-NK cells display longer telomeres and acquire features of CD56dim NK cells upon activation. J Immunol 178(8):4947–4955.

[49] Sadhu C, Harris EA, Staunton DE (2007) Enhancement of natural killer cell cytotoxicity by a CD18 integrin-activating antibody. Biochem Biophys Res Commun 358(3):938.

[50] Savas B, Kerr PE, Pross HF (2006) Lymphokine-activated killer cell susceptibility and adhesion molecule expression of multidrug resistant breast carcinoma. Cancer Cell Int 6:24.

[51] Sinkovics JG, Horvath JC (2005) Human natural killer cells: a comprehensive review. Int J Oncol 27(1):5–47.

[52] Strand S, Galle PR (2001) Immune evasion by tumours: involvement of the CD95 (APO-1/Fas) system and its clinical implications. Mol Med Today 1998; 4(2):63–68.

[53] Street SE, Cretney E, Smyth MJ Perforin and interferon-γ activities independently control tumor initiation, growth, and metastasis. Blood 97(1):192–197.

[54] Stutman O (1974) Tumor development after 3-methylcholanthrene in immunologically deficient athymic-nude mice. Science 183(124):534–536.

[55] Subauste CS, Dawson L, Remington JS (1992) Human lymphokine-activated killer cells are cytotoxic against cells infected with toxoplasma gondii. J Exp Med 176(6):1511–1519.

[56] Taga K, Mostowski HS, Bloom ET (1996) Target cell-induced apoptosis of interleukin-2-activated human natural killer cells: roles of cell surface molecules and intracellular events. Blood 87(12):5127–5135.

[57] Takeda K, Smyth MJ, Cretney E et al. (2002) Critical role for tumor necrosis factor-related apoptosis-inducing ligand in immune surveillance against tumor development. J Exp Med 195(2):161–169.

[58] Takeda K, Okumura K (2004) CAM and NK Cells. eCAM 1(1):17–27.

[59] Tanaka K, Yoshioka T, Bieberich C, Jay C (1988) Role of major histocompatibility complex class I antigens in tumor growth and metastasis. Annu Rev Immunol 6:359–680.

[60] Thomas LD, Shah H, Bankhurst AD, Whalen MM (2005) Effects of interleukins 2 and 12 on the levels of granzyme B and perforin and their mRNAs in tributyltin-exposed human natural killer cells. Arch Toxicol 79(12):711–720.

[61] Trinchieri G, Matsumoto-Kobayashi M, Clark SC et al. (1984) Response of resting human peripheral blood natural killer cells to interleukin 2. J Exp Med 160:1147–1169.

[62] Trinchieri G (1989) Biology of natural killer cells. Adv Immunol 47:187–376.

[63] Verma V, Sharma V, Shrivastava SK, Nadkarni JJ (2000) IL-12 and IL-2 potentiate the in vitro tumor-specific activity of peripheral blood cells from cervical cancer patients. J Exp Clin Cancer Res 19(3):367–374.

[64] Vitale M, Della Chiesa M, Carlomagno S et al. (2004) The small subset of CD56^{bright}CD16$^-$ natural killer cells is selectively responsible for both cell proliferation and interferon-γ production upon interaction with dendritic cells. Eur J Immunol 34(6):1715–1722.

[65] Vollenweider I, Moser R, Groscurth P (1994) Development of four donor-specific phenotypes in human long-term lymphokine-activated killer cell cultures. Cancer Immunol Immunother 39(5):305–312.

[66] Wodnar-Filipowicz A, Kalberer CP (2007) Function of natural killer cells in immune defence against human leukaemia. Swiss Med Wkly 137 (Suppl 155):25S–30S.

[67] Yamamoto T, Yoneda K, Osaki T et al. (1995) Longer local retention of adoptively transferred T-LAK cells correlates with lesser adhesion molecule expression than NK-LAK cells. Clin Exp Immunol 100(1):13–20.

[68] Young HA, Ortaldo JR (2006) Cytokines as critical co-stimulatory molecules in modulating the immune response of natural killer cells. J Cell Res 16(1):20–24.

4. CD4$^+$/CD25$^+$ T-regulatory cells

IRINA ZH. SHUBINA, NADEZHDA P. VELIZHEVA
AND MIKHAIL V. KISELEVSKY
NN Blokhin Russian Cancer Research Center RAMS
Laboratory of Cell Immunity Moscow
Russia

Keywords: Treg, CD4$^+$/CD25$^+$ cells, suppressor

Abstract

CD4$^+$/CD25$^+$ T-regulatory cells are a suppressive subpopulation of lymphocytes that play a key role in auto-tolerance development. T-regulatory cells in cancer patients can inhibit proliferation and killer activity of cytotoxic lymphocytes and suppress anti-tumor immune response. T-suppressor number increases with the long-term cultivation of lymphocytes in the presence of interleukine-2 and leads to down-regulation of the anti-tumor activity of lymphokine-activated killers. Therefore, activated lymphocytes obtained from an early period culture with IL-2 are preferable to include in adoptive immunotherapy.

CD4$^+$/CD25$^+$ T-regulatory cells (Treg) in humans account for approximately 5% of total peripheral CD4$^+$T-lymphocytes and they function to maintain the homeostasis of peripheral auto-tolerance by suppressing the auto-reactive T-cells [31]. Tregs originate in thymus and have an IL-2 receptor (CD25) α-chain, express cytotoxic T-lymphocyte associated antigen-4 (CTLA-4), glucocorticoid-induced TNF-receptor (GITR) and transcriptional factor FOXP3 – being the main determinant of Treg suppressive function [1, 5, 10, 12, 13, 23, 33, 35]. Treg lymphocytes play the key role in mediating auto-tolerance [11, 15] that was shown in cases with genetic susceptibility to immune dysfunctions associated with FOXP3 mutations [9] and decreased numbers of CD4$^+$/CD25$^+$ T-lymphocytes [16, 19]. CD4$^+$/CD25$^+$Tregs have a lower proliferative activity than CD4$^+$/CD25$^-$ T-cells and can inhibit *in vitro* CD8$^+$ and CD4$^+$/CD25$^-$ T-cell activation [21, 32, 43]. CD4$^+$/CD25$^+$Tregs can also inhibit CD4$^+$ T-helper ability to generate cytokines [4]. Experiments on murine tumor models demonstrated that the presence of Tregs might reduce tumor response to active immunization by transferred T-cells [29, 35]. Tregs are found in peripheral blood and in sites of metastatic nodes in cancer patients [15, 19, 40, 44]. Tregs secrete IL-10 and may suppress proliferation of CD4$^+$/CD25$^-$, CD8$^+$ T lymphocytes and tumor-infiltrating lymphocytes (TIL) activity [7, 10, 20, 38, 42] and lead to inhibition of anti-tumor immunity [2, 3, 10, 18, 20, 24, 28, 36].

M.V. Kiselevsky (ed.), Atlas Effectors of Anti-tumor Immunity, 65–72.
© Springer Science+Business Media B.V. 2008

Treg cells down-regulate lytic and secretory activity of natural killer (NK) cells and control their proliferation [6]. Interaction between NKG2D and Treg membrane associated TGF-β results in inhibiting the NK function [24]. Depletion of CD4$^+$/CD25$^+$ Treg cells in homeostasis conditions results in enhancement of NK proliferation as well as their cytotoxicity [8].

Other studies searched for enhancing anti-tumor immunity by the selective depletion of the Tregs from peripheral blood mononuclear cells (PBMCs). The inhibiting immune effects of Treg lymphocytes can partly be responsible for the lower effectiveness of immunotherapy in cancer patients. When PBMCs are activated *in vitro* in the presence of IL-2, CD4$^+$/CD25$^+$Tregs may be registered in the population of activated lymphocytes. This can be considered as the result of the ambiguous effect of IL-2 on lymphocytes *in vitro* and on the tolerance and anti-tumor immunity or self-antigens *in vivo* [2, 4, 34].

Firstly, IL-2 was identified as a T-cell growth factor since it stimulated T-lymphocyte proliferation in culture [25]. This special feature has then become the grounds for anti-tumor immunotherapy [26]. However, recent studies on mice deficient in IL-2Rα or IL-2 production have significantly changed the understanding of this cytokine's role. Mice deficient in IL-2 production or that had mutant gene encoding IL-2Rα developed an auto-immune syndrome with an increased number of activated CD4$^+$ T-cells, antibodies production and inflammation [22, 41, 37]. These facts led to a hypothesis of a paradoxal role of IL-2 as a factor in auto-tolerance processes as well as a T-cell growth factor [26]. Moreover, IL-2 regulates the Treg lymphocytes balance that plays a key role in the peripheral tolerance to self-antigens [3, 32] and as shown recently, suppresses the anti-tumor immune response [9, 12, 13, 34]. Thymic Tregs highly express CD25 molecule that is part of the high-affinity receptor IL-2Rα [17]. Cytokine IL-2 up-regulates CD25 expression in almost all T-lymphocyte subpopulations although it is especially important for CD4$^+$/CD25$^+$Treg homeostasis, proliferation and function [45].

The IL-2 mechanism of action mediating suppressive CD4$^+$/CD25$^+$Treg function is associated with CD25 and FOXP3 expression [13, 14, 27, 39].

Studies on CD25 deficient mice (CD25$^{-/-}$) showed no difference in the suppressive function of FOXP3$^+$ T-cells and the control of lymphocytes of wild type in CD25$^{-/-}$ mice. This may be associated with the lack of an IL-2 signal and CD25 expression [12]. Within some period CD25$^{-/-}$ mice developed auto-immune diseases in spite of the normal rate of FOXP3 expression in Tregs [14, 30]. The high rate of CD25 expression increases the sensitivity of the IL-2Rα affinity to IL-2 almost 100-fold as compared to the low-affine receptor. This feature helps Treg cells to compete for IL-2 and thus enhances their survival in non-lymphoid tissues with low cytokine expression [24].

To support normal self-tolerance processes, Treg lymphocytes involve an IL-2 binding to their high-affinity receptor IL-2Rα that causes FOXP3 expression necessary for the Treg suppressive function. The essential role of IL-2 for FOXP3 ^{high}- Treg maturation was demonstrated in experiments with the adoptive transfer of this cell population in a lymphopenic environment. Despite a high CD25 expression on the isolated Tregs, CD25 expression rate decreased significantly after the cell transfer to the tumor-bearing hosts RAG-1$^{-/-}$. Simultaneously, FOXP3 was down-regulated but restored after an additional transfer of wild-type T-lymphocytes producing IL-2 [24].

Obviously, IL-2 stimulation, high CD25 expression rate and FOXP3 expression are required to determine Tregs and to support their function and homeostasis. However, IL-2 is also a crucial factor for inducing killer activity and proliferation of T-lymphocyte effectors [18, 30].

These findings seem to be very important when immunotherapy is involved since an increased IL-2 concentration, during a long-term period both in the case of IL-2 infusion in patients and generating *in vitro*, activated lymphocytes with an enhanced killer activity. There may occur a compensatory increase in the Treg number due to a prolonged IL-2 effect on the high-affinity receptor IL-2Rα with the following FOXP3 expression. This phenomenon may probably explain the inefficient response (15%–20%) of cancer patients to IL-2/LAK immunotherapy.

Therefore, considering the revealed ambiguous IL-2 effect on *ex vivo* activated PBMCs, and depression of suppressive Tregs may lead to increased immunotherapy effectiveness [8, 17]. Since lymphokine-activated killers are one of the key elements in anti-cancer adoptive immunotherapy, the role of Tregs in the population of *ex vivo* generated LAKs becomes an important issue for discussion.

A modern technique of immunomagnetic separation that has 95%–99% sensitivity helps to select definite cell subpopulations for various purposes.

A study was performed to estimate the CD4$^+$/CD25$^+$Treg subpopulation in LAK culture generated from PBMCs of patients with advanced colon cancer, disseminated renal cancer and melanoma, as well as that of the PBMC of healthy donors. The results showed that the Treg percentage varied dependent on the LAK cultivating period.

PBMCs were isolated by a standard gradient-density methodology and then cultured in complete RPMI in the presence of IL-2 (10000 IU/ml) for 3, 7 and 10 days. CD4$^+$/CD25$^+$T-cells were selected by immunomagnetic separation at different periods of cell culture and their number was calculated and registered as percentage

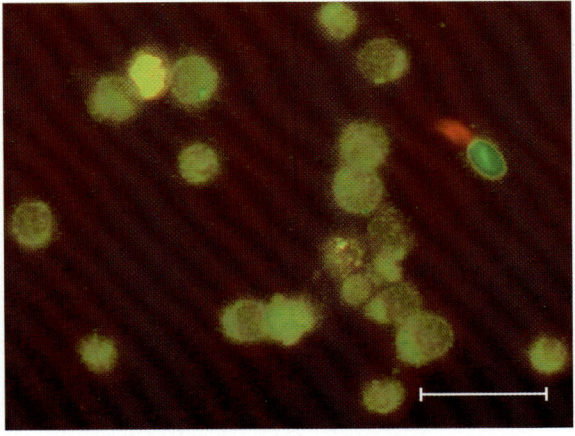

Figure 4.1. Blood mononuclear cells of healthy donors stained fluorescent antibodies to CD4/CD25 antigens Microphotographs of double marker stained cells in culture meal; stained fluorescein isothiocyanat (FITS) and phycoerithrin (PE). Scale bar: 20 μm

of LAK population. CD4$^+$/CD25$^+$T-cell percentage in the LAK population generated from the PBMC of patients with advanced colon cancer, disseminated renal cancer and melanoma increased gradually, correlating with the culture period. But CD4$^+$/CD25$^+$T-cell number in generated LAKs from the PBMC of healthy donors remained virtually constant (1.5%–4.3%) up to the 10th culture day. Within the first 3 days of culture CD4$^+$/CD25$^+$T-cell percentage in the LAKs generated from the PBMC of patients (2.3%–4.0%) and donors (1.5%) had no significant difference. However, prolonged PBMC cultivation in the presence of IL-2 led to a growing number of Tregs in the LAK culture generated from the PBMC of patients with advanced cancer, reaching 20% of the total activated lymphocyte population by day 20. The number of CD4$^+$/CD25$^+$T-lymphocytes in the cell culture generated from the PBMC of healthy donors increased less rapidly and reached 7.8%–10.4% by day 20 (Figures 4.1 and 4.2).

The morphological examination of CD4$^+$/CD25$^+$T-lymphocytes isolated from

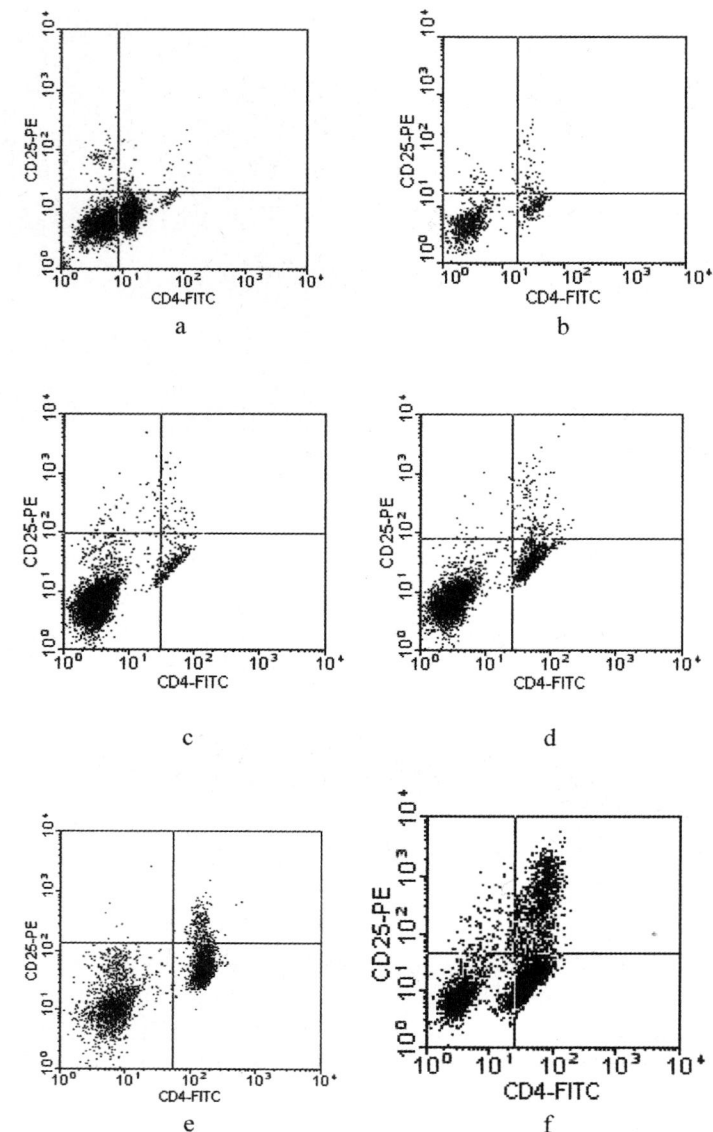

Figure 4.2. Expression rate of CD4/CD25 molecules in culture of MNLs and LAKs depending on culture period **a** – Expression rate of CD4/CD25 molecules in culture of initial blood mononuclear cells of a healthy donor; **b** – Expression rate of CD4/CD25 molecules in culture of initial blood mononuclear cells of a disseminated melanoma patient; **c** – Expression rate of CD4/CD25 molecules in culture of healthy donor LAKs (3 days); **d** – Expression rate of CD4/CD25 molecules in culture of disseminated melanoma patient LAKs (3 days); **e** – Expression rate of CD4/CD25 molecules in culture of healthy donor LAKs (10 days); **f** – Expression rate of CD4/CD25 molecules in culture of disseminated melanoma patient LAKs (10 days)

the LAK culture by immunomagnetic separation on days 7–10 describes large prolymphocyte-like cells (Figure 4.3).

Immunophenotype analysis of the PBMC of healthy donors and patients with disseminated melanoma showed that 1%–3% of PBMCs express Treg CD4/CD25 antigens. During the period of MNL cultivation in the presence of IL-2 CD4$^+$/CD25$^+$ lymphocyte the percentage increased gradually, correlating with the source of PBMCs and the culture period. CD4$^+$/CD25$^+$ Tregs

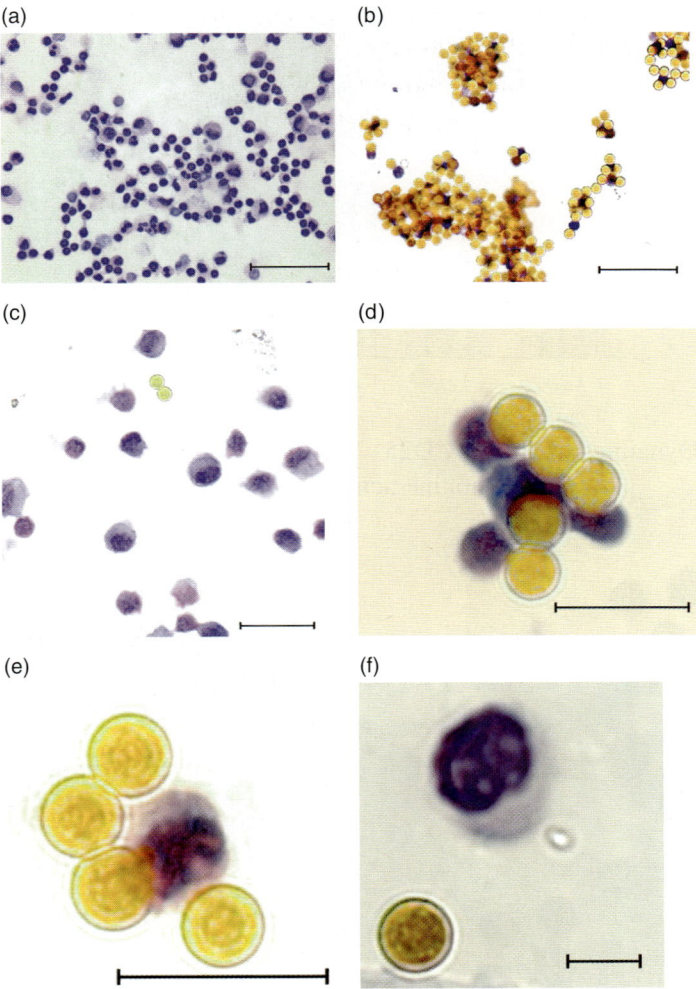

Figure 4.3. CD4 + /CD25+ lymphocytes separation scheme by magnetic beads with monoclonal antibodies Microphotographs of lymphocytes bearing magnetic beads: **a** – Initial culture of lymphokine-activated killers; Scale bar: 50 μm; **b** – Immunomagnetic separation of CD19$^+$, CD16$^+$, CD8$^+$ cells — lymphocytes form rosettes with beads bearing antibodies (lymphocytes dominate in rosette complexes); Scale bar: 50 μm; **c** – Remained lymphocytes after depletion of CD19$^+$, CD16$^+$, CD8$^+$ cells from LAK culture (mainly blast forms and large prolymphocyte-like cells); Scale bar: 20 μm; **d–e** – Immunomagnetic separation of CD4$^+$/25$^+$ cells — Lymphocytes remaining after depletion of CD19$^+$, CD16$^+$, CD8$^+$ cells from LAK culture form rosettes with beads bearing antibodies to CD4/CD25 antigens (mainly blast forms and large prolymphocyte-like cells); Scale bar: 20 μm; **f** – CD4$^+$/CD25$^-$cells in culture after depletion of CD4$^+$/CD25$^+$ lymphocytes — remaining lymphocytes do not form rosettes with beads bearing antibodies to CD4/CD25 antigens; stained Asur II-Eosin; Scale bar: 10 μm

were found in the 5 day culture of both donors' and melanoma patients' LAKs and reached 2 and 6%, respectively. On day 10, the proportion of CD4$^+$/CD25$^+$Treg comprised 21% of the LAKs generated from the PBMC of patients with disseminated melanoma and 7% of healthy donors' LAKs (Figure 4.4).

CD4$^+$/CD25$^+$T-lymphocytes selected by immunomagnetic separation from lymphokine-activated lymphocytes suppress NK-activity of LAKs (Figure 4.5). Figure 4.6 demonstrates

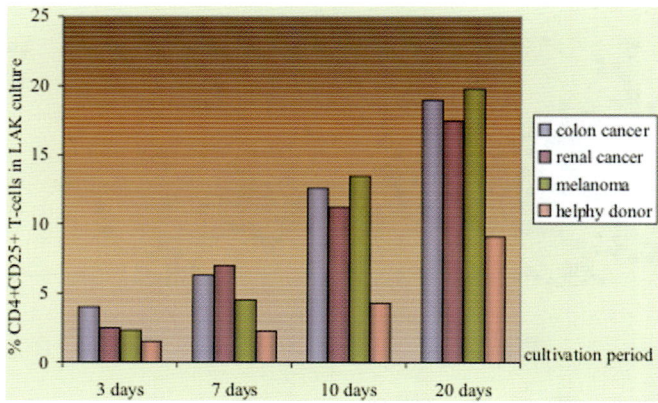

Figure 4.4. Dynamics of CD4$^+$/CD25$^+$ T-lymphocyte subpopulation in culture of lymphokine-activated killer cells

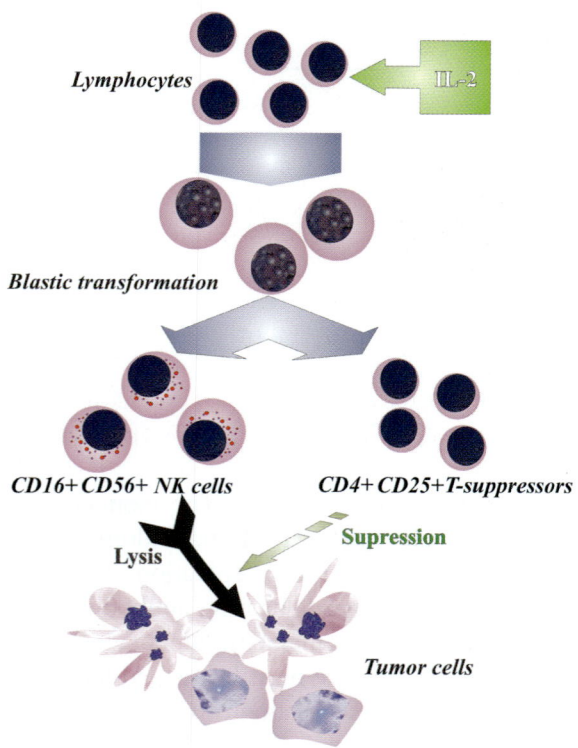

Figure 4.5. Mechanism of suppression of NK-activity by Treg (Refs. [6, 8, 10, 20, 42])

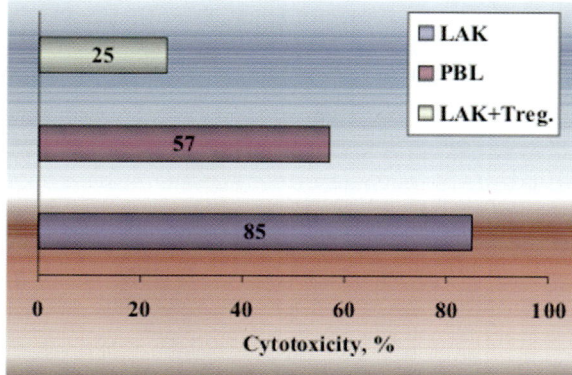

Figure 4.6. Comparative cytotoxicity of LAKs and LAKs co-cultured with CD4$^+$/CD25$^+$ T-cells

a significantly lower NK-activity of LAKs incubated with regulatory CD4$^+$/CD25$^+$ T cells than that of LAKs alone.

These results suggest that the depletion of Tregs from LAKs generated *ex vivo* may be a way to enhance efficacy of the cell-based adoptive immunotherapy of cancer.

References

[1] Allan SE, Passerini L, Baccheta R (2005) The role of 2 FOXP 3 isoforms in the generation of human CD4$^+$ tregs. J Clin Invest 115(11): 3276–3284

[2] Antony PA, Paulos CM, Ahmadzadeh M et al (2006) Interleukin-2-Dependent Mechanisms of Tolerance and Immunity *In Vivo*. J Immunol 176(9):5255–5266

[3] Antony PA, Piccirillo CA, Akpinarli A et al (2005) CD8$^+$ T cell immunity against a tumor/self-antigen is augmented by CD4$^+$ T helper cells and hindered by naturally occurring T regulatory cells. J Immunol 174(5):2591–2601

[4] Antony PA, Restifo NP (2005) CD4$^+$CD25$^+$ T regulatory cells, immunotherapy of cancer, and interleukin-2. J Immunother 28(2):120–1283

[5] Bennett CL, Christie J, Ramsdell F et al (2001) The immune dysregulation, polyendocrinopathy, enteropathy, X-linked syndrome (IPEX) is caused by mutations of FOXP3. Nat Genet 27(1):20–21

[6] Bauer S, Groh V, Wu J et al (1999) Activation of NK cells and T cells by NKG2D, a receptor for stress-inducible MICA. Science 285(5428): 727–729

[7] Curiel TJ, Coukos G, Zou L et al (2004) Specific recruitment of regulatory T cells in ovarian carcinoma fosters immune privilege and predicts reduced survival. Nat Med 10(9):942–949

[8] Chen A, Liu S, Park D et al (2007) Depleting intratumoral CD4$^+$CD25$^+$ Regulatory T cells via FasL protein transfer enhances the therapeutic efficacy of adoptive T cell transfer. Cancer Res 67(3):1291–1298

[9] D'Cruz LM, Klein L (2005) Development and function of agonist-induced CD25$^+$Foxp3$^+$ regulatory T cells in the absence of interleukin 2 signaling. Nat Immunol 6(11):1152–1159

[10] Dieckmann D, Plottner H, Berchtold S et al (2001) *Ex vivo* isolation and characterization of CD4(+)CD25(+) T cells with regulatory properties from human blood. J Exp Med 193(11):1303–131031

[11] Fehervari Z, Sakaguchi S (2004) CD4$^+$Tregs and immune control. J Clin Invest 114(9): 1209–1217

[12] Fontenot JD, Rasmussen JP, Gavin MA et al (2005) A function for interleukin 2 in Foxp3-expressing regulatory T cells. Nat Immunol 6(11):1142–1151

[13] Fontenot JD, Rasmussen JP, Williams LM et al (2005) Regulatory T cell lineage specification by the forkhead transcription factor foxp3. Immunity 22(3):329–341

[14] Furtado GC, de Lafaille Curotto MA, et al (2002) Interleukin 2 signaling is required for CD4$^+$ regulatory T cell function. J Exp Med 196(6):851–857

[15] Gattinoni L, Powell DJ Jr, Rosenberg SA et al (2006) Adoptive immunotherapy for cancer: building on success. Nat Rev Immunol 6(5): 383–393

[16] Ghiringhelli F, Ménard C, Terme M et al (2005) CD4$^+$CD25$^+$ regulatory T cells inhibit natural killer cell functions in a transforming growth factor-beta-dependent manner. J Exp Med 202(8):1075–1085

[17] Hoffmann P, Boeld TJ, Eder R et al (2006) Isolation of CD4$^+$CD25$^+$ regulatory T cells for clinical trials. Arch Immunol Ther Exp (Warsz) 54(1):33–43

[18] Ichihara F, Kono1 K, Takahashi A et al (2003) Copyright notice and disclaimer increased populations of regulatory T cells in peripheral blood and tumor-infiltrating lymphocytes in patients with gastric and esophageal cancers. Clin Cancer Res 9(12):4404–4408

[19] Javia LR, Rosenberg SA (2003) CD4$^+$CD25$^+$ suppressor lymphocytes in the circulation of patients immunized against melanoma antigens. J Immunother 26(1):85–93

[20] Jonuleit H, Schmitt E, Stassen M et al (2001) Identification and functional characterization of human CD4(+)CD25(+) T cells with regulatory properties isolated from peripheral blood. J Exp Med 193(11):1285–1294

[21] Kullberg MC, Jankovic D, Gorelick PL et al (2002) Bacteria-triggered CD4$^+$ T regulatory cells suppress *Helicobacter hepaticus*-induced colitis. J Exp Med 196(4): 505–515

[22] Kundig TM, Schorle H, Bachmann MF et al (1993) Immune responses in interleukin-2-deficient mice. Science 262 (5136):1059–1061

[23] Leung DT, Morefield S, Willerford DM (2000) Regulation of lymphoid homeostasis by IL-2 receptor signals *in vivo*. J Immunol 164(7): 3527–3534

[24] Ling KL, Pratap SE, Bates GJ et al (2007) Increased frequency of regulatory T cells in peripheral blood and tumour infiltrating lymphocytes in colorectal cancer patients. Cancer Immunity 7:7–14

[25] Morgan DA, Ruscetti FW, Gallo R (1976) Selective *in vitro* growth of T lymphocytes from normal human bone marrows. Science 193 (4257):1007–1008

[26] Mule JJ, Shu S, Schwarz SL et al (1984) Adoptive immunotherapy of established pulmonary metastases with LAK cells and recombinant interleukin-2. Science 225(1): 1487–1489

[27] Nelson BH (2004) IL-2, regulatory T cells, and tolerance. J Immunology 172(7):3983– 3988

[28] Overwijk WW, Theoret MR, Finkelstein SE et al (2003) Tumor regression and autoimmunity after reversal of a functionally tolerant state of self-reactive CD8$^+$ T cells. J Exp Med 198(4): 569–580

[29] Ralainirina N, Poli A, Michel T et al (2007) Control of NK cell functions by CD4$^+$CD25$^+$ regulatory T cells. Journal of Leukocyte Biology 81(4):144–153

[30] Sadlack B, Merz H, Schorle H et al (1993) Ulcerative colitis-like disease in mice with a disrupted interleukin-2 gene. Cell 75(2): 253–261

[31] Sakaguchi S (2004) Naturally Arising CD4$^+$ regulatory T cells for immunologic self-tolerance and negative control of immune responses. Annu Rev Immunol 22:531–562

[32] Sakaguchi S (2005) Naturally arising Foxp3-expressing CD25$^+$CD4$^+$ regulatory T cells in immunological tolerance to self and non-self. Nat Immunol 6(3–4):345–352

[33] Setoguchi R, Hori S, Takahashi T et al (2005) Homeostatic maintenance of natural Foxp3$^+$CD25$^+$CD4$^+$ regulatory T cells by interleukin (IL)-2 and induction of autoimmune disease by IL-2 neutralization. J Exp Med 201(5):723–735

[34] Sharfe N, Dadi HK, Shahar M et al (1997) Human immune disorder arising from mutation of the α-chain of the interleukin-2 receptor. Proc Natl Acad Sci USA 94(7):3168–3171

[35] Simon AK, Jones E, Richards H et al (2007) Regulatory T cells inhibit Fas ligand-induced innate and adaptive tumour immunity. Eur J Immunol 37(3):758–767

[36] Somasundaram R, Jacob L, Swoboda R et al (2002) Inhibition of cytolytic T lymphocyte proliferation by autologous CD4$^+$/CD25$^+$ regulatory T cells in a colorectal carcinoma patient is mediated by transforming growth factor-ß. Cancer Res 62(18):5267–5272

[37] Suzuki H, Kunding TM, Furlonger C et al (1995) Deregulated T cell activation and autoimmunity in mice lacking interleukin-2 receptor β. Science 268(5216):1472–1476

[38] Takahashi T, Tagami T, Yamazaki S et al (2000) Immunologic self-tolerance maintained by CD25$^+$CD4$^+$ regulatory T cells constitutively expressing cytotoxic T lymphocyte-associated antigen 4. J Exp Med 192(2):303–309

[39] Thornton AM, Donovan EE, Piccirillo CA et al (2004) Cutting edge: IL-2 is critically required for the *in vitro* activation of CD4$^+$CD25$^+$ T cell suppressor function. J Immunol 172(11): 6519–6523

[40] Wang HY, Lee DA, Peng G et al (2004) Tumor-specific human CD4$^+$ regulatory T cells and their ligands: implications for immunotherapy. Immunity 20(1):107–118

[41] Willerford DM, Chen J, Ferry JA et al (1995) Interleukin-2 receptor α-chain regulates the size and content of the peripheral lymphoid compartment. Immunity 3(4):521–530

[42] Woo EY, Chu CS, Goletz TJ et al (2001) Regulatory CD4(+)CD25(+) T cells in tumors from patients with early-stage non-small cell lung cancer and late-stage ovarian cancer. Cancer Res 61(12):4766–4772

[43] Woo EY, Yeh H, Chu CS et al (2002) Cutting edge: regulatory T cells from lung cancer patients directly inhibit autologous T cell proliferation. J Immunol 168(9):4272–4276

[44] Viguier M, Lemaitre F, Verola O et al (2004) Foxp3 expressing CD4$^+$CD25(high) regulatory T cells are overrepresented in human metastatic melanoma lymph nodes and inhibit the function of infiltrating T cells. J Immunol 173(2): 1444–1453

[45] de Visser KE, Eichten A, Coussens LM (2006) Paradoxical roles of the immune system during cancer development. Nat Rev Cancer 6(1):24–37

5. CD8$^+$ CD57$^+$ T cells in tumor immunology

MARÍA I. SADA-OVALLE

Research Unit, Biochemistry Department
National Institute of Respiratory Diseases
Calzada de Tlalpan 4502, Col. Sección XVI
Delegación Tlalpan, Mexico D.F

Keywords: CD8$^+$ T Cells, CD57, cytotoxicity, perforin, granzyme

Abstract

The proportion of human peripheral blood CD8$^+$ T cells that express CD57 is lower at birth but increases with age as well as in patients with several pathologies such as the human immunodeficiency virus infection (HIV), cytomegalovirus infection (CMV), myeloma multiple, colorectal cancer and gastric cancer. This T cell subset has been shown to be an effector phenotype characterized by IFN-γ production as well as being an important perforin and granzyme-A expression. It has been hypothesized that this results from continuous stimulation, however, this phenotype may be due to direct tumoral effects on CD8$^+$ T cells. CD8$^+$CD57$^+$ T cells have been shown to infiltrate tumors in different stages, suggesting that they play a role in tumor immunology. In this chapter we analyze some basic aspects about how CD8$^+$CD57$^+$ T cells behave in tumor immunology.

5.1. CD8$^+$ T Cells

One of the responses that the immune system develops against tumors is based on CD8$^+$ T cells activity, mainly, memory CD8$^+$ T cells. Memory CD8$^+$ T cells can be classified into two categories, named central memory T cell (TCM) and effector memory T cells (TEM), according to their phenotypic markers, effector functions and homing capabilities. In 1999, Sallusto F et al. proposed this classification where TCM cells that express CD62L and CCR7 can migrate to the secondary lymph node but lacks of cytotoxic function. TEM, characterized by the absence of CD62L and CCR7 expression, are antigen-primed cells that function as sentinels and mediate diverse effector functions [43]. Klebanoff C et al. showed in a mouse adoptive transfer model that after an established cancer, CD8$^+$ TCM were superior mediators of immunity than CD8$^+$ TEM. This was due mainly to their important proliferative capacity. As a consequence, large numbers of these effector cells were reached and mediated antigen or tumor clearance [27]. A summary of these phenotypic markers is shown in Table 5.1. This could be one of the most important findings to consider for the future development of cancer immunotherapies and tumor-antigen vaccine trials. However, how is the differentiation of CD8$^+$ T cells that are chronically

M.V. Kiselevsky (ed.), Atlas Effectors of Anti-tumor Immunity, 73–80.
© Springer Science+Business Media B.V. 2008

Table 5.1. Surface markers on naive and memory T cell subsets. Per-GraA-: Perforine (−) and Granzyme A (−)

Naive	T cell memory	T cell effector	T effector
CD62L +++	CD62L ++	CD62L−	CD62L−
CCR7 +++	CCR7 ++	CCR7−	CCR7−
CD28 +++	CD28 ++	CD28 +/−	CD28−
CD45RA +++	CD45RA−	CD45RA− /+	CD45RA+
CD57−	CD57	CD57 − /+	CD57+
Per-GraA−		Perlow GraA+	PerhighGraA+

stimulated by pathogens or tumors and how much of its effector function is modified? CD8$^+$ T cells that have been exposed to antigens (viral, tumoral or bacterial) for an extensive period tend to express some well characterized phenotypic markers such as: CD28−, CD45RA+, CD57$^+$ and short telomers [8, 35] (Figures 5.1 and 5.2 CD45RA). There are two physiopathological consequences for this cell surface expression profile. Firstly, CD8$^+$ T cells with a decrease in telomere length have a very poor proliferative capacity. Secondly, the number of

epitopes that are normally recognized by CD8$^+$ T cells is decreased due to a selective production of TEM cells over TCM cells. The logical result of this is that we do not have a suitable CD8$^+$ T cell repertoire to eliminate tumors or pathogens.

The main function of the CD8+ T cells (TCM or TEM) is to kill infected or tumoral cells. The mechanisms involved in the destruction of their targets are multifaceted. The most important death pathways are related to: (1) cytokine and chemokine secretion (2) Fas/Fas ligand interactions and (3) perforin/granzyme-mediated cell lysis after recognition of cognate antigens.

5.2. Cytokines

Cytokines are important mediators of innate and adaptive immunity. Their beneficial effects in stimulating T-cell mediated immunity, antigen presentation and T cell proliferation are interesting for antitumor vaccine adjuvants. It has been demonstrated that an important variety of cytokines, chemokines and growth factors are produced in the local tumor environment by different immune and tumor cells [13]. There is a long list of tumor derived cytokines that include:

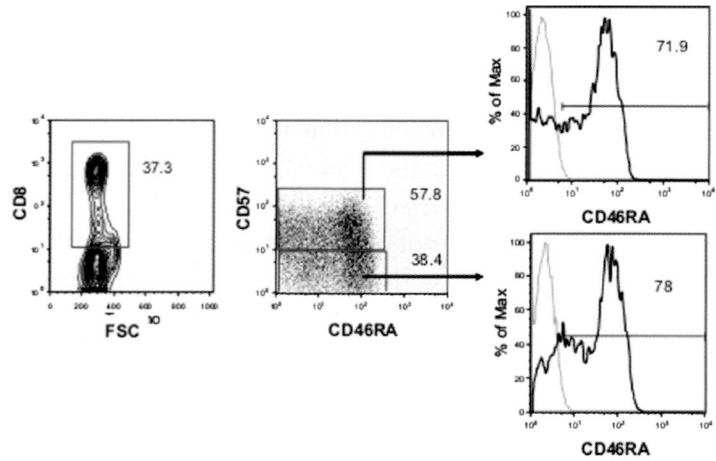

Figure 5.1. CD57 and CD45RA are co expressed on a subset of peripheral blood human CD8 T cells. Lymphocytes were stained with monoclonal antibodies of CD8, CD45RA and CD57. The percentage of the bright cells is indicated

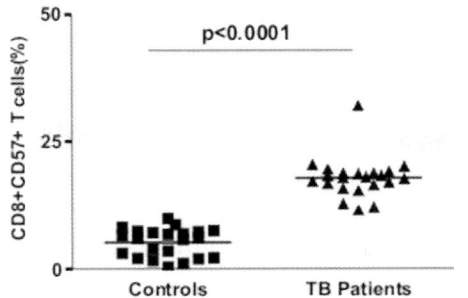

Figure 5.2. Proportion of CD8+CD57+ T cells. Peripheral blood mononuclear cells were stained with monoclonal antibodies of CD8 and CD57 and analyzed by flow cytometry. Results are expressed as median using the Wilcoxon rank-sum (Mann-Witney); the p value of the difference between controls and TB patients is indicated. n = 20

IL-1, IL-2, IL-4, IL-6 IL-10, IL-15, TGF-β and TNF-α and the list is still increasing [5, 12, 24]. Some of the best characterized tumor cytokines are IL-10 and TGF-β. Both of them are known as immunosuppressive cytokines. IL-10 is a cytokine that is mainly produced by T cells, monocytes, macrophages and tumor cells by the downregulation of HLA classes I and II molecules. They inhibit IFN-γ secretion and T cell proliferation [54]. On the other hand, TGF-β is a cytokine that is produced by T cells and macrophages and is considered to be a regulator of the maturation and activity of different cells [29]. This cytokine mediates suppression of cytotoxic T lymphocytes and the production of IL-2 as well as inhibiting the activation of the response to different kinds of stimuli [30]. One of the most novel cytokines with antitumor activity is IL-27, which is an early product of activated antigen presenting cells and is part of the IL-12 family [37]. IL-27 is produced by antigen presenting cells (APC) and synergizes with IL-12 to trigger the production of IFN-γ by naïve CD4 T cells but its potent antitumor activity is mainly mediated by CD8 T cells which act directly on the CD8 T cell or through T-bet [18, 46].

5.3. CD95/CD95L System

Apoptosis is one of the most important immune mechanisms for the maintenance of tissue homeostasis and is also the mechanism that mediates the destruction of damaged cells. Therefore, the balance between pro-apoptotic and anti-apoptotic mechanisms should be well regulated. There is, however, inhibition of the apoptotic process in several diseases such as cancer [16]. CD95 (member of the tumor necrosis factor (TNF)-receptor family) on the surface of activated T cells mediates apoptosis when triggered by its cognate ligand, CD95L. CD95L (FasL) belongs to the TNF family and is expressed in two different forms: on cell membranes or as a soluble factor [25, 51]. Upon the binding of CD95L, CD95 signaling through the adaptor molecule Fas-associated death domain protein (FADD), procaspase-8, procaspase-10 and FLIP [36].

The induction of apoptosis through CD95 is the main mechanism that regulates tumor proliferation. However, tumor cells have developed some strategies to evade apoptosis induction. One of these strategies is the upregulated activity of metalloproteinase-7 (MMP-7) that mediates Fas cleavage from the tumor cells. The consequence of this is an increased resistance to the FasL induced apoptosis [53]. Another alteration in this pathway has been associated with the amount of the Bcl-2 antiapoptotic protein. An overexpression of the Bcl-2 gene has been found in several pathologies such as lymphomas, leukaemias and some solid tumors [6, 50]. At the same level the inverse situation has been observed; a decreased expression of pro-apoptotic proteins has been found in some cancers such as colon cancer [39].

5.4. Granule-Exocytosis Pathway

The third mechanism mediated by CD8+ T cells against infected cells and tumors is the granule-exocytosis pathway. Perforin is a pore-forming protein that is stored together with several granzymes (serine proteases) in granules of the CD8+ T cells and NK cells. Exocytosis of granules is presented after the CD8+ T cell or NK cell establishes contact with a target cell. This allows the release of the granules content, activation of the apoptotic pathway and the elimination of the infected or transformed cell [7, 49]. In 1994 the importance of this pathway was demonstrated by the use of perforin-deficient mice, which showed a rapid growth and spread of some experimental tumors [11]. Even though perforin alone can mediate membrane damage, granzymes are necessary to induce apoptosis.

5.5. Antigen Recognition of CD8 T Cells

Generally, CD8+ T cells recognize cytosolic antigens, which are presented on MHC class I molecules. Tumoral and viral antigens can get access to the antigen presentation class I pathway to CD8+ T cells through a novel mechanism named cross-presentation [17]. Cross-presentation is a process where the cell (antigen presenting cell, APC) that contains the antigen is unable to present it to the T cell, so the antigen should be transferred to another APC, which is then able to present it to the T cells. Cross-priming is the name for the activation of T cells by cross-presented antigens [3]. There are some hypotheses for this process. One of them suggests that MHC class I molecules, located in the endoplasmic reticulum (ER), join the new phagosomes loaded with antigens derived from apoptotic vesicles to acquire the new antigens [14, 20]. It is not well known whether tumor antigens are cross-presented by apoptotic vesicles but it has been described as a relationship between apoptosis and the activation of T cells in mice that were transfected with AB1 tumors and after that treated with the apoptosis-inducing reagent gemcitabine [32].

5.6. CD8$^+$ T Cells that Express the NK Cell Marker CD57

Some of the CD8+ T cells may express NK receptors (NKRs) such as CD56, CD57 or CD244 and have been correlated with T cell activation and may regulate their effector functions against tumor antigens [33, 38]. CD161 T cells have been widely described, therefore, we are going to focus on CD8+ T cells that express the CD57 marker. CD57, also known as HNK-1, is a glycan expressed on some cell-surface glycoproteins, glycolipids and on unconventional T cells [22, 23, 44]. The increased expression of CD57 on CD4+ and CD8+ T cells has been associated with an effector/memory phenotype in several pathologies such as citomegalovirus infection, chronic lymphocytic leukaemia, colorectal cancer, gastric cancer and tuberculosis. This is probably a result of the chronic antigenic stimulation [10, 31, 34, 40, 52]. Figure 5.3 (box) and Figure 5.4 (histograms) show examples of the increased percentage of the CD8+ CD57+ T cells in an infectious disease such as pulmonary tuberculosis compared with healthy controls.

The phenotypic profile of this T cell subset is mainly characterized by the differential expression of some markers such as CD28, CD62L, CCR7, CD45RA, CD57, perforine and granzimes as well as spontaneous cytotoxic activity against autologous monocytes [28, 40]. Although CD8+CD57+ T cells are not frequent in children and younger adults, the number of CD57+ T cells increases with age or after some viral infections, suggesting that the accumulation of these T cells is the result of the clonal expansion after chronic antigen exposition [26, 45]. However, Hoji A et al., have recently described that the differentiation of effector CD8+CD57+ T cells is impaired in some cases of chronic HIV infection, suggesting a failure in the control of the cellular immune response against HIV [19]. In healthy donors,

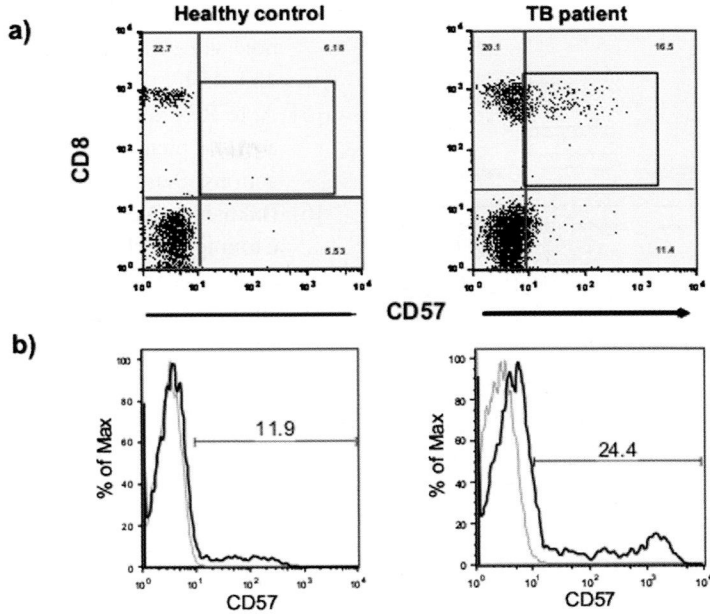

Figure 5.3. Expression of CD8 and CD57 on peripheral blood mononuclear cells (**a, b**). Representative staining from a healthy control and from a tuberculosis patient

the CD57 marker is expressed in less than 10% of the peripheral blood mononuclear cells (PBMC) [1]. However, almost 90% of the CD57+ T cells are CD8 T cells and it has been observed that this percentage increases with age thus suggesting their extrathymic origin [2]. CD8+ CD57+ T cells have the capacity to produce large amounts of IFN-γ compared to regular αβT cells [33] and have been shown to kill tumor cells when activated with cytokines or superantigens [4]. Garland et al. described that CD8+CD57+ T cells are able to spontaneously lyse allogenic uninfected cell lines [15], whereas Mollet et al., reported that CD8 +CD57+ T cells can mediate spontaneous cytotoxic activity, which may be downregulated by a recognized lectin-binding soluble factor [41, 42]. We previously described that CD8 +CD57+ T cells from tuberculosis patients had spontaneous cytotoxic activity against autologous monocytes when they were analyzed in an ex-vivo assay (Figure 5.4). This suggests that they are effector cells that may be found in peripheral blood [40]. A large number of

studies have tried to elucidate the reason for the expanded populations of T cell subsets with the phenotype of cytotoxic T cells in infectious (HIV, CMV and EBV) and tumoral pathologies (myeloma multiple and colorectal cancer) [21, 41, 47]. The expression of CD57 on CD8+ T cells and why they are part of the infiltrating lymphocytes in different tumors suggest that they play a role in the Th1 immune response. In 2003 Chochi, K. et al., stated that CD8 +CD57+ T cells were significantly higher in the early stages of gastric cancer compared to a significant decrease found in advanced gastric cancer. They also stated that the IFN-γ production did not correlate with the proportion of CD8 +CD57+ T cells in patients [10]. Other recent works have described how the CD57 immunostaining on epithelial cells is a useful adjunct to the diagnosis or prognosis of papillary thyroid carcinoma and cutaneous malignant melanoma [9, 48]

All these results suggest that CD8 +CD57+ T cells may contribute or regulate the final immune response against tumors or infections

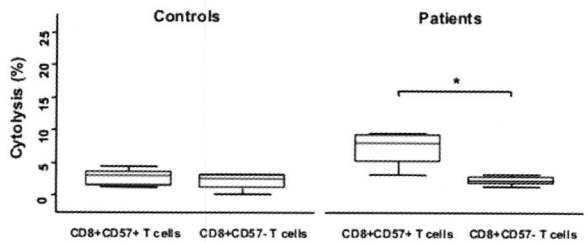

Figure 5.4. Cytotoxic activity of CD8+ T cells subsets. CD8+CD57+ and CD8+CD57− T cells from controls and TB-patients were tested for cytotoxicity in a colorimetric LDH *ex-vivo* assay. Non-stimulated CD8+CD57+ and CD8+CD57− T cells were incubated with autologous monocytes in a 4-h cytotoxicity assay. Results represent the median from triplicate wells from 6 individual donors. $*p < 0.05$

and it will depend on diverse factors such as age, infection nature (viral, bacterial or tumoral) or the elapsed time since the antigen exposition began. We might consider that the infiltration of CD8+ and CD57+ cells in tumors is an important prognostic factor. However, their interaction with tumor cells is not completely understood. Recent evidence indicates that CD8+ T cells that express NK markers play an important role in the immune surveillance in tumors. However, more clinical trails will be necessary to elucidate the final function of this T cell subset.

References

[1] Abo T and Balch C M (1981) A differentiation antigen of human NK and K cells identified by a monoclonal antibody (HNK-1) J Immunol 127(3): 1024–1029

[2] Abo T, Watanabe H et al (1995) Extrathymic T cells stand at an intermediate phylogenetic position between natural killer cells and thymus-derived T cells. Nat Immun 14(4): 173–187

[3] Ackerman A L and Cresswell P (2004) Cellular mechanisms governing cross-presentation of exogenous antigens. Nat Immunol 5(7): 678–684

[4] Ami K, Ohkawa T et al (2002) Activation of human T cells with NK cell markers by staphylococcal enterotoxin A via IL-12 but not via IL-18. Clin Exp Immunol 128(3): 453–459.

[5] Apte R N and Voronov E (2002) Interleukin-1 – a major pleiotropic cytokine in tumor-host interactions. Semin Cancer Biol 12(4): 277–290

[6] Bakhshi A, Jensen J P et al (1985) Cloning the chromosomal breakpoint of t(14;18) human lymphomas: clustering around JH on chromosome 14 and near a transcriptional unit on 18. Cell 41(3): 899–906

[7] Barry M and Bleackley R C (2002) Cytotoxic T lymphocytes: all roads lead to death. Nat Rev Immunol 2(6): 401–409

[8] Brenchley J M, Karandikar N J et al (2003) Expression of CD57 defines replicative senescence and antigen-induced apoptotic death of CD8+ T cells. Blood 101(7): 2711–2720

[9] Chandan V S, Faquin W C et al (2006) The role of immunolocalization of CD57 and GLUT-1 in cell blocks in fine-needle aspiration diagnosis of papillary thyroid carcinoma. Cancer 108(5): 331–336

[10] Chochi K, Ichikura T et al (2003) The increase of CD57+ T cells in the peripheral blood and their impaired immune functions in patients with advanced gastric cancer. Oncol Rep 10(5): 1443–1448

[11] Clark W R (1994) Immunology. The hole truth about perforin. Nature 369(6475): 16–17

[12] Culig Z (2005) Interleukin-6 polymorphism: expression and pleiotropic regulation in human prostate cancer. J Urol 174(2): 417

[13] Dinarello C A (2006) The paradox of pro-inflammatory cytokines in cancer. Cancer Metastasis Rev 25(3): 307–313

[14] Gagnon E, Duclos S et al (2002) Endoplasmic reticulum-mediated phagocytosis is a mechanism of entry into macrophages. Cell 110(1): 119–131

[15] Garland R J, El-Shanti N et al (2002) Human CD8+ CTL recognition and *in vitro* lysis of herpes simplex virus-infected cells by a non-MHC restricted mechanism. Scand J Immunol 55(1): 61–69

[16] Hanahan D and Weinberg R A (2000) The hallmarks of cancer. Cell 100(1): 57–70

[17] Heath W R and Carbone F R (2001) Cross-presentation in viral immunity and self-tolerance. Nat Rev Immunol 1(2): 126–134

[18] Hisada M, Kamiya S et al (2004) Potent antitumor activity of interleukin-27. Cancer Res 64(3): 1152–1156

[19] Hoji A, Connolly N C et al (2007) CD27 and CD57 expression reveals atypical differentiation of human immunodeficiency virus type 1-specific memory CD8+ T cells. Clin Vaccine Immunol 14(1): 74–80

[20] Houde M, Bertholet S et al (2003) Phagosomes are competent organelles for antigen cross-presentation. Nature 425(6956): 402–406

[21] Ibegbu C C, Xu Y X et al (2005) Expression of killer cell lectin-like receptor G1 on antigen-specific human CD8+ T lymphocytes during active, latent, and resolved infection and its relation with CD57. J Immunol 174(10): 6088–6094

[22] Jimenez-Martinez M C, Linares M et al (2004) Intracellular expression of interleukin-4 and interferon-gamma by a Mycobacterium tuberculosis antigen-stimulated CD4+ CD57+ T-cell subpopulation with memory phenotype in tuberculosis patients. Immunology 111(1): 100–106

[23] Jungalwala F B (1994) Expression and biological functions of sulfoglucuronyl glycolipids (SGGLs) in the nervous system – a review. Neurochem Res 19(8): 945–957

[24] Kay N E and Pittner B T (2003) IL-4 biology: impact on normal and leukemic CLL B cells. Leuk Lymphoma 44(6): 897–903

[25] Kayagaki N, Kawasaki A et al (1995) Metalloproteinase-mediated release of human Fas ligand. J Exp Med 182(6): 1777–1783

[26] Khan N, Shariff N et al (2002) Cytomegalovirus seropositivity drives the CD8 T cell repertoire toward greater clonality in healthy elderly individuals. J Immunol 169(4): 1984–1992

[27] Klebanoff C A, Gattinoni L et al (2005) Central memory self/tumor-reactive CD8+ T cells confer superior antitumor immunity compared with effector memory T cells. Proc Natl Acad Sci U S A 102(27): 9571–9576

[28] Klebanoff C A, Gattinoni L et al (2006) CD8+ T-cell memory in tumor immunology and immunotherapy. Immunol Rev 211:214–224

[29] Kulkarni A B, Thyagarajan T et al (2002) Function of cytokines within the TGF-beta superfamily as determined from transgenic and gene knockout studies in mice. Curr Mol Med 2(3): 303–327

[30] Letterio J J (2005) TGF-beta signaling in T cells: roles in lymphoid and epithelial neoplasia. Oncogene 24(37): 5701–5712

[31] Linn Y C and Hui K M (2003) Cytokine-induced killer cells: NK-like T cells with cytotolytic specificity against leukemia. Leuk Lymphoma 44(9): 1457–1462

[32] Nowak A K, Lake R A et al (2003) Induction of tumor cell apoptosis in vivo increases tumor antigen cross-presentation, cross-priming rather than cross-tolerizing host tumor-specific CD8 T cells. J Immunol 170(10): 4905–4913

[33] Ohkawa T, Seki S et al (2001) Systematic characterization of human CD8+ T cells with natural killer cell markers in comparison with natural killer cells and normal CD8+ T cells. Immunology 103(3): 281–290

[34] Okada T, Iiai T et al (1995) Origin of CD57+ T cells which increase at tumour sites in patients with colorectal cancer. Clin Exp Immunol 102(1): 159–166

[35] Papagno L, Spina C A et al (2004) Immune activation and CD8+ T-cell differentiation towards senescence in HIV-1 infection. PLoS Biol 2(2): E20

[36] Peter M E and Krammer P H (2003) The CD95(APO-1/Fas) DISC and beyond. Cell Death Differ 10(1): 26–35

[37] Pflanz S, Timans J C et al (2002) IL-27, a heterodimeric cytokine composed of EBI3 and p28 protein, induces proliferation of naive CD4(+) T cells. Immunity 16(6): 779–790

[38] Pittet M J, Speiser D E et al (2000) Cutting edge: cytolytic effector function in human circulating CD8+ T cells closely correlates with CD56 surface expression. J Immunol 164(3): 1148–1152

[39] Rampino N, Yamamoto H et al (1997) Somatic frameshift mutations in the BAX gene in colon cancers of the microsatellite mutator phenotype. Science 275(5302): 967–969

[40] Sada-Ovalle I, Torre-Bouscoulet L et al (2006) Characterization of a cytotoxic CD57+ T cell subset from patients with pulmonary tuberculosis. Clin Immunol 121(3): 314–323

[41] Sadat-Sowti B, Debre P et al (1991) A lectin-binding soluble factor released by CD8+CD57+ lymphocytes from AIDS patients inhibits T cell cytotoxicity. Eur J Immunol 21(3): 737–741

[42] Sadat-Sowti B, Debre P et al (1994) An inhibitor of cytotoxic functions produced by CD8+ CD57+ T lymphocytes from patients suffering from AIDS and immunosuppressed bone marrow recipients. Eur J Immunol 24(11): 2882–2888

[43] Sallusto F, Lenig D et al (1999) Two subsets of memory T lymphocytes with distinct homing potentials and effector functions. Nature 401(6754): 708–712

[44] Schachner M and Martini R (1995) Glycans and the modulation of neural-recognition molecule function. Trends Neurosci 18(4): 183–191

[45] Sze D M, Giesajtis G et al (2001) Clonal cytotoxic T cells are expanded in myeloma and reside in the CD8(+)CD57(+)CD28(−) compartment. Blood 98(9): 2817–2827

[46] Takeda A, Hamano S et al (2003) Cutting edge: role of IL-27/WSX-1 signaling for induction of T-bet through activation of STAT1 during initial Th1 commitment. J Immunol 170(10): 4886–4890

[47] Tan L C, Mowat A G et al (2000) Specificity of T cells in synovial fluid: high frequencies of CD8(+) T cells that are specific for certain viral epitopes. Arthritis Res 2(2): 154–164

[48] Thies A, Schachner M et al (2004) The developmentally regulated neural crest-associated glycotope HNK-1 predicts metastasis in cutaneous malignant melanoma. J Pathol 203(4):933–939

[49] Trapani J A and Smyth M J (2002) Functional significance of the perforin/granzyme cell death pathway. Nat Rev Immunol 2(10): 735–747

[50] Tsujimoto Y, Yunis J et al (1984) Molecular cloning of the chromosomal breakpoint of B-cell lymphomas and leukemias with the t(11;14) chromosome translocation. Science 224(4656): 1403–1406

[51] Wallach D, Kovalenko A V et al (1998) Death-inducing functions of ligands of the tumor necrosis factor family: a Sanhedrin verdict. Curr Opin Immunol 10(3): 279–288.

[52] Wang E C, Taylor-Wiedeman J et al (1993) Subsets of CD8+, CD57+ cells in normal, healthy individuals: correlations with human cytomegalovirus (HCMV) carrier status, phenotypic and functional analyses. Clin Exp Immunol 94(2): 297–305

[53] Wang W S, Chen P M et al (2006) Matrix metalloproteinase-7 increases resistance to Fas-mediated apoptosis and is a poor prognostic factor of patients with colorectal carcinoma. Carcinogenesis 27(5): 1113–1120

[54] Yue F Y, Dummer R et al (1997) Interleukin-10 is a growth factor for human melanoma cells and down-regulates HLA class-I, HLA class-II and ICAM-1 molecules. Int J Cancer 71(4): 630–637

6. Natural killer T (NKT) cells: Immunophenotype, functional characteristics and significance in clinical practice

OLGA V. LEBEDINSKAYA

EA Vagner Perm Medical Academy Department of Histology
Embryology and Cytology
Perm
Russia

NELLY K. AKCHMATOVA

II Metchnikov Research Institute of Vaccines and Serum Laboratory
of Therapeutic Vaccines Moscow
Russia

IRINA O. CHIKILEVA

NN Blokhin Russian Cancer Research Center RAMS
Laboratory of Cell Immunity
Moscow
Russia

IRINA ZH. SHUBINA

NN Blokhin Russian Cancer Research Center RAMS
Laboratory of Cell Immunity
Moscow
Russia

MIKHAIL V. KISELEVSKY

NN Blokhin Russian Cancer Research Center RAMS
Laboratory of Cell Immunity
Moscow
Russia

Keywords: NKT cells, IL-12, cytokines, immunophenotype

Abstract

Natural killer T cells are lymphocytes that express both T-cell and natural killer-cell markers. Natural killer T cells are found in parenchymal organs such as liver, lungs, spleen etc and a small number are found in peripheral blood. Natural killer T cells comprise a significant part of leukocyte infiltrates that occur in liver and other organs of patients with cancer or infectious diseases. These cells have a large impact on the functional activity of effectors of anti-tumor and anti-infectious immunity.

M.V. Kiselevsky (ed.), Atlas Effectors of Anti-tumor Immunity, 81–99.
© Springer Science+Business Media B.V. 2008

Recent research studies revealed a particular lymphocyte subpopulation called natural killer T (NKT) cells. This is a unique T lymphocyte subtype involved in immune response regulation and associated with a number of diseases including cancer, autoimmune disorders and infections. NKT cells can either have a stimulating or an inhibiting effect on the immune response by the activation of Th1 or Th2 cells to produce regulatory cytokines. Therefore they may be regarded as effectors for different types of cell-based immunotherapy [20, 21, 55, 65].

NKT cells express on surface membrane both T-cell (CD3) and natural killer-cell markers (CD16, CD57, CD161 or NK1.1 in mice) [19, 28, 33]. According to immunophenotype, NKT cells are divided into two subsets: $CD4^+$ and $CD4^-$ although they can also express CD8 antigen in humans and monkeys [13, 19, 28, 29, 33, 41].

NKT cells recognize glycolipid antigens more readily than peptide ones. They bind non-polymorphic MHC I-like glycolipid antigen-presenting molecules CD1d, known to be expressed on cells of hematopoietic origin (dendritic cells, B cells, T cells and macrophages) as well as hepatocytes [36, 58]. Considering the immunophenotype characteristics some authors distinguish between "classical" (CD1d–restricted) NKT-cells and "non-classical" ones that express different surface T-cell receptors and their generation does not depend on CD1d expression on the cell surface membrane [41, 49, 51]. Obviously NKT cells include a heterogenic T-lymphocyte population.

Hepatic NKT cells have been most widely characterized. The liver presents the major components of innate immunity (NKT cells, dendritic cells and macrophages etc.) as well as a part of adaptive immunity effectors such as T lymphocytes [19, 28, 39, 51, 67, 68]. During the hepatolineal period of embryonic development the liver plays the main hemopoietic role, however in a number of conditions it still keeps its hemopoietic function after birth [1, 22]. The human liver includes stem cells ($c-kit^+$) and develops as an organ of ex-thymic generation of T cells, NK cells and granulocytes. In childhood the ex-thymic T-cell number is low but it increases with age. The ex-thymic T-lymphocyte generation in liver involves the formation of cells expressing T-cell receptors (TCR) as well as markers of NKT cells ($NK1.1^+$ TCR) [13, 22].

Most data on hepatic NKT-cell activation and NKT-cell interaction with other immune effectors has been obtained from experiments on mice [33, 46, 63]. NKT cells present the major part of hepatic T lymphocytes in mice although in thymus, bone marrow, lymph nodes and peripheral blood the NKT-cell number only reaches 1% of the T-cell population [15, 19, 28, 41, 46]. Mouse NKT cells are defined as $CD4^+CD8^-$ or $CD4^-CD8^-$ (double negative) cells which display a restricted $TCR\alpha\beta$ repertoire ($V\alpha14/V\beta8$, $\beta7$ or $\beta2$ TCR) [28, 46]. These TCR molecules bind the nonclassical MHC class I-like molecule CD1d. In mice, NKT cells comprise 30–50% of the total hepatic T lymphocytes and have a potential anti-tumor activity [15, 28, 46].

NKT cell activation in liver is mediated by interleukin (IL)-12 which is produced by antigen-presenting cells (APCs) such as macrophages, Kupfer and dendritic cells (DCs) in response to bacterial and viral factors such as endotoxins as well as to malignant cell transformation [28, 33, 46, 63] (Figure 6.1). Hepatic NKT-cell activation is associated with the expression of CD69 activating molecule, enhanced NKT-cell cytotoxicity and IFN-γ secretion [69].

Another stimulating factor for NKT-cell activation is glycosphingolipid (isolated from the oceanic sponge *Agelas mauritianus*) α-galactosylceramide (α-GalCer) that leads to hepatic damage when administered systemically [15, 25, 26, 31, 46, 57]. Injection of α-GalCer in mice results in the formation of

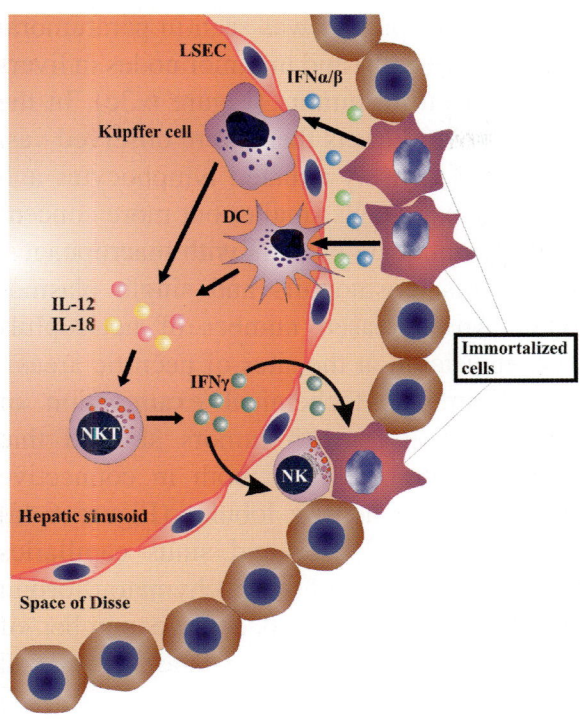

Figure 6.1. Scheme of hepatic immunocompetent cells distribution (Refs. [15, 19, 28, 41, 46])

venous fibrin clots and multi-focal infarctions. A similar picture can be seen in the case of super-acute (mediated by antibodies) or acute (cellular) rejection of hepatic allotransplants. Such disorders with hepatocellular damage and inflammatory foci, consisting MNLs were registered in the HBV transgenic mice. The authors assigned the above-mentioned processes with NKT-cell activation by α-GalCer resulting in a release of TNF-α and INF-γ [15, 28, 33, 68, 69]. α-GalCer NKT-cell activation has a therapeutic effect in diseases caused by *Cryptococcus neoformans* or in viral encephalomyocarditis and prevents the development of the intra-heptocytic stage of *Plasmodium yoelii* and *Plasmodium bergheri* in mice [30]. Therefore α-GalCer NKT-cell activation may be of clinical significance in infections and cancer [8, 23, 64].

A proposed mechanism of action for α-GalCer NKT-cell activation may be the following: α-GalCer binds to CD1d and the glycolipid-CD1d complex interacts with restricted TCR molecules expressed by NKT cells thus leading to activation of these cells [44, 56]. There is a suggestion that α-GalCer-activated NKT cells can not act as immune system effectors and directly lyse tumor cells. However, they can recruit and stimulate other effectors such as NK cells and cytotoxic T lymphocytes (CTLs) through INF-γ secretion [21, 24, 54, 61].

The activation of NKT cells by different glycolipids and lipopolysaccharides was registered. TCR-ligand activated NKT cells responded by a marked production of cytokines within 1–2 hours [5, 19, 37].

Effective NKT-cell stimulation requires direct contact between NKT cells and DCs via CD40-CD40-ligand interaction and IL-12 produced by DCs [2, 17, 35]. In particular, lipopolysaccharide derivatives were shown to reduce hepatic metastases in mice after systemic treatment [63]. This anti-metastatic effect was assigned to hepatic NK-cell activation in response to increasing IL-12 secretion due to a hepatic DC stimulation by lipopolisaccharides [63].

DC-secreted IL-12 is the most important cytokine inducing interferon (INF)-γ production by NKT cells. There are certain data demonstrating that IL-12-activated NKT cells function as effectors of type 1 that produce INF-γ, while α-GalCer-activated NKT cells may function as innate immunity effectors of type 2 producing IL-4 and IL-13 as well as INF-γ [27, 60, 62, 71].

The NKT-cell function to secrete immuno-suppressive or type 2 (humoral immune response) cytokines such as IL-10, IL-4 and IL-13 suggests that these cells can suppress cellular immune response. Experimental studies have shown that NKT cells can induce tolerance towards allotransplant [10, 21, 42, 43, 52, 60, 71].

The hepatic NKT-cell lifetime is short: they are activated, perform their effector functions and die within several hours mainly as the result of apoptosis. This fact may partly explain the decreasing number of NKT cells in the liver relative to the CD8$^+$ T-cell decrease. There might be other mechanisms for NKT-cell down-regulation including generation disorders due to CD1d modulation, alterations in ligand binding or cytokine homeostasis imbalance [68].

A number of studies on mice demonstrated an important role of the hepatic NKT cells in anti-tumor immunity. In particular, NKT cells were found to infiltrate liver tissue affected by the malignant process, especially parametastatic liver sites [15, 28, 33, 46, 63, 67, 68, 69].

The infiltration of mononuclear leukocytes in the liver was studied in CBA mice with inoculated ovarian carcinoma CAO-1 into the liver [3, 38]. On day 14, after tumor cell implantation into the murine liver, oval shaped tumor nodules of 3–5 mm, in diameter were seen to invade surrounding tissue (Figure 6.2).

The morphological examination of the slide series revealed leukocyte infiltrations in intact liver sites that concentrated mainly in connective tissue layers around vessels of portal tract (Figure 6.3a). The infiltrations were rather small and included a moderate number of leukocytes.

A different picture was seen in paratumoral sites (Figure 6.3b) and in tumor nodes in livers of mice bearing tumors (Figure 6.3c). In the areas of portal tracts there were observed vast clusters of densely situated lymphocytes and among hepatic cells smaller but more concentrated lymphocyte clusters with macrophages, neutrophils, eosinophils and single plasmocytes. An increased number of neutrophils were registered at the sites of necrotic areas.

An immunocytochemical examination of the murine liver with tumors showed that all the infiltrating cells, both in connective tissue between hepatic lobules (Figure 6.4a) and inside lobules around sinus capillaries (Figure 6.4b), were of mesenchymatous origin (WIM$^+$). They included a large number of NK (CD16$^+$) cells (Figure 6.4c). Stem cell antigen CD10 was determined on the surface of the cells infiltrating connective tissue and those in sinusoid lumens (Figures 6.4d,e). A T-and B-lymphocyte progenitor marker (Tdt) was also revealed on numerous cells of leukocyte infiltrations (Figure 6.4f). A high rate of positive reaction with pan-T-marker (CD3) was observed on the cell surface in all liver sites of mice with tumors (Figure 6.4g). Antigen CD68 expression was noted on macrophages found in connective tissue infiltrates (Figure 6.4h) as well as on leukocytes adjacent to tumor cells (Figure 6.4i). The infiltrates of paratumoral liver sites comprised a large number of proliferating cells that stained intensively by proliferation marker (Ki-67) (Figures 6.4j,k).

Lymphocytes isolated from a tumor-affected liver comprise two subsets; one of them is represented mostly by T lymphocytes and the other consists of lymphocytes expressing NK- and NKT-cell markers (Figures 6.5a–d). Spleen lymphocytes from intact and tumor-bearing mice express mainly CD3 surface marker while NK cells are shown to comprise less than 2.5% (Figure 6.5e) [52]. Mononuclear leukocytes (MNLs) from murine tumor-bearing liver had a high spontaneous

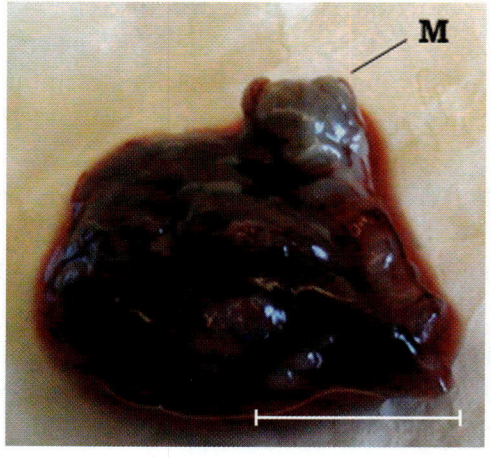

Figure 6.2. Ovarian carcinoma CaO-1 implant in a CBA mouse liver M – tumor implant; Scale bar: 1sm

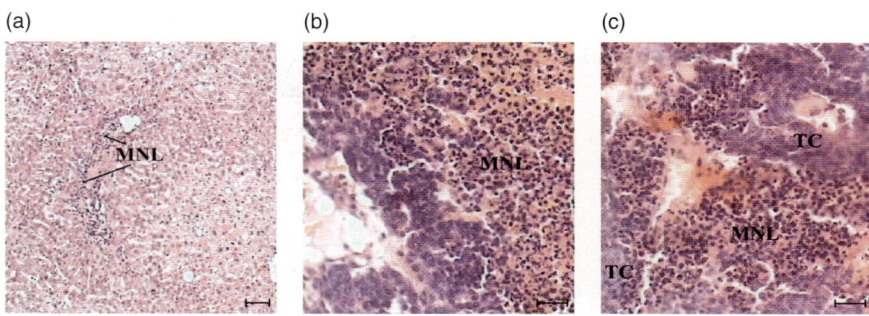

Figure 6.3. Microphotographs of histologic slides of intact **a**, paratumoral **b** and metastatic **c** liver sites of CBA mice challenged with ovarian carcinoma CaO-1 **a** – leukocyte infiltrates in an intact murine liver; **b** – leukocyte infiltrates in paratumoral site of a murine liver; **c** – leukocyte infiltrates in metastatic site of a murine liver; stained by hematoxylin-eosin; Scale bar: **a** – 80 μm; **b,c** – 20 μm; MNL – mononuclear leucocytes, TC – tumor cells

NK-activity and a 2-fold higher killer activity than that of spleen lymphocytes. Hepatic MNLs lysed autologous tumor cells more effectively than spleen MNLs (Figure 6.6). The intact control mice displayed a scarce number of hepatic lymphocytes.

Therefore, when a tumor node in a mouse liver develops it stimulates parenchyma infiltration with MNLs including WIM$^+$, CD3$^+$, CD10$^+$, CD16$^+$, CD68$^+$, Tdt$^+$ and Ki67$^+$-cells. Thus the lymphocyte hepatic parenchyma infiltration seems to be a response by local immunity to cell malignant transformation [6, 11, 53]. The tissue NKT-cell distribution in humans has been intensively studied but unlike that of mice, a healthy human liver has a low number of NKT cells (0.5% of CD3$^+$) and even less in peripheral blood (0.02%) [34, 41].

So far, studies have revealed that a major NKT-cell subset from a healthy and tumor-affected human liver includes Vα24/Vβ11$^+$ NKT cells [13, 19, 29, 32, 41, 49, 51]. Human hepatic NKT cells differ from blood NKT cells by expression of Vβ11-chain. NKT-cell variants display the following profiles of T-cell marker expression: CD4$^+$CD8$^-$, CD4$^-$CD8$^-$; they also possess high levels of NK-cell antigens CD56, CD161 and/or CD69 [7, 13, 19, 51].

Many authors suggest that human hepatic NKT cells, as those of mice, have an anti-tumor function. The activation of these cells may significantly enhance their cytotoxic potential. The problem is especially important since the liver is one of the main organs of metastases of various cancer types. About 20% of patients with colorectal cancer after surgery develop liver metastases that cause the patient's death due to hepatic failure [1, 15]. M. A. Exley and M. J. Koziel's review also presents data on the protective role of NKT cells in acute hepatitis and their importance in the pathogenesis of chronic hepatotropic infection and the fibroid process in liver [14].

The examination of hepatic tissue from cancer patients showed that the sites, located far from metastases, consist of excessive fibrous connective tissue with moderate combined lymphoid - macrophage infiltrates (Figure 6.7a). Practically no leukocytes were found inside lobules (Figure 6.7b) while in paratumoral sites around vessels of the portal tract large leukocyte infiltrates were revealed. They consisted mostly of lymphoid cells but included macrophages and single granular leukocytes (Figures 6.7c,d). Similar cells infiltrate the area around sinusoid capillaries (Figure 6.7e). Immunocytochemical examination of slides with cancer patients'

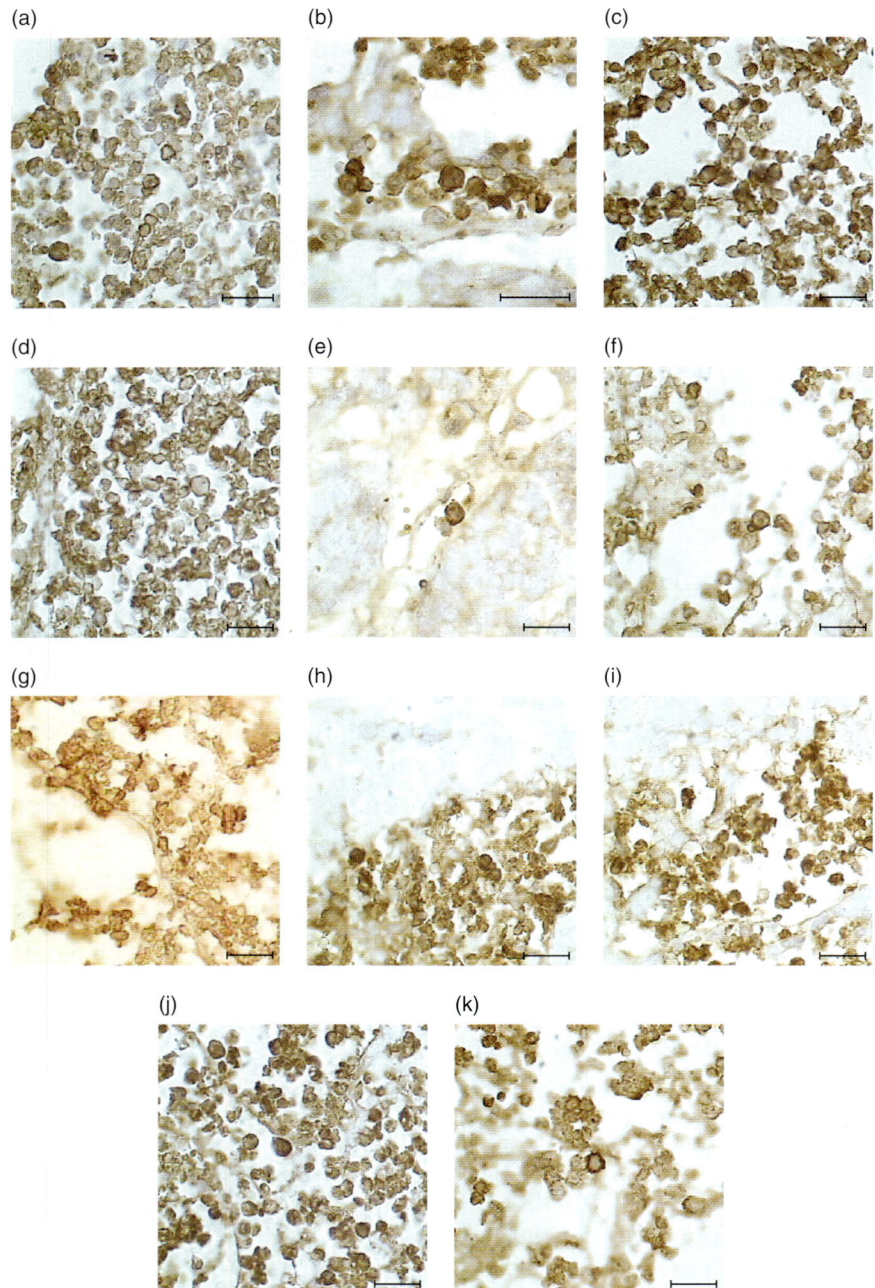

Figure 6.4. Microphotographs of histologic slides of leukocyte hepatic infiltrates stained by monoclonal antibodies obtained from CBA mice challenged with ovarian carcinoma CaO-1 **a,b** – WIM$^+$ cells; **c** – CD16$^+$ cells; **d,e** – CD10$^+$ cells; **f** – Tdt$^+$ cells; **g** – CD3$^+$ cells; **h,i** – CD68$^+$ cells; **j,k** – Ki67$^+$ cells; nuclei additional staining by hematoxylin; Scale bar: 30 μm

liver samples, using monoclonal antibodies, revealed leukocyte infiltrates WIM$^+$-cells of mesenchymatous origin (Figure 6.8a). The leukocyte infiltrates of paratumoral sites include T cells (CD3$^+$) with moderate intensity of staining (Figure 6.8f) and a significant number of CD16$^+$ cells (Figure 6.8b,c). Inside sinusoid capillaries there are single light positive CD10$^+$ cells (Figure 6.8d) and bright positive TdT$^+$ cells, which present

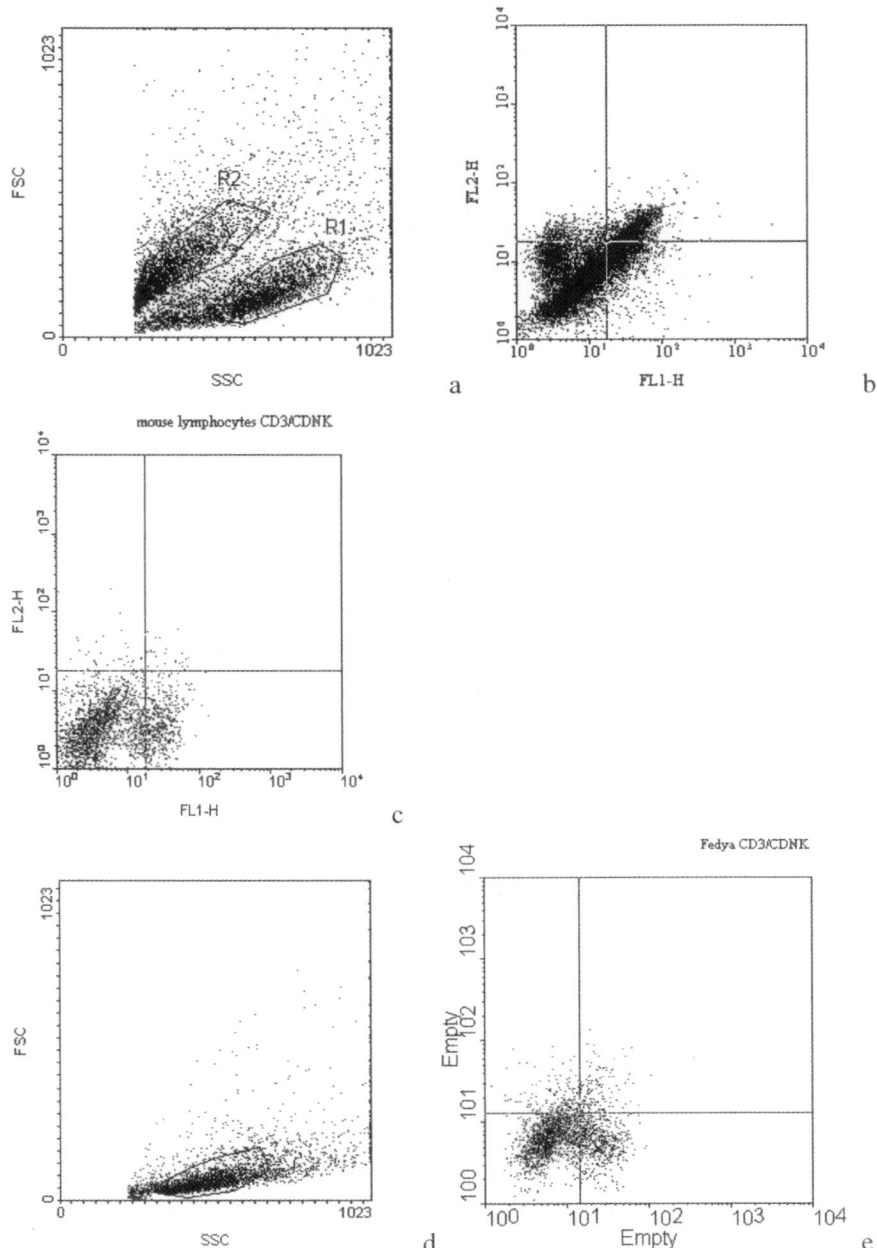

Figure 6.5. DotPlot of flow cytometry analysis reflecting expression of cell-surface markers CD3(FITC), NK (PE) of mononuclear lymphocytes (MNL), isolated from the liver (**a–c**) and spleen (**d,e**) of CBA mice challenged with ovarian carcinoma CaO-1 **a** – hepatic MNL distribution; **b** – hepatic MNL distribution with double staining (CD3/NK) in R2; **c** – hepatic MNL distribution with double staining (CD3/NK) in R1; **d** – spleen MNL distribution; **e** – spleen MNL distribution with double staining (CD3/NK)

blast precursors of B and T lymphocytes (Figure 6.8e). The antigen CD68 is expressed in macrophages found in the wall of sinusoid capillaries (Figure 6.8g). The proliferation marker Ki-67 stains wall cells of paratumoral sites (Figure 6.8h). The hepatic lymphoid infiltrates have practically no B lymphocytes (CD20[+]).

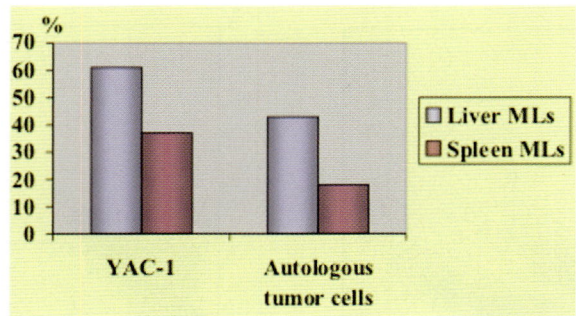

Figure 6.6. NK-activity and cytotoxicity of MNL isolated from liver and spleen of tumor-bearing mice against tumor cell line YAC-1 and autologous tumor cells (%)

Hepatic leukocyte infiltrates, from different liver sites of patients with various primary cancer types, were studied to describe their morphological, functional and immunophenotypic characteristics [40, 70] (Figure 6.9). The number of MNLs isolated from livers of patients who had no previous radio or chemotherapy accounted for $5-6 \times 10^6$ cells per cm^3 of the liver samples. The number of isolated MNLs from pararumoral sites was 1.5–2 fold higher than that of intact liver sites. The number of MNLs isolated from livers of patients who had received previous radiation or chemotherapy accounted for less than 1×10 cells per cm^3 of the liver samples. Patients with breast cancer and metastases in the liver who had previously received 4–6 chemotherapy courses

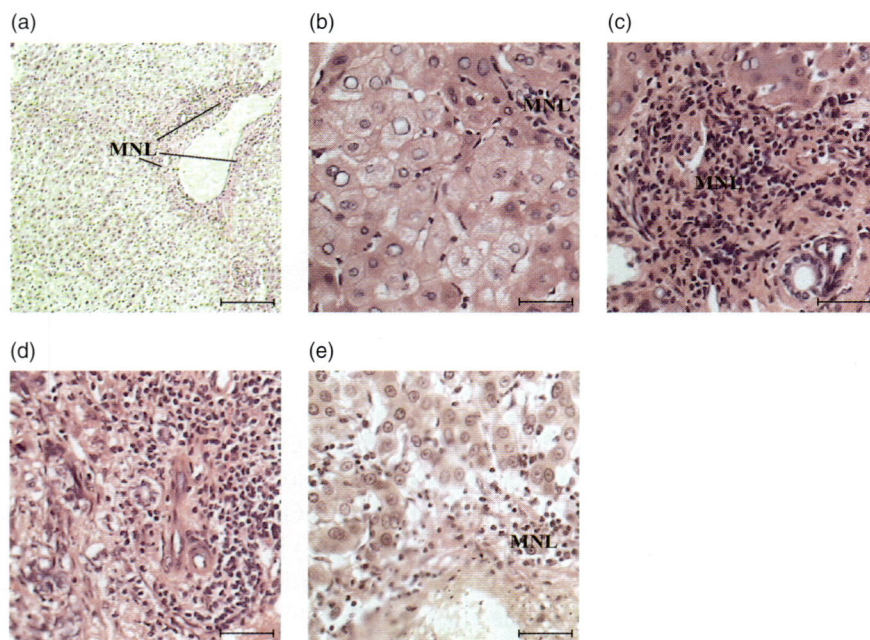

Figure 6.7. Microphotographs of histologic slides of intact (**a,b**) and paratumoral (**c,d,e**) sites of a colorectal cancer patient's liver with a metastatic process **a,b** – leukocyte infiltrates in intact liver sites; **c,e** – leukocyte infiltrates in paratmetastatic liver sites; **a** – stained by Van Gison; **b–e** – stained by hematoxylin-eosin; Scale bar: **a** – 80 μm; **b** – 30 μm; **c,d** – 50 μm; **e** – 30 μm; MNL – mononuclear leucocyte

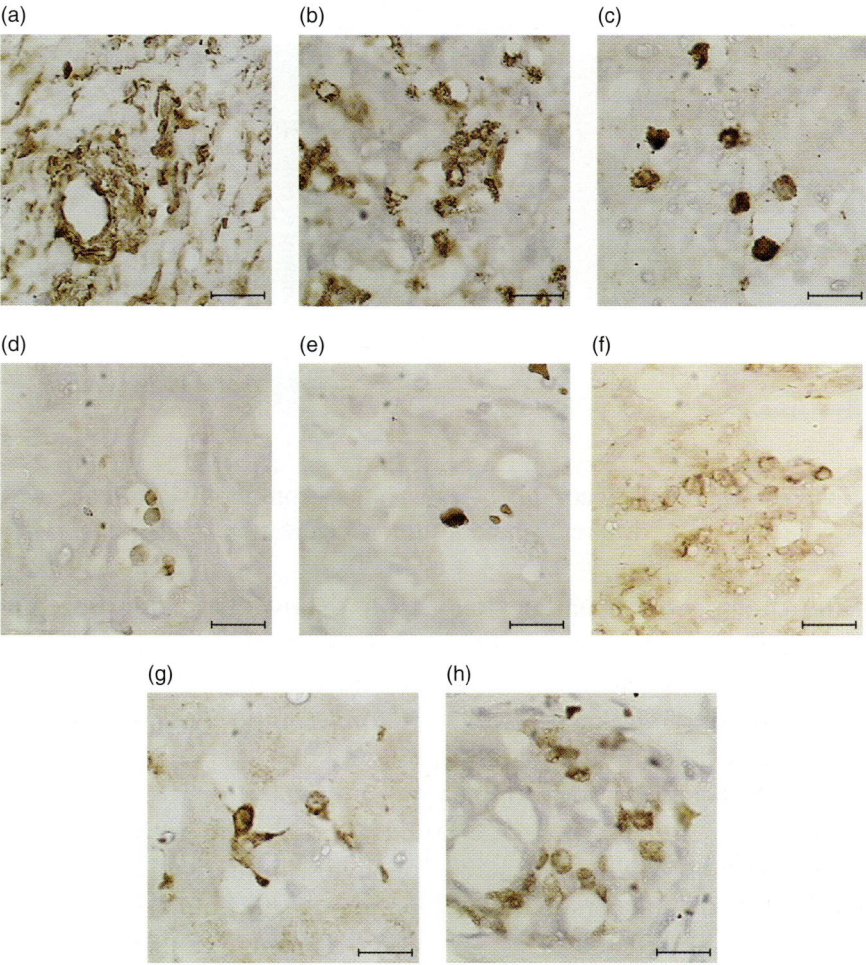

Figure 6.8. Microphotographs of histologic slides of leukocyte hepatic infiltrates stained by monoclonal antibodies obtained from the liver sample of a colorectal cancer patient **a** – WIM$^+$ cells; **b,c** – CD16+ cells; **d** – CD10+ cells; **e** – Tdt+ cells; **f** – CD3+ cells; **g** – CD68+ cells; **h** – Ki67+ cells; additional nulei staining with hematoxylin; Scale bar: 30 μm

(CAF+ radiation therapy) had practically no hepatic MNLs while the number of MNLs isolated from patients' livers who had received immunotherapy (Intron A) prior to surgery accounted for 10–15 × 10^6 cells per 1cm^3 of the liver samples. Thus, the number of hepatic MNLs depends on the type of pre-surgery treatment: after radio and chemotherapy the MNL number is minimal while after immunotherapy it increases significantly, as compared to untreated patients. The control examination was performed with MNLs isolated from the liver of patients who had hepatic trauma.

Morphological histochemical analysis showed that the intact liver presented mostly small and medium lymphocytes that had average pyroninophilic component in cytoplasm when stained by Brachet (Figure 6.10). Examination of MNLs isolated from tumor-affected liver showed that it was infiltrated by lymphoid cells of prolymphocyte and immunoblast types (most numerous in paratumoral sites). The interaction between lymphocytes, macrophages and dendritic cells was noted (Figures 6.11a,b). A significant number of lymphocytes with a bright pyroninophilic staining of cytoplasm and nucleoli was

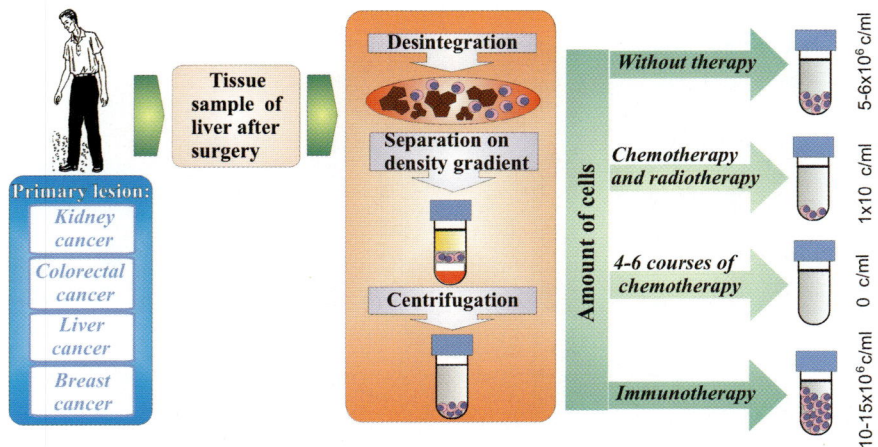

Figure 6.9. Scheme of mononuclear leukocytes isolation from the liver of cancer patients with different primary tumor localization

registered and the staining disappeared after treatment with RNAse, which showed their high synthesizing function (Figures 6.11c,d). Activated pyroninophilic lymphocytes were seen in large numbers both in the paratumoral sites and in the metastatic node tissue (Figures 6.11e,f).

A comparative study of MNLs of intact and paratumoral sites of cancer patients'

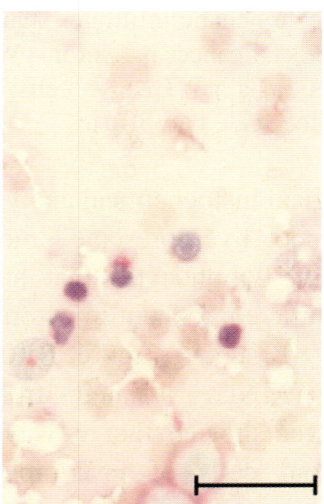

Figure 6.10. Mononuclear leukocytes (MNL) isolated from an intact hepatic sample of a patient with liver trauma MNL microphotographs in cytospins; stained with methyl green-pyronin by Brachet; Scale bar: 20 μm

liver showed that prolymphocytes and immunoblasts accounts for 24.7% of MNLs in intact liver sites and the number of pyroninophilic lymphocytes reached 15.7% (Figure 6.12a) while in paratumoral sites most of MNLs (91.3%) were presented by activated lymphoid cells such as prolymphocytes, immunoblasts and pyroninophilic lymphocytes (Figure 6.12b).

A comparative study of the cytotoxic activity of MNLs isolated from intact or paratumoral liver sites, peripheral blood of cancer patients and healthy donors revealed that lymphocytes isolated from the paratumoral liver sites of cancer patients had the highest killer activity against allogeneic (NK-sensitive tumor cells K562) and autologous tumor cells (90 and 62% respectively). The cancer patients' peripheral blood mononuclear cells (PBMCs) had a lower rate of cytotoxic activity compared to that of hepatic MNLs and it was similar to the cytotoxicity of healthy donors'. The cancer patients' PBMCs had practically no killer function against autologous tumor cells.

The lymphocyte population from the paratumoral and metastatic sites of cancer patients' liver presents three main subsets: NK cells, T lymphocytes and NKT cells expressing both NK- and T-cell markers (Figures 6.13

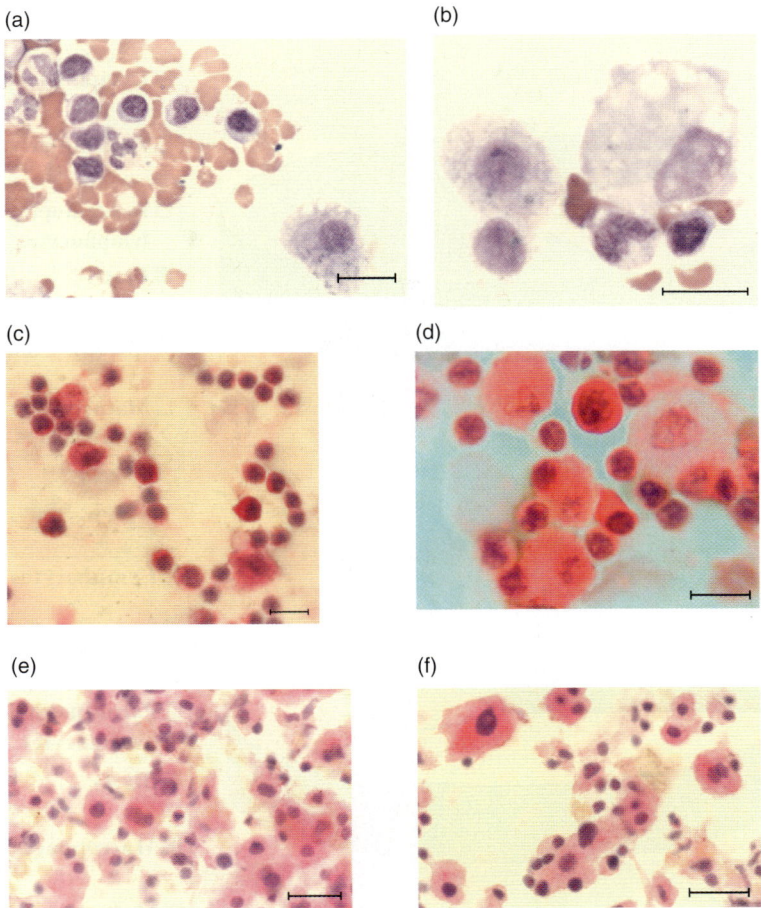

Figure 6.11. Mononuclear leukocytes in cytospins obtained from paratumoral **a–d** and metastatic **e,f** liver sites of a patient with colorectal cancer **a–d** – microphotographs of pyroninophylic lymphocytes, blast cells and macrophage-like cells in cytospins of a parametastatic liver site of a cancer patient; **a,b** – stained by azur II –eosin by Romanovsky-Gimsa; **c,d** – stained with methyl green-pyronin by Brachet; **e,f** – microphotographs of pyroninophylic lymphocytes, blast cells and macrophage-like cells in cytospins of a hepatic metastasis of a cancer patient; stained with methyl green-pironin by Brachet; Scale bar: **a** – 20 μm; **b** – 20 μm; **c** – 10 μm; **d** – 10 μm; **e** – 20 μm; **f** – 20 μm; MNL – mononuclear leucocytes

and 6.14). The comparative immunophenotype analysis of MNLs isolated from the different liver sites of cancer patients showed that the percentage of MNLs expressing surface antigens CD4, CD8, CD3 and CD16 were approximately the same in intact and pararumoral sites. However, the fluorescence intensity characterizing levels of expression of these CD markers was 1.2–1.3 fold higher on the surface of MNLs isolated from paratumoral sites than that of MNLs from intact sites.

The immunophenotype difference in expression of antigens such as CD25, CD38 and CD56 and MNLs isolated from two studied liver sites is insignificant. However, the number of MNLs expressing adhesion molecules (CD58) from the paratumoral site is almost 3 fold higher than that of the intact liver site. The most significant difference is observed between the immunophenotype of lymphocytes isolated from PBMCs of cancer patients and the MNLs of the paratumoral liver site. MNLs from the metastatic liver

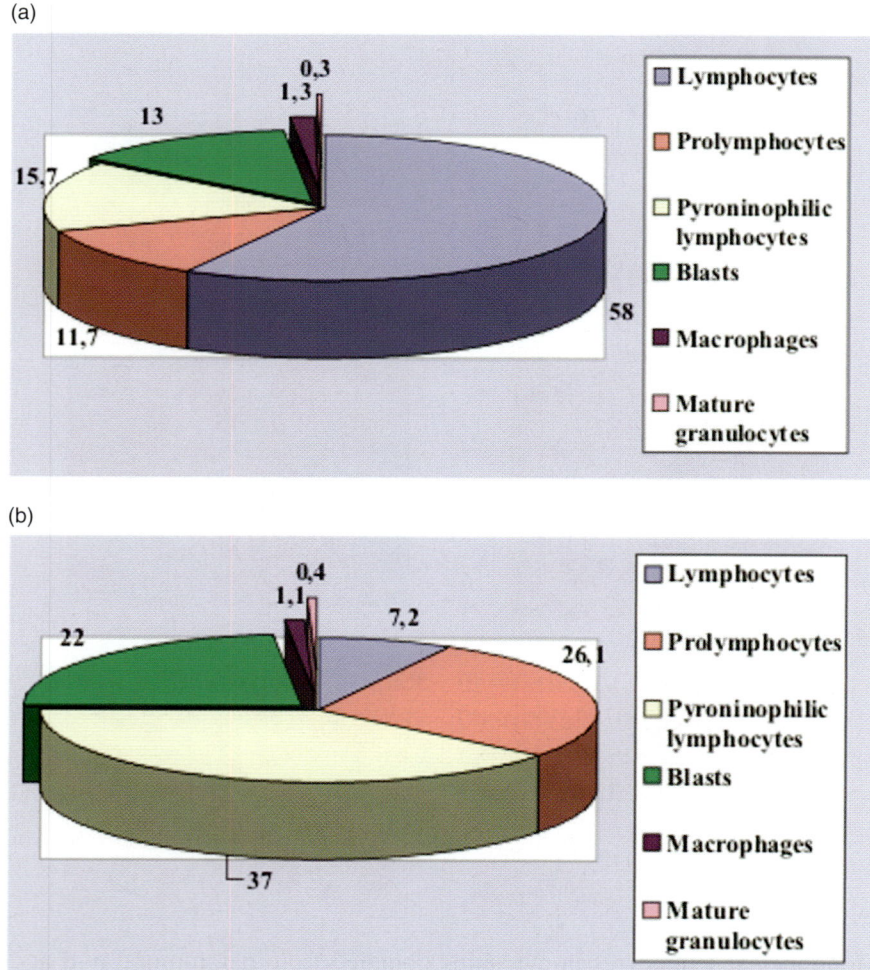

Figure 6.12. Cellular contents of mononuclear leukocytes isolated from intact **a** and parametastatic **b** sites of cancer patients' liver (%)

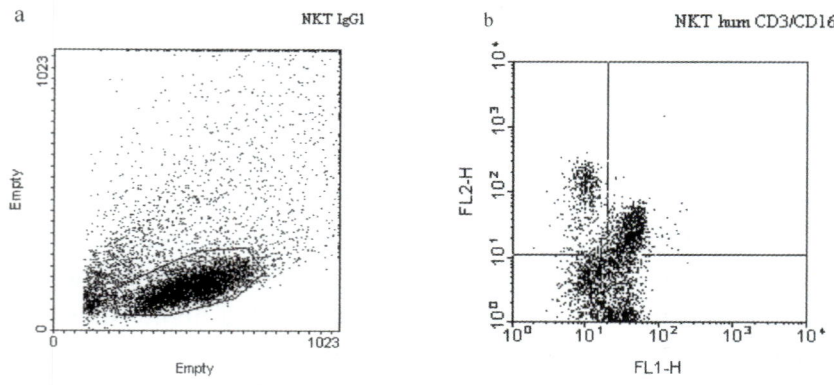

Figure 6.13. DotPlot flow cytometry analysis of cell-surface markers CD3(FITC), NK (PE) of mononuclear leukocytes (MNL) isolated from parametastatic site of a colorectal cancer patient's liver **a** – hepatic MNL distribution; **b** – hepatic MNL distribution with double staining (CD3/CD16)

(a) (b)

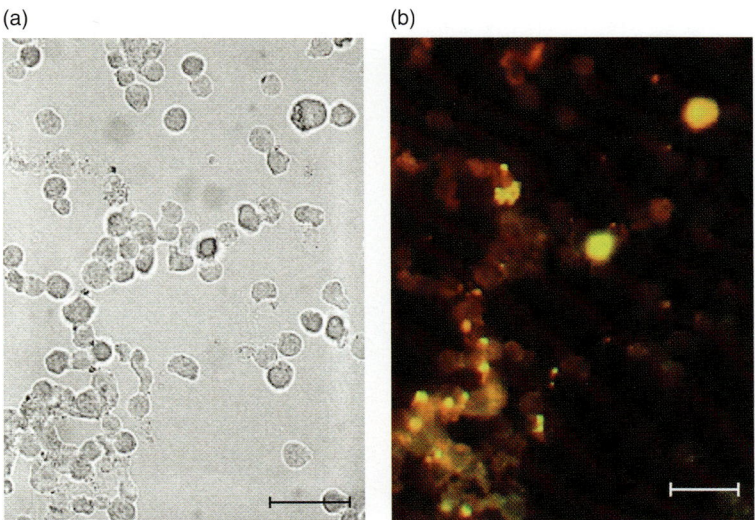

Figure 6.14. Mononuclear leukocytes (MNL) isolated from a paratumoral site of a colorectal cancer patient's liver **a** – microphotographs of MNL cytospins stained by fluorescent monoclonal antibodies CD3/CD16 in bright field; **b** – microphotographs of MNL cytospins stained by fluorescent monoclonal antibodies CD3/CD16 in dark field; 20 μm

have a much higher expression of CD8 antigen, CD38 activation antigen, NK-cell markers (CD16 and CD56) and adhesion molecule CD58 although the percentage of CD4$^+$-cells from PBMCs is 4 times higher than that of hepatic MNLs. The obtained data shows that MNLs from a tumor-affected liver consists mainly of CD3$^+$ T lymphocytes but unlike PBMCs they also express NK-cell antigens (CD16, CD56).

The morphological examination of MNLs from the metastatic liver, particularly from paratumoral sites, revealed mostly immature and synthesizing lymphoid cells, which is characteristic for the processes of lymphocyte blast-transformation, differentiation and activation that may result in NKT cell subset development. This subset has a high NK-activity and an enhanced expression of adhesion molecules that increases their fixation in tumor sites and interaction with antigen-presenting DCs as well as with tumor cells. Hepatic lymphocytes have a higher cytotoxic activity against autologous tumor cells than that of lymphocytes of cancer patients' peripheral blood. Therefore the

results of the studies support previous experimental data presenting a definite NKT cell subset in a tumor-affected liver. Their specific characteristics may be used in the development of immunotherapy methods for cancer patients with metastases in liver.

Similar results were obtained through morphologic and immunophenotypic analysis of liver samples from patients with hepatitis B and C (Figures 6.15 and 6.16). Histological slides present a marked leukocyte infiltration in the connective tissue around the vessels of the portal tract (Figures 6.15a,b,e) as well as hepatic parenchyma (Figures 6.15b,c,f,g). The infiltrating lymphocytes displayed the immunophenotype of CD3$^+$/CD16$^+$/CD56$^+$-cells (Figure 6.16). The studies also revealed lymphocytes of the same immunophenotype in the lymphoid infiltrates of submucous gastric tissue (Figure 6.17) in patients with cancer of the gastric body (Figure 6.18).

Thus, in tumor-affected liver and infection processes, a similar leukocyte infiltration is observed that includes NK and NKT cells. Some approaches to involve NKT cells in anti-

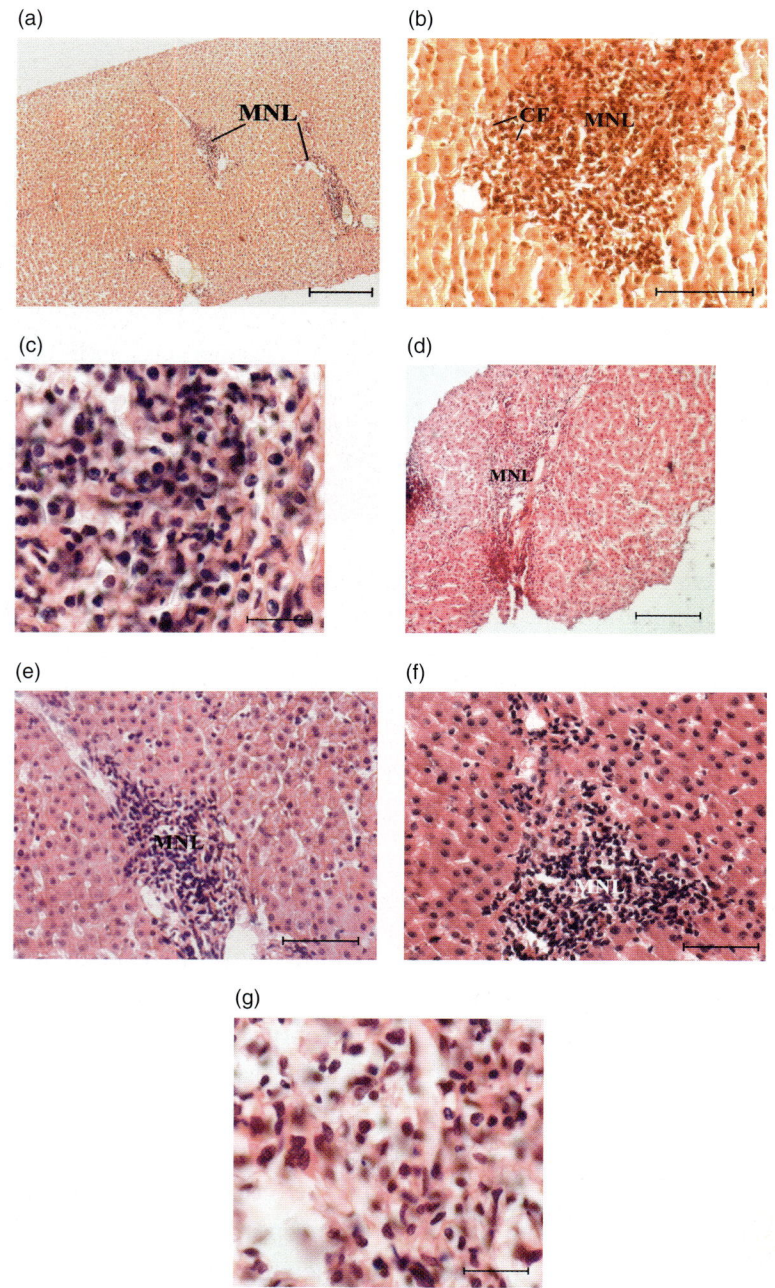

Figure 6.15. Microphotographs of histologic slides of liver samples of patients with hepatitis B and C
a–c – leukocyte infiltrates in a liver of a patient with hepatitis B; **a,b** – stained by Van Gison;
c – stained by hematoxylin-eosin; **d–g** – leukocyte infiltrates in a liver of a patient with hepatitis C;
stained by hematoxylin-eosin; Scale bar: **a** – 100 μm; **b** – 70 μm; **c** – 30 μm; **d** – 100 μm; **e** – 70 μm;
f – 70 μm; **g** – 30 μm; MNL – mononuclear leucocytes

tumor immunotherapy on mouse models are under investigation as well as in clinical studies.

The study on NKT-deficient Ja18 −/− mice showed that the incidence of methylholantren-induced sarcomas in NKT-deficient mice was much higher than in the wild type [59]. Tumor regression was registered in NKT-deficient mice when NKT cells were

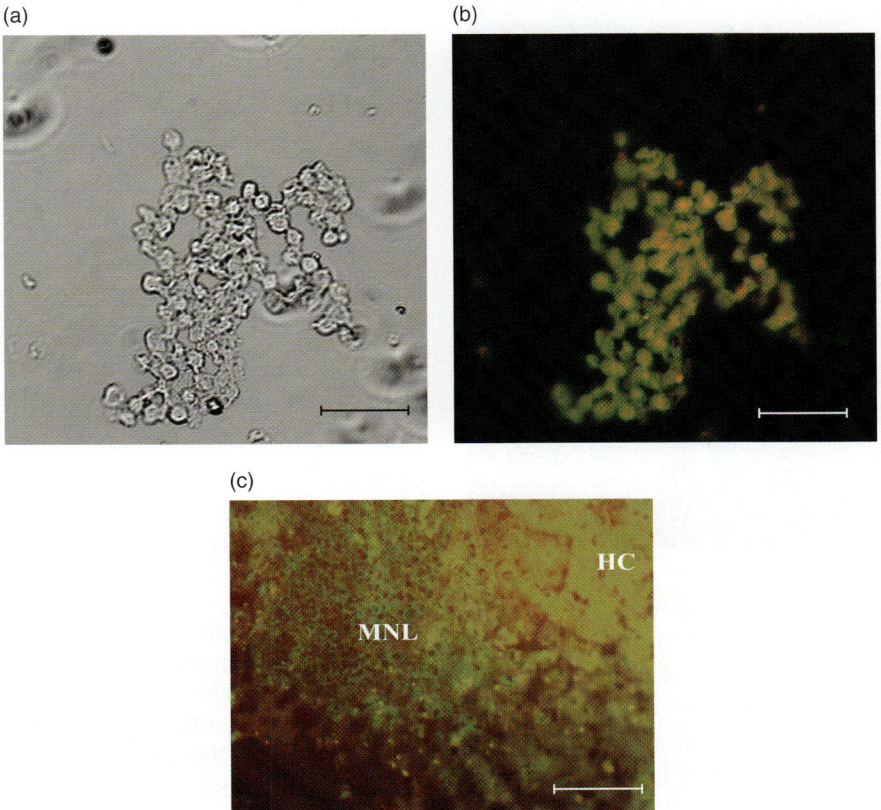

Figure 6.16. Mononuclear leukocytes (MNL) of leukocyte infiltrates in a liver of a patient with viral hepatitis BMicrophotographs of MNLs stained by fluorescent monoclonal antibodies: **a,b** – mAb to cell-surface markers CD3/CD16 in cytospins in bright **a** and dark **b** fields; Scale bar: 50 μm; **c** – mAb to cell-surface markers CD3/CD56 in frozen section; mAb conjugated with FITC or PE; Scale bar: 80 μm

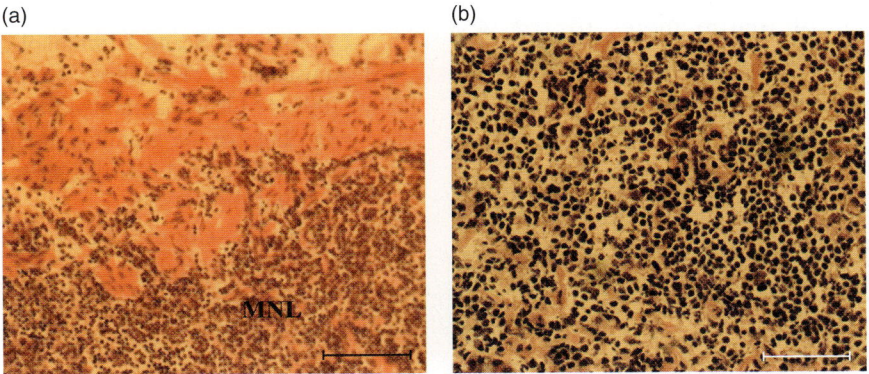

Figure 6.17. Microphotographs of histologic slides of parametastatic sites of a pyloric part of the stomach of a patient with gastric cancer **a,b** – leukocyte infiltrates in parametastatic site of a submucosal layer of a pyloric part of the stomach of a patient with gastric cancer; stained by hematoxylin-eosin; Scale bar: **a** – 100 μm; **b** – 70

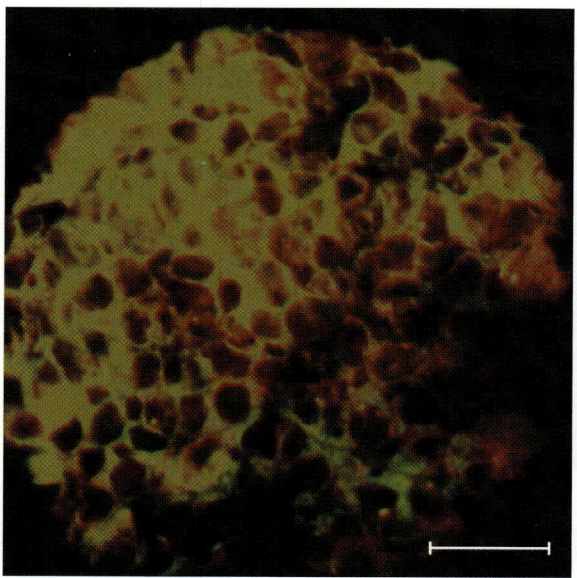

Figure 6.18. Mononuclear leukocytes (MNL) of leukocyte infiltrates in parametastatic sites of a pyloric part of the stomach of a patient with gastric cancerMicrophotographs of MNLs stained by fluorescent monoclonal antibodies to cell-surface markers CD3/CD56 in frozen section; Scale bar: 30 μm

adoptively transferred from wild-type mice [9]. Similar data were obtained on the models of sarcoma lung metastases where tumor regression was induced with α-GalCer stimulation [9, 16, 48, 50, 66].

Deficiencies in the NKT cell number or functions are registered in many but not in all of the types of malignancies [4, 12, 45] although it is unclear whether such disorders occur prior to tumor development or as the result of cancer progression. Clinical phase I trials studied the effect of α-GalCer or autologous DCs loaded with α-GalCer in cancer patients [18]. The results showed a good tolerance to such immunotherapy [47]. The patients with the background transient decrease of NKT and NK cell percentage presented an augmentation in IFN-γ and IL-12 rate in the peripheral blood and as a consequence, increased NK-cell cytotoxicity. In addition, the patients developed an inflammation process at the tumor site that was considered to be an enhancement of the immune response [47].

Thus, NKT cells present a distinguished subset of lymphocytes that has a high immunoregulatory potential. They play an important role in the local anti-tumor and anti-infectious immune responses. This lymphocyte subset comprises a significant part of tumor-infiltrating lymphocytes and leukocyte infiltrates of paratumoral sites. Considering their functional characteristics, NKT cells may be involved in the adoptive immunotherapy of cancer and infectious diseases.

References

[1] Abo T, Kawamura T, Watanabe H (2000) Physiological responses of extrathymic T cells in the liver. Immunol Rev 174(2):135–149

[2] Akhmatova NK, Kuzovlev EN, Lebedinskaya OV et al. (2006) Cytotoxic activity of natural killer T-(NKT) cells in mice with tumor-affected liver. Bull Exp Biol and Med 141(1):76–79.

[3] Ali Tahir SM, Cheng O, Shaulov A et al. (2001) Loss of IFN-gamma production by invariant NK T cells in advanced cancer. J Immunol 167: 4046–4050.

[4] Ananias RZ, Rodrigues EG, Braga EG et al. (2007) Modulatory effect of killed Propionibacterium acnes and its purified soluble polysaccharide on peritoneal exudate cells from C57Bl/6 mice: major NKT cell recruitment and increased cytotoxicity. Scand J Immunol 65(6):538–548.

[5] Apostolou I, Takahama Y, Belmant C et al. (1999) Murine natural killer T (NKT) cells contribute to the granulomatous reaction caused by mycobacterial cell walls. Proc Natl Acad Sci USA 96(9):5141–5146.

[6] Arrunategui-Correa V, Lenz L, Kim HS (2004) CD1d-independent regulation of NKT cell migration and cytokine production upon Listeria monocytogenes infection. Cell Immunol 232(1–2):38–48.

[7] Carlens S, Gilljam M, Chambers BJ et al. (2001) A new method for *in vitro* expansion of cytotoxic human CD3-CD56+ natural killer cells. Human Immunol 62(4):1092–1098.

[8] Chang YJ, Huang JR, Tsai YC et al. (2007) Potent immune-modulating and anticancer

effects of NKT cell stimulatory glycolipids. Proc Natl Acad Sci USA 104(25):10299–304.

[9] Crowe NY, Smyth MJ, Godfrey DI (2002) A critical role for natural killer T cells in immunosurveillance of methylcholanthrene-induced sarcomas. J Exp Med 196(1): 119–127.

[10] Crowe NY, Uldrich AP, Kyparissoudis K et al. (2003) Glycolipid antigen drives rapid expansion and sustained cytokine production by NK T Cells. J Immunol 171:4020–4027.

[11] Davydov MI, Normantovich VA, Kiselevsky MV et al. (2000) Adoptive immunotherapy in malignant effusions: clinical laboratory study. Russian Oncol J 6:14–17.

[12] Dhodapkar MV, Geller MD, Chang DH et al. (2003) A reversible defect in natural killer T cell function characterizes the progression of premalignant to malignant multiple myeloma. J Exp Med 197(12):1667–1676.

[13] Emoto M, Kaufmann SH (2003) Liver NKT cells: an account of heterogeneity. Trends Immunol 24(7):368–369.

[14] Exley MA, Koziel MJ (2004) To be or not to be NKT: Natural Killer T Cells in the Liver. Hepatol 40(5):1033–1040.

[15] Fuji N, Ueda Y, Fujiwara H et al. (2000) Antitumor effect of α-galactosylceramide (KRN7000) on spontaneous hepatic metastases requires endogenous interleukin 12 in the liver. Clin Cancer Res 6(8):3380–3387.

[16] Fujii S, Shimizu K, Kronenberg M, Steinman RM (2002) Prolonged IFN-gamma-producing NKT response induced with alpha-galactosylceramide-loaded DCs. Nature Immunol 3:867–874.

[17] Fujii S, Shimizu K, Smith C et al. (2003) Activation of natural killer T cells by alpha-galactosylceramide rapidly induces the full maturation of dendritic cells in vivo and thereby acts as an adjuvant for combined CD4 and CD8 T cell immunity to a co-administered protein. J Exp Med 198(2):267–279.

[18] Giaccone G, Punt SJ, Ado Y et al. (2002) A phase I study of the natural killer T-cell ligand alpha-Galactosylceramide (KRN7000) in patients with solid tumors. Clin Cancer Res 8:3702–3709.

[19] Godfrey DI, Hammond KJ, Poulton LD et al. (2000) NKT cells: facts, functions and fallacies. Immunol Today 21:573–583.

[20] Godfrey DI, MacDonald HR, Kronenberg M et al. (2004) NKT cells: what's in a name? Nature Rev Immunol 4(3):231–237.

[21] Godfrey DL, Kronenberg M (2004) Going both ways: Immune regulation via CD1dp-dependent NKT cells. Clin Invest 114:1379–1388.

[22] Golden-Mason L, O'Farrely C (2002) Having it all? Stem cells, haematopoiesis and lymphopoiesis in adult human liver. Immunol Cell Biol 80(1):45–51.

[23] Gonzalez-Aseguinolaza G, Van Kaer L, Bergmann CC et al. (2002) Natural killer T cell ligand alpha-galactosylceramide enhances protective immunity induced by malaria vaccines. J Exp Med 195(5):617–624.

[24] Hayakawa Y, Takeda H, Yagita H et al. (2001) Critical contribution of IFN-gamma and NK cells, but not perforin- mediated cytotoxicity, to anti-metastatic effect of alpha-galactosylceramide. Eur J Immunol 31(6): 1720–1727.

[25] Hayakawa Y, Godfrey DI, Smyth MJ (2004) Alpha-galactosylceramide: potential immunomodulatory activity and future application. Curr Med Chem 11(2):241–252.

[26] Hong SM, Scherer DC, Singh N et al. (1999) Lipid antigen presentation in the immune system: lessons learned from CD 1 d knockout mice. Immunol Rev 169(1):31–44.

[27] Ikeda H, Chamoto K, Tsuji T et al. (2004) The critical role of type-1 innate and acquired immunity in tumor immunotherapy. Cancer Sci 95(9):697–703.

[28] Kakimi K, Guidotti LG, Koezuka Y, Chisari FV (2000) Natural killer T cell activation inhibits hepatitis B virus replication in vivo. J Exp Med 192(7):921–930.

[29] Kasper HU, Drebber U, Zur Hausen A et al. (2003) Dominance of CD4+ alpha/beta T-cells and inferior role of innate immune reaction in the liver metastases. Anticancer Res 23(4): 3175–3181.

[30] Kawakami K, Kinjo Y, Uezu K et al. (2001) Monocyte chemoattractant protein-1-dependent increase of V alpha 14 NKT cells in lungs and their roles in Th1 response and host defense in cryptococcal infection. J Immunol (Baltimore, Md.: 1950) 167(11):6525–6532.

[31] Kawano T, Cui J, Koezuka Y et al. (1997) CD1d-restricted and TCR-mediated activation of Va14 NKT cells by glycosylceramides. Science 278(5343):1626–1629.

[32] Kawano T, Nakayama T, Kamada N et al. (1999) Antitumor cytotoxicity mediated by ligand-activated human V alpha24 NKT cells. Cancer Res 59:5102–5105.

[33] Kenna T, Mason LG, Porcelli SA et al. (2003) NKT cells from normal and tumor-bearing human liver are phenotypically and functionally distinct from murine NKT cells. J Immunol 166(11):6578–6584.

[34] Kenna T, O'Brien M, Hogan AE et al. (2007) CD1 expression and CD1-restricted T cell activity in normal and tumour-bearing human liver. Cancer Immunol Immunother 56(4): 563–572.

[35] Kitamura H, Iwakabe K, Yahata T et al. (1999) The natural killer T (NKT) cell ligand alpha-galactosylceramide demonstrates its immunopotentiating effect by inducing interleukin (IL)-12 production by dendritic cells and IL-12 receptor expression on NKT cells. J Exp Med 189(7):1121–1127.

[36] Kronenberg M (2005) Toward an understanding of NKT cell biology: progress and paradoxes. Annual rev Immunol 23:877–900.

[37] Kronenberg M, Gapin L (2002) The unconventional lifestyle of NKT cells. Nature Rev Immunol 2(8):557–568.

[38] Lebedinskaya OV, Kiselevsky MV, Lebedinskaya EA, Donenko FV (2006) Cytoimmunochemical characteristics of leukocyte infiltrates in different sites of murine liver with metastatic process. Curr Sci Technol 5:32–33.

[39] Lebedinskaya OV, Patlusova ES, Lebedinskaya EA, et al. (2006) Morphological characteristics and reaction of hepatic lymphoid tissue of patients with metastatic process and hepatitis B. Achiev Curr Nat Sci 5:52.

[40] Lebedinskaya OV, Patutko Yu I, Zabezhinsky DA et al. (2005) Morphological functional characteristics of natural killer T-cells (NKT) in patients with tumor-affected liver. Siberian Oncol J 3:24–31.

[41] Lucas M, Gadola S, Meier U et al. (2003) Frequency and phenotype of Circulating $V\alpha24/V\beta11$ double-positive natural killer cells during hepatitis C infection. J Virol 77(3): 2251–2257.

[42] Matsuda JL, Gapin L, Baron JL et al. (2003) Mouse V14i natural killer T cells are resistant to cytokine polarization *in vivo*. Proc Natl Acad Sci USA 100(14):8395–8400.

[43] Matsuda JL, Naidenko OV, Gapin L et al. (2000) Tracking the Response of Natural Killer T Cells to a Glycolipid Antigen Using CD1d Tetramers. J Exp Med 192(5):205–212.

[44] Metelitsa LS, Naidenko OV, Kant A et al. (2001) Human NKT cells mediate antitumor cytotoxicity directly by recognizing target cell CD1d with bound ligand or indirectly by producing IL-2 to activate NK cells. J Immunol 167: 3114–3122.

[45] Motohashi S, Kobayashi S, Ito T et al. (2002) Preserved IFN-alpha production of circulating V alpha 24 NKT cells in primary lung cancer patients. Int J Cancer 102(2):159–165.

[46] Nakagawa R, Nagafune I, Tazunoki Y et al. (2001) Mechanisms of the antimetastatic effect in the liver and of the hepatocyte injury induced by α-galactosylceramide in mice. J Immunol 166(11):6578–6584.

[47] Nieda M, Okai M, Tazbirkova A et al. (2004) Therapeutic activation of V{alpha}24 + V{beta}11+ NKT cells in human subjects results in highly coordinated secondary activation of acquired and innate immunity. Blood 103(2):383–389.

[48] Nishikawa H, Kato T, Tanida K et al. (2003) CD4 + CD25+ T cells responding to serologically defined autoantigens suppress antitumor immune responses. Proc Natl Acad Sci USA 100(19):10902–10906.

[49] Norris S, Doherty DG, Collins C et al. (1999) Natural T cells in the human liver: cytotoxic lymphocytes with dual T cell and natural killer cell phenotype and function are phenotypically heterogeous and include $V\alpha24$-$J\alpha Q$ and $\gamma\delta T$ cell receptor bearing cells. Human Immunol 60:20–31.

[50] Ostrand-Rosenberg S, Clements VK, Terabe M et al. (2002) Resistance to metastatic disease in STAT6-deficient mice requires hemopoietic and nonhemopoietic cells and is INF-gamma dependent. J Immunol 169: 5796–5804.

[51] Park SH, Kyin T, Bendelas A, Carnaud C (2003) The contribution of NKT cells, NK cells, and other gamma-chain-dependent non-T non-B cells to IL-12-mediated rejection of tumors. J Immunol 170(3):1197–1201.

[52] Paschenkov MV, Pinegin BV (2001) Major features of dendritic cells. Immunology 22:7–16.

[53] Pillai AB, George TI, Dutt S et al. (2007) Host NKT cells can prevent graft-versus-host disease and permit graft antitumor activity after bone marrow transplantation. J Immunol 178(10):6242–6251.

[54] Schmieg J, Yang G, Franck RW, Tsuji M (2003) Superior protection against malaria and melanoma metastases by a C-glycoside analogue of the natural killer T cell ligand

alpha-Galactosylceramide. J Exp Med 198(11): 1631–1641.

[55] Seino K, Motohashi S, Fujisawa T et al. (2006) Natural killer T cell-mediated antitumor immune responses and their clinical applications. Cancer Sci 97(9):807–812.

[56] Sidobre S, Naidenko OV, Sim BC et al. (2002) The V14 NKT Cell TCR Exhibits High-Affinity Binding to a Glycolipid/CD1d Complex. J Immunol 169:1340–1348.

[57] Singh AK, Yang JQ, Parekh VV et al. (2005) The natural killer T cell ligand alpha-galactosylceramide prevents or promotes pristane-induced lupus in mice. Eur J Immunol 35(4):1143–1154.

[58] Smiley ST, Lanthier PA, Couper KN et al. (2005) Exacerbated susceptibility to infection-stimulated immunopathology in CD1d-deficient mice. J Immunol 174(12):7904–7911.

[59] Smyth MJ, Thia KY, Street SE et al. (2000) Differential tumor surveillance by natural killer (NK) and NKT cells. J Exp Med 191(4):661–668.

[60] Smyth MJ, Godfrey DI (2000) NKT cells and tumor immunity–a double-edged sword. Nature Immunol 1:459–460.

[61] Smyth MJ, Crowe NY, Takeda K et al. (2002) NKT cells - conductors of tumor immunity? Curr Opin Immunol 14:165–171.

[62] Spadaro M, Curcio C, Varadhachary A et al. (2007) Requirement for IFN-gamma, CD8+ T lymphocytes, and NKT cells in talactoferrin-induced inhibition of neu+ tumors. Cancer Res 67(13):6425–6432.

[63] Stober D, Jomantaite I, Schirmbeck R, Peimann J (2003) NKT cells provide help for dendritic cell-dependent priming of MHC class I-restricted CD8+ T cells in vivo. J Immunol 170(5): 2540–2548.

[64] Su Z, Segura M, Morgan K et al. (2005) Impairment of protective immunity to blood-stage malaria by concurrent nematode infection. Inf and immunity 73(6):3531–3539.

[65] Swann JB, Coquet JM, Smyth MJ, Godfrey DI (2007) CD1-restricted T cells and tumor immunity. Curr Top Microbiol Immunol 314:293–323.

[66] Terabe M, Matsui S, Noben-Trauth N et al. (2000) NKT cell-mediated repression of tumor immunosurveillance by IL-13 and the IL-4R-STAT6 pathway. Nature immunol 1(6): 515–520.

[67] Trobonjaca Z, Leithauser F, Moller P et al. (2001) Activating immunity in the liver. I. Liver dendritic cells (but not hepatocytes) are potent activators of IFN-γ release by liver NKT cells. J Immunol 167(3):1413–1422.

[68] Trobonjaca Z, Kroger A, Stober D et al. (2002) Activating immunity in the liver. II. IFN-β attenuates NK cell-dependent liver injury triggered by liver NKT cell activation. J Immunol 168(8):3763–3770.

[69] Varma TK, Lin CY, Toliver-Kinsky TE et al. (2002) Endotoxin-induced gamma interferon production: contributing cell types and key regulatory factors. Clin Diagn Lab Immunol 9(3):530–554.

[70] Vershinina MYu, Khalturina EO, Donenko FV et al. (2004) Comparative functional and immunophenotype characteristics of lymphokine-activated killers (LAK), generated from natural killer T- (NKT) cells from patients with tumor-affected liver. Vestnik RAMS 12:32–36.

[71] Wilson SB, Delovitch TL (2003) Janus-like role of regulatory iNKT cells in autoimmune disease and tumour immunity. Nature Rev Immunol 3:211–222.

7. LAK immunotherapy in clinical studies

IRINA ZH. SHUBINA
NN Blokhin Russian Cancer Research Center RAMS
Laboratory of Cell Immunity
Moscow
Russia

LEV V. DEMIDOV
NN Blokhin Russian Cancer Research Center RAMS
Department of Biotherapy
Moscow
Russia

IRINA O. CHIKILEVA
NN Blokhin Russian Cancer Research Center RAMS
Laboratory of Cell Immunity
Moscow
Russia

OLGA V. LEBEDINSKAYA
EAVagner Perm Medical Academy
Department of Histology
Embryology and Cytology
Perm
Russia

MIKHAIL V. KISELEVSKY
NN Blokhin Russian Cancer Research Center RAMS
Laboratory of Cell Immunity
Moscow
Russia

Keywords: interleukin-2(IL-2), lymphokine-activated killers (LAK), adoptive immunotherapy

M.V. Kiselevsky (ed.), Atlas Effectors of Anti-tumor Immunity, 101–110.
© Springer Science+Business Media B.V. 2008

Abstract

Adoptive immunotherapy of cancer involving activated cells of the immune system has been used on a extended basis in clinical oncology. Randomized studies showed that the combination of IL-2 with LAKs was most effective as compared with the IL-2 therapy alone. Despite the fact that the immunotherapy basic research is focused on melanoma, renal cancer, colorectal cancer and lymphomas, there are published data related to an effective use of IL-2/LAK-therapy in patients with other localizations. Adminstration of IL-2 and LAKs for effusion forms of cancer led to clinical effects in 88–94% of cases. A maximum cytoreduction of tumor is an additional way to enhance the efficacy of immunotherapy; it ensures the establishment of maximum correlation between tumor cells and killers. A combination of methods for activation of specific and non-specific immunity should be regarded as the most promising trend in the development of anti-tumor biotherapy. A promising approach in immunotherapy involves simultaneous treatment with LAKs and DCs that can stimulate both innate and adaptive anti-tumor immunity.

Current chemotherapy schemes for cancer treatment often result in poor effectiveness, particularly in cases of so-called immuno-sensitive (melanoma, renal carcinoma, etc.) or chemo-resistant malignancies such as non-small cell lung cancer, gastric cancer and others [7, 9, 12]. Therefore a search for biotherapy methods that stimulate anti-tumor immunity may lead to the improvement of anticancer therapy. One of the biotherapy approaches involves adoptive transfer of lymphokine-activated killer (LAK) cells [6, 7, 11, 15, 23] and has been translated into clinical studies after a number of successful experimental results [15, 16, 17, 20]. Over the last few years, biotherapy has developed yet some other methods based on generating anti-tumor vaccines and antigen specific cytotoxic T-lymphocytes (CTL). However, the main problem for achieving higher effectiveness by these methods is lack or low expression of MHC I on tumor cells.

Although natural killers (NK) can recognize and lyse MHC I-negative tumor cells, this lymphocyte subpopulation is limited and insufficient to completely eliminate them [3, 9, 11]. *Ex vivo* generation of LAKs gives an opportunity to obtain a significant number of lymphoid cells with a high rate of NK-activity and then include them in adoptive immunotherapy techniques. Systemic administration of LAKs results in an average 10% clinical effect in cancer patients, which is apparently due to the adhesive function of activated T-cells in the parenchymal organs (lungs and liver) and inefficient LAK accumulation at the tumor site [8]. On the other hand, when locoregional administration was performed, in particular, in case of malignant effusions or ascitis, a higher rate of marked effect reached 77%–94% [12, 17, 21]. The results of several studies demonstrated that the efficiency of IL-2/LAK anti-metastatic immunotherapy correlates with the method of agent administration, i.e., intra-portal for liver metastases or systemic i.v. injection for lung metastases, as well as with the LAK numbers necessary to lyse tumor cells [12, 13].

Kimura et al. performed a randomized controlled clinical study of IL-2/LAK immunotherapy in adjuvant schemes combined with chemotherapy or radiotherapy on 174 lung carcinoma patients to assess 5- and 9-year survival rate. The results showed that the suggested scheme of adoptive immunotherapy with IL-2 and LAK cells improved the survival of patients after surgical resection of primary lung carcinoma [10]. Similar results were obtained in some other studies evaluating the effectiveness of adoptive locoregional immunotherapy in

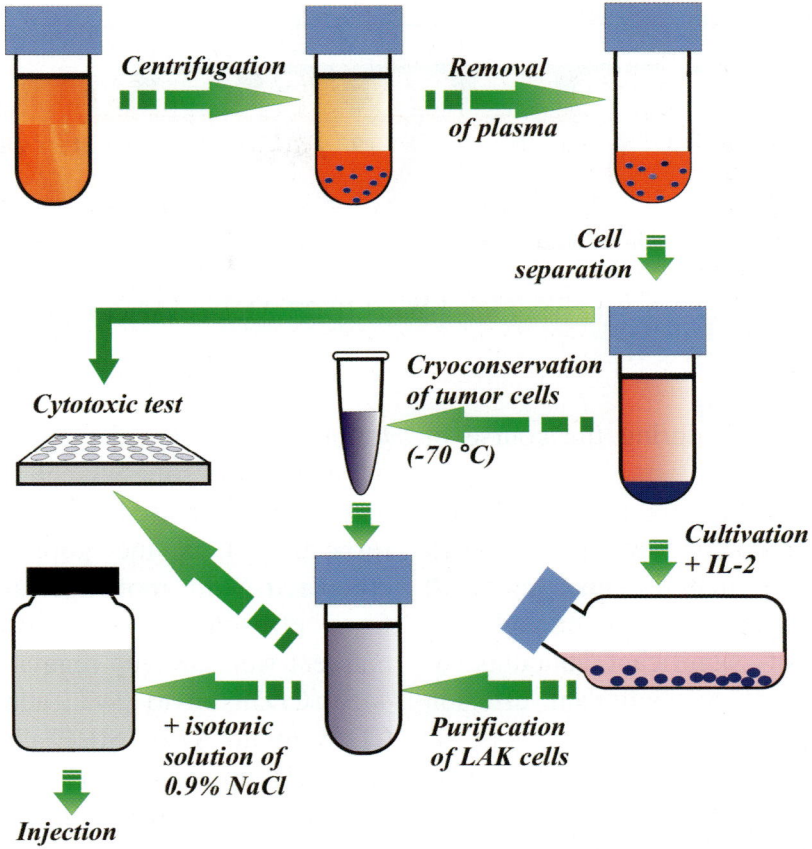

Figure 7.1. Scheme of *ex vivo* LAK generation

esophageal cancer patients [18, 19, 22] and in patients with recurrent glioblastoma [2].

A long-term clinical trial was performed at the Russian Cancer Research Center to study the effectiveness of IL-2/LAK immunotherapy for malignant effusions [1, 3, 4, 5, 6, 11].

The study involved 85 patients with malignant pleural effusions: 31 lung cancer (37%), 26 breast cancer (30%), 6 mesothelioma of pleura (7%) and 22 other cancer types (26%). Prior to immunotherapy, malignant pleural was evacuated and an appropriate catheter was installed and drainage of the cavity was performed for 2–3 weeks. The MNLs isolated from the effusion were used to generate LAKs *ex vivo* (Figure 7.1). All patients received 1–3 IL-2/LAK immunotherapy courses. Every course included 5–20 intrapleural injections of IL-2 in the dose of 0.5–1.0×10^6 IU and 2–8 injections of 50–100×10^6 LAK-cells. Each course continued for 2 weeks (Figure 7.2).

The clinical effectiveness of IL-2/LAK immunotherapy reached 88% with complete reduction of malignant effusion in 60 patients and partial reduction in 15 patients, which was registered by x-ray analysis (Figure 7.3). Moreover, x-ray analysis and CT-examination showed the absence of rough formations on the pleura after immunotherapy that had been common features of pleurodesis resulting from cytostatic or sclerosing agent effects.

Determining cell quantity and composition of malignant effusions is of great importance for validation of treatment efficacy

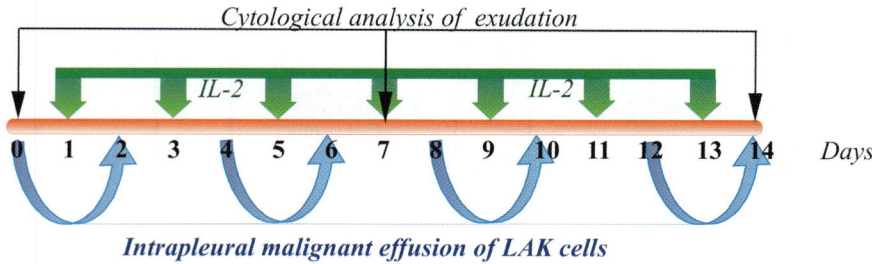

Figure 7.2. Scheme of intrapleural IL-2/LAK immunotherapy

and disease prognosis during the course of immunotherapy.

Pleural or peritoneal malignant effusions of cancer patients before treatment contain small numbers of mature (not activated) lymphocytes, which are not enough for effective lysis of significant amounts of tumor cells present in malignant effusion (Figure 7.4).

We observed the process of LAK generation *in vitro* from mononuclear cells separated from malignant effusions [14]. IL-2 activated the proliferation of lymphocytes (Figure 7.5). Our observations showed the formation of lymphoid elements at different stages of maturity, we registered single mitotic events. The quantity of large activated lymphocytes and prolymphocytes mounted.

Immunoblast-like cells appeared. The level of expression of NK-cell markers CD16 and CD56 increased (up to 30% and 47%, respectively) in the population of LAKs compared with mononuclear cells isolated from effusions. The following activation markers were also up-regulated: CD25 up to 44%, CD38 up to 24%, adhesion molecule CD58 up to 87%, MHC class II molecule HLA-DR up to 49% (Figure 7.6). Freshly isolated mononuclear cells almost completely lacked expression of all the markers (0–15%). By the end of the first week of immunotherapy, a lot of activated and immature lymphoid cells surrounding single degrading tumor cells were observed in patients' malignant effusions (Figure 7.7). By the end of the immunotherapy course

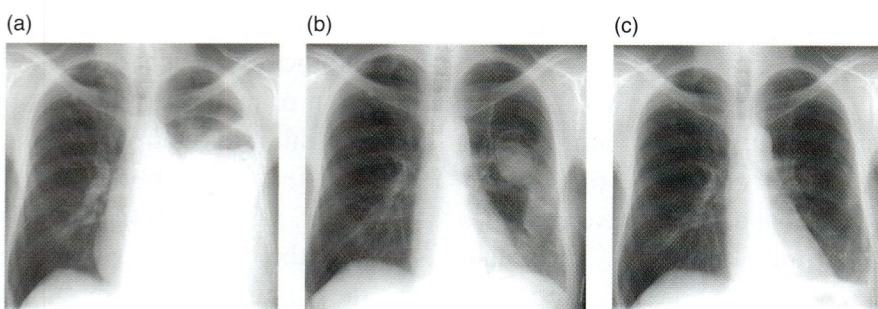

Figure 7.3. Images of x-ray examination of patient with malignant effusion
a – Prior to immunotherapy (malignant effusion in the left hemithorax); **b** – In the middle of immunotherapy (residual malignant effusion); **c** – After immunotherapy (complete regression of malignant effusion)

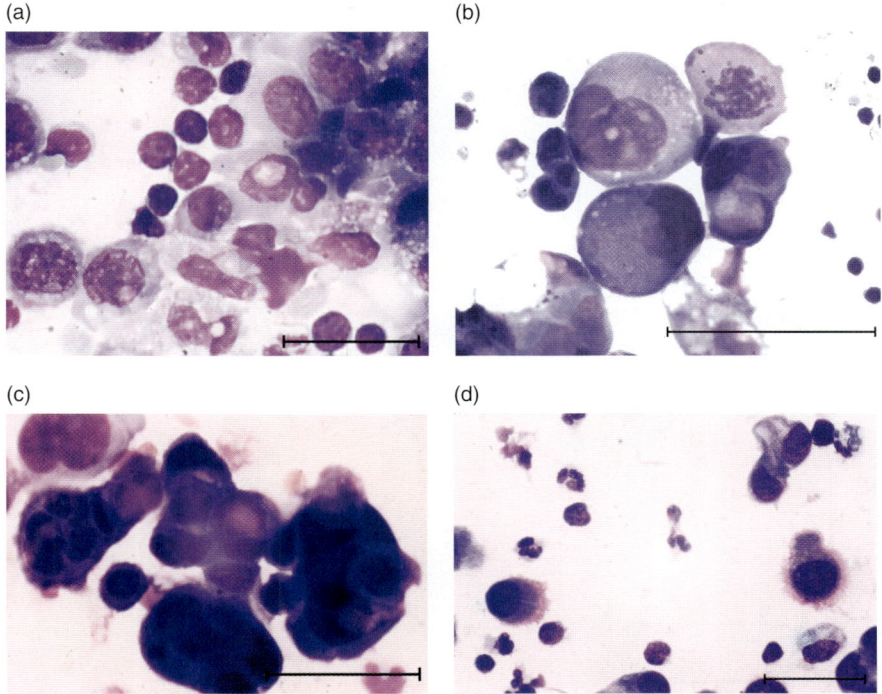

Figure 7.4. Cytological picture of malignant effusions of cancer patients prior to intrapleural IL-2/LAK immunotherapy Microphotographs of cytospins of effusions from patients with: **a** – Breast cancer; **b** – Non-small cell lung cancer; **c** – Mesothelioma of pleura; **d** – Ovarian cancer; stained with azur II-eosin

(14th day) we observed a practical absence of tumor cells (Figure 7.8). The remaining tumor cells were undergoing apoptotic death (Figure 7.9).

Complete or partial reduction of pleural effusion was achieved in those cases where morphological examination of the effusion showed a significant number of

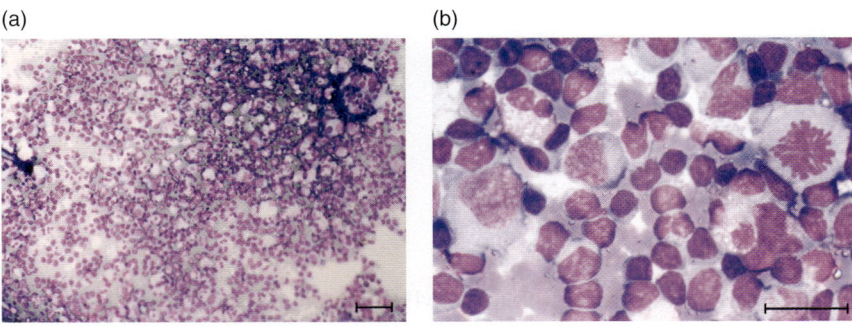

Figure 7.5. IL-2 activated mononuclear leukocytes of pleural effusion of a patient with breast cancer (incubation day 5) Microphotographs of LAK-cell cytospins generated from mononuclear leukocytes of a cancer patient's effusion; stained with azur II-eosin. **a** – Scale bar 40 μm; **b** – Scale bar 20 μm

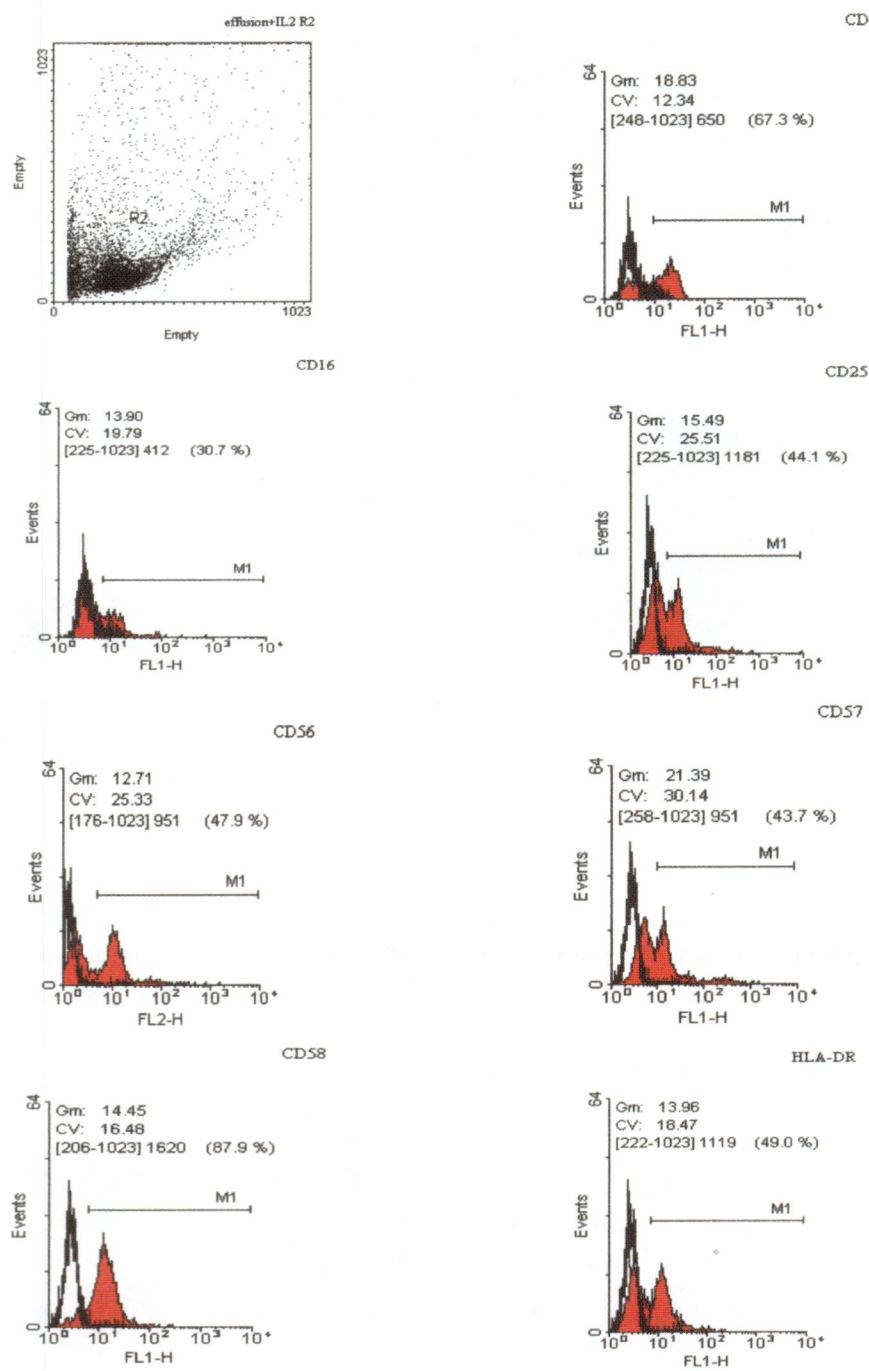

Figure 7.6. Expression of cell-surface antigens of MNLs isolated from malignant effusion of a patient with breast cancer and incubated in the presence of IL-2 (incubation day 3) Upper line: Dot-Plot of MNL in the selected region, histograms present: left peak cells stained with isotype control, right peak cell fluorescence after staining with monoclonal antibodies conjugated with FITC or R-PE. Y-axis – number of analyszed cells, x-axis – fluorescence intensity in relative units. CD — differentiation antigens (CD34, CD14, CD80, CD83, CD86,CD1a, CD11c)

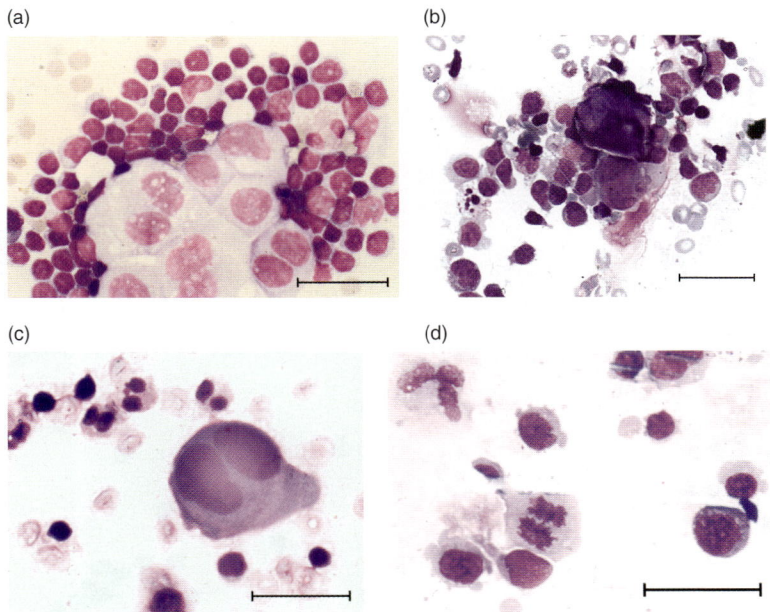

Figure 7.7. Cytological picture of malignant effusions of cancer patients in the middle of intrapleural IL-2/LAK immunotherapy (day 7) Microphotographs of cytospins of effusions from patients with: **a** – Breast cancer; **b** – Non-small cell lung cancer; **c** – Mesothelioma of pleura; **d** – Ovarian cancer; stained with azur II-eosin; **a** – Scale bar 20 μm

activated lymphoid immunoblast-like cells (Figures 7.6–7.8). In some cases, immunological pleurodesis was associated with the decreasing rate of tumor markers and reduction of size and density of metastatic lymph nodes. Elimination of pleural effusion was a necessary condition to successfully performing further radiation therapy (one patient) or chemotherapy (15 patients) and continue dynamic follow up examination for a period of 2 months to over 1 year *when the disease was characterized by other than effusion clinical symptoms*.

In case of concomitant pleural effusion and ascitis, a simultaneous drainage of pleural and the abdominal cavity was performed with daily elimination of malignant liquid followed by 1.0×10^6 IU IL-2 and 100×10^6 LAK-cells intrapleural and intraperitoneal injection. A 2-week immunotherapy course led to complete reduction of malignant effusion and ascitis in these patients.

Therefore, IL-2/LAK immunotherapy was shown to be an effective method of treatment for malignant effusions and those with concomitant ascitis. Intrapleural and intraperitoneal immunotherapy was well tolerated by cancer patients, even by those with severe disease conditions, who could not receive conventional anti-cancer therapy.

7.1. Beneficial Areas for IL-2/LAK Immunotherapy in Clinical Practice

So far, various approaches have been made to establish the most effective mode of

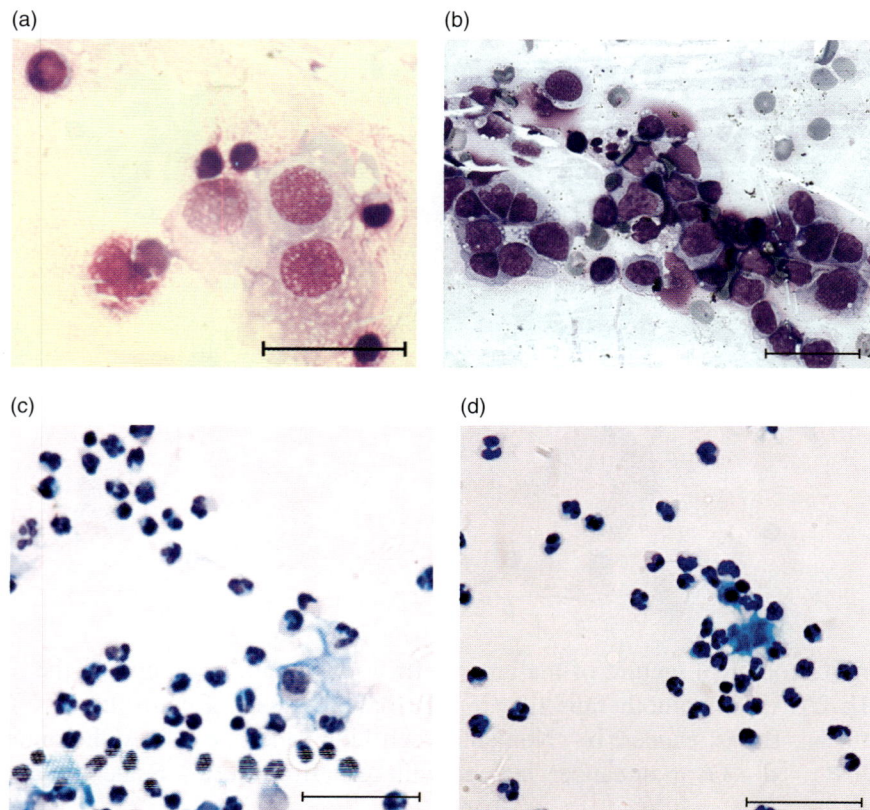

Figure 7.8. Cytological picture of malignant effusions of cancer patients at the end of intrapleural IL-2/LAK immunotherapy (day 14) Microphotographs of cytospins of effusions from patients with: **a** – Breast cancer; **b** – Non-small cell lung cancer; **c** – Mesothelioma of pleura; **d** – Ovarian cancer; stained with azur II-eosin; **a, b** – Scale bar 40 μm; **c, d** – Scale bar 50 μm

immunotherapy in cancer. The results of the studies suggest that enhanced effectiveness of IL-2/LAK immunotherapy may be achieved with locoregional or intrapleural or intraperitoneal administration of LAK-cells when cell concentration reaches its highest rate at the tumor site.

Another way for achieving the highest effective ratio between LAKs and tumor cells is performing maximal cytoreduction of malignant lesions. Therefore, IL-2/LAK immunotherapy can be effective for relapsed prophylactics after radical surgery. Such treatment should have a continuous course, including the whole period of possible recurrences.

The systemic method of LAK administration (considering the LAK special characteristics described above) can be effective for prophylactics and treatment of tumors and metastases in lungs only.

In addition, the efficiency of cell immunotherapy may be increased by including enriched a NK population and its subsequent activation in the presence of IL-2.

A promising approach in immunotherapy involves simultaneous treatment with LAKs and DCs, which can stimulate both innate and adaptive anti-tumor immunity.

(a)

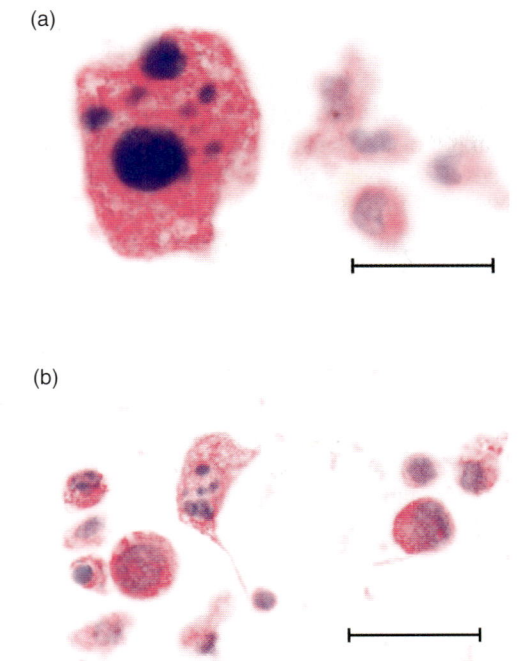

(b)

Figure 7.9. Cellular content of malignant pleural effusion of a patient with non-small cell lung cancer after completion of intrapleural IL-2/LAK immunotherapy (day 16) Microphotographs of tumor cells in apoptosis with surrounding macrophages and lymphocytes: **a** – Initial stage of apoptosis; **b** – Final stage of apoptosis – Stained with methyl green-pironin by Brachet Scale bar 20 μm

References

[1] Blymenberg AG, Kiselevski MV, Gorbunova VA et al. (2002) Immunotherapy IL-2/LAK for the treatment of platinum and taxman-resistant advanced. Int J Gynecol Cancer 12(5): OV070.

[2] Boiardi A, Silvani A, Ruffini P et al. (1994) Loco-regional immunotherapy with recombinant interleukin-2 and adherent lymphokine-activated killer cells (A-LAK) in recurrent glioblastoma patients. Cancer Immunol Immunother 39(3): 193–197.

[3] Chikileva IO, Khalturina EO, Kiselevsky MV (2003) Current approaches and trends in immunotherapy and immuno-prophylactics of cancer. Mol Med 2: 40–50.

[4] Davydov MI, Normantovich VA, Polotsky BE et al. (1996) Adoptive immuno-lympho-chemotherapy of non-small cell lung cancer. Vestnik AMN 3: 3–9.

[5] Davydov MI, Normantovich VA, Kiselevsky MV et al. (2000) Adoptive immunotherapy in malignant effusions: clinical and laboratory study. Russian Oncol J 6: 14–17.

[6] Davydov MI, Normantovich VA (2003) New approaches to combined anti-cancer treatment. Moscow, Publisher Medicine: 211–223.

[7] Davydov MI, Aksel EM (2006) Statistics of cancer in Russia and CIS countries in 2004. Vtstnic RCCR 17(3 Suppl 1): 1–132.

[8] Goldfarb RH, Brunson KW (2002) Antimetastatic therapy. Biologic Therapy of Cancer Vincent T. DeVita Jr., Samuel Hellman, Ateven A. Rosenberg (eds) Moscow, Publisher Medicine: 878–887.

[9] Hishii M, Andrews D, Boyle L A et al. (1997) *In vivo* accumulation of the same anti-melanoma T cell clone in two different metastatic sites. Proc Natl Acad Sci 94(4): 1378–1383.

[10] Kimura H, Yamaguchi Y (1997) A phase III randomized study of interleukin-2 lymphokine-activated killer cell immunotherapy combined with chemotherapy or radiotherapy after curative or noncurative resection of primary lung carcinoma. Cancer 80(1): 42–49.

[11] Kiselevsky MV (2003) Adoptive immunotherapy in cancer. Vestnik RAMS 1: 40–44.

[12] Kjaergaard J, Marianne E, Agger R et al. (2000) Biodistribution and tumor localization of lymphokine-activated killer T cells following different routes of administration into tumor-bearing animals. Cancer Immunol Immunother 48(10): 550–560.

[13] Kobari M, Egawa S, Shibuya K et al. (2000) Effect of intraportal adoptive immunotherapy on liver metastases after resection of pancreatic cancer. Br J Surg 87(1): 43–48.

[14] Muranski P, Boni A, Wrzesinski C, Citrin DE, Rosenberg SA et al. (2000) Increased intensity lymphodepletion and adoptive immunotherapy – how far can we go? Nat Clin Pract Oncol 3(12): 668–681.

[15] Porgador A, Mandelboim O, Restifo NP, Strominger JL (1997) Natural killer cell lines kill autologous β_2-microglobulin-deficient melanoma cells: implications for cancer immunotherapy. Proc Natl Acad Sci U S A 94(24): 13140–13145.

[16] Rosenberg SA (2002) Adoptive immunotherapy: clinical application. Biologic Therapy of Cancer Vincent T. DeVita Jr., Samuel Hellman,

Steven A. Rosenberg (eds) Moscow, Publisher Medicine.

[17] Savas B, Arslan G, Gelen T, Karpuzoglu G, Ozkaynak C (1999) Multidrug resistant malignant melanoma with intracranial metastasis responding to immunotherapy. Anticancer Res 9(5C): 4413–4420.

[18] Semino C, Martini L, Queirolo P, et al. (1999) Adoptive immunotherapy of advanced solid tumors: an eight year clinical experience. Anticancer Res 19(6C): 5645–5649.

[19] Toh U, Yamana H, Sueyoshi S et al. (2000) Locoregional cellular immunotherapy for patients with advanced esophageal cancer. Clin Cancer Res 6(12): 4663–4673.

[20] Topalian SL (2002) Adoptive cell therapy: preclinical studies. Biologic Therapy of Cancer

Vincent T. DeVita Jr., Samuel Hellman, Ateven A. Rosenberg (eds) Moscow, Publisher Medicine: 484–503.

[21] Tresoldi M, Chies G (1994) Intrapleural administration of interleukine-2 and LAK cells in locally advanced non-small-cell lung cancer. Tumori 80(3): 246–250.

[22] Ueda Y, Sonoyama T, Itoi H et al. (2000) Locoregional adoptive immunotherapy using LAK cells and IL-2 against liver metastases from digestive tract cancer. Gan To Kagaku Ryoho 27(12): 1962–1965.

[23] Yamaguchi Y, Ohshita A, Kawabuchi Y et al.(2003) Adoptive immunotherapy of cancer using activated autologous lymphocytes – current status and new strategies. Hum Cell 16(4): 183–189.

8. Major properties of dendritic cells and their actual and potential applications in cancer therapy and infectious disease prophylaxis

IRINA O. CHIKILEVA
NN Blokhin Russian Cancer Research Center RAMS,
Laboratory of Cell Immunity, Moscow, Russia

NATALIA YU. ANISIMOVA
NN Blokhin Russian Cancer Research Center RAMS,
Laboratory of Cell Immunity, Moscow, Russia

OLGA V. LEBEDINSKAYA
EAVagner Perm Medical Academy, Department of Histology,
Embryology and Cytology, Perm, Russia

MIKHAIL V. KISELEVSKY
NN Blokhin Russian Cancer Research Center RAMS, Laboratory of Cell Immunity,
Moscow, Russia

VYACHESLAV M. ABRAMOV
Institute of Immunological Engineering, Moscow Region, Russia

Keywords: dendritic cells, morphology, functions, Phenotype, Vaccines

Abstract

Dendritic cells are generally considered to be the most powerful and important among other antigen-presenting cells. Their major functions consist of capturing and processing different microbial antigens and the subsequent activation of naïve and resting memory antigen-specific T cells. There exist multiple dendritic cell subtypes expressing different sets of receptors, recognizing antigens and "danger signals" (lectins, receptors for constant fragments of antibodies, Toll-like receptors for conserved pathogen-associated molecular patterns and even natural killer receptors targeting virus-infected or tumour cells). Due to their variability and functional plasticity, dendritic cells are able to execute multiple functions including the initiation of immune reactions favourable for protection against different infectious agents or the induction of tolerance towards self-antigens and allergens. It is obvious that dendritic cell physiology should be considered in the design and production of new, more effective vaccines. Several methods of generation of dendritic cells *in vitro* were developed. Vaccines based on such dendritic cells were used successfully in mice to elicit protective T-cell immunity against pathogens and tumours. Their usefulness in the prevention and treatment of human infectious diseases and cancer is currently under investigation.

M.V. Kiselevsky (ed.), Atlas Effectors of Anti-tumor Immunity, 111–159.

Antigen presentation is a key process of adaptive immunity reactions. It is well known that any cells of mammalian organism are capable of presenting antigen to CD8$^+$ cytotoxic T lymphocytes (CTL) in the context of major histocompatibility complex class I (MHC-I) molecules. The effective induction of immune reactions requires the participation of so-called "professional" antigen-presenting cells (APCs) (B cells, macrophages and the most important among them – dendritic cells (DCs)). "Professional" APCs are capable of presenting antigen not only in the context of MHC-I but also in the context of MHC-II molecules to CD4$^+$ T-helper (Th) cells. Moreover, they express on their surface costimulatory molecules (B7-1 (CD80), B7-2 (CD86), CD40, etc.). The interaction of these molecules with the receptor for the costimulatory signal on the T-cell surface (CD28) is necessary, as well as the ligation of the T-cell receptor (TCR) with MHC-antigen complex, for the successful activation of T lymphocytes.

DCs are considered to be the most powerful "professional" APCs possessing a unique capability to prime naïve T cells and initiate primary immune reactions [10, 65, 80, 136]. DCs also interact directly with the B cells and lymphocytes of the innate immune system [133]. Activated DCs can directly induce B-cell proliferation, immunoglobulin isotype switching, plasma cell differentiation through the production of B-cell activation and survival molecules (BAFF (B-cell-activating factor belonging to the TNF family) and APRIL (a proliferation-inducing ligand)) and cytokines such as interleukin (IL)-6 and interferon (IFN)-α/β. DCs can also activate and induce the expansion of the resting natural killer (NK) cells through the cytokines secreted or cell-bound (IL-12,-15) and cell-contact-dependent mechanisms [53, 54].

8.1. Morphology and Functions of Dendritic Cells

Skin DCs (unusual cells with multiple membrane protrusions: "branches"/"den-drites") were first described by Langerhans in 1868 [88]. However, nothing was known for a long period of time about their actual functions. They were even supposed to be special skin nerve cells.

R. Steinman and Z. Cohn identified DCs in murine spleen in 1973 [172]. According to their observations, DCs adhered to the glass surface along with macrophages after a 0.5–1 hour incubation in a foetal calf serum (FCS) containing medium. They differed greatly from them, however. First of all, they possessed numerous membrane protrusions (pseudopodia and dendrites). The authors remarked on the variability of such protrusions, their motility and the rapid changes in their form. Most pseudopodia were long, uniform in width and had blunt terminations but smaller spine-like processes were also evident. The cell shapes ranged from bipolar elongated cells to elaborate stellate or dendritic ones. We also observed cells of variable peculiar shapes in our DC cultures (Figure 8.1). The DC nuclei were very large, contorted in shape and refractile [172]. Their cytoplasm contained numerous large circular mitochondria. The macrophages appeared to be much more static in comparison to the DCs.

In contrast to the macrophages DCs lacked active endocytosis [172]. Thus, the cell surface was not ruffled. The macrophages had a ruffled surface because of the active endocytosis. The DCs in contrast to the macrophages had few lysosomes and endosomes. However, immature DCs are capable to endocytize antigens (both by phagocytosis and pinocytosis) [65, 93, 109]. Steinman and Cohn probably observed the population of mature DCs with suppressed endocytosis. During maturation, DCs lose their ability for endocytosis and the processing of antigens [153]. According to our data, immature DCs actively phagocytized *Staphylococcus aureus* cells but they completely lost the ability after maturation during a 24 hour incubation in the presence of the tumour necrosis factor α (TNF-α) (Figure 8.2) [4].

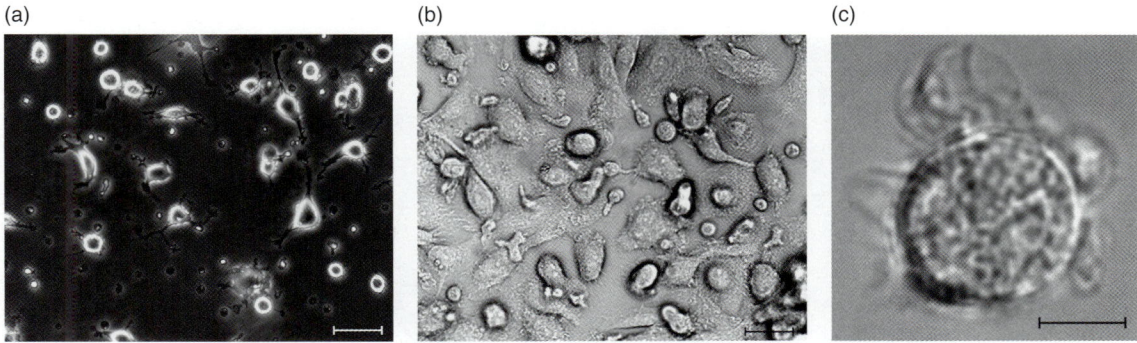

(a)　　　　　　(b)　　　　　　(c)

Figure 8.1. The morphology of human cultured monocyte-derived DCs. **a** Phase-contrast micrograph in dark field of floating immature DCs. (Original magnification (OM) × 400). **b** Phase-contrast micrograph in bright field of adherent immature DCs, OM × 400. **c** Phase-contrast micrograph in bright field of floating mature DCs, OM × 400 Scale bar: a, b − 20 μm; c − 5 μm

However, mature DCs have recently been shown to restart endocytosis under the action of constitutive lymph node chemokines CC-ligand (CCL)19 and CCL21, which bind CC-receptor (CCR)7 expressed exclusively by mature DCs [200].

R. Steinman and Z. Cohn also identified DCs in lymph nodes and Peyer's patches [172]. They found cells similar in outline to DCs in thymus but their mitochondria were rod-like in shape. The authors also noticed features of active endocytosis (membrane ruffles, lysosomes, etc.) and considered that the cells were not DCs but rather macrophages [172]. They concluded that DCs were absent in thymus. It is well known however, that there is a specialized population of thymus DCs which participates in the negative selection of T cells [6, 65]. It clearly shows that the morphological criterion is not sufficient for a precise DC definition.

For a better illustration let us compare the electron micrographs of monocyte-derived immature human DCs and macrophages obtained in our laboratory. In contrast to the spleen DCs identified by Steinman R. M. & Z. A. Cohn [172] most of the immature monocyte-derived DCs are a rounded shape, but not elongated cells (Figures 8.3 and 8.4a). They have long and thin membrane

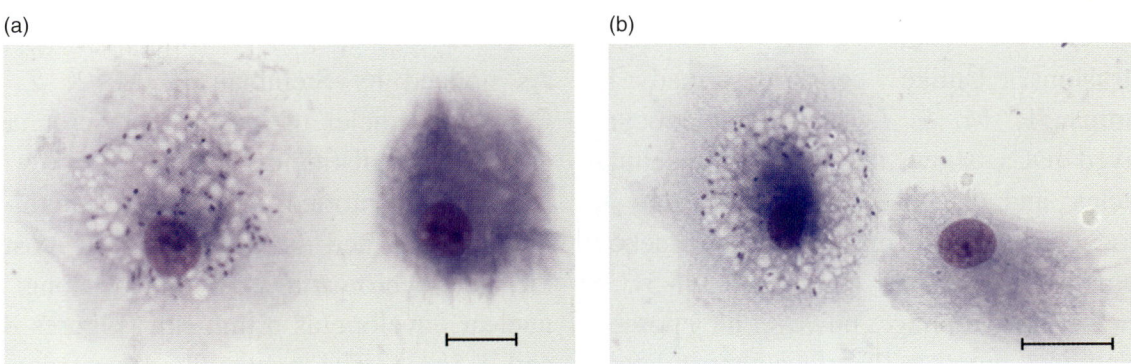

(a)　　　　　　(b)

Figure 8.2. Phagocytosis of *S. aureus* cells by immature (left) and mature (right) DCs. Micrographs of DCs phagocytizing *S. aureus* during a 1.5 hour coincubation. DC maturation was achieved with a 24 hour incubation in the presence of TNF-α (20 ng/ml). (Romanovsky-Giemsa azure-eosin staining, OM × 900 Scale bar: 5 μm)

(a)   (b)

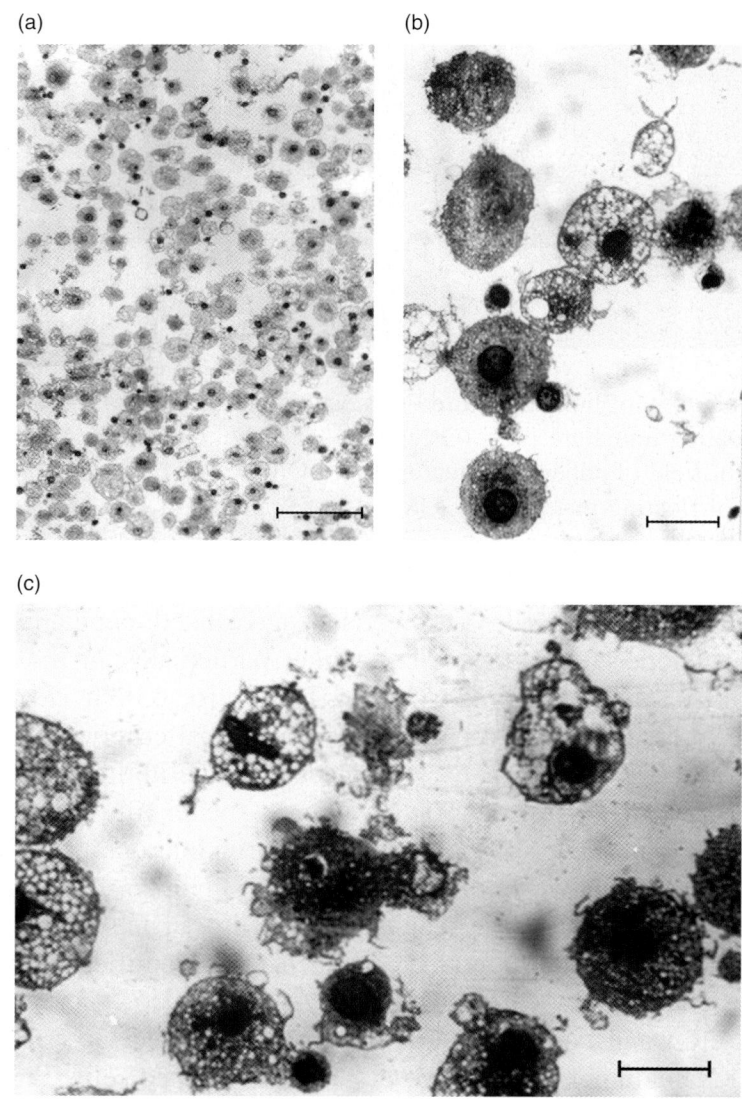

(c)

Figure 8.3. Micrographs of ultrathin sections of human monocyte-derived DCs. **a** OM × 100, **b** and **c** OM × 900 Scale bar: a − 50; b,c − 10 μm

protrusions. Unlike cells described by Steinman R. M. & Z. A. Cohn monocyte-derived DCs show numerous intracellular vesicles and vacuoles, apparently due to endocytosis, which makes them somehow resemble macrophages (Figures 8.3–8.5). In contrast to macrophages however they possess a relatively smooth cell surface almost devoid of microprojections and surface lacunae (Figure 8.4a). The macrophage surface exhibits numerous lacunae and microvilli as a result of membrane ruffling (Figure 8.5a).

As noticed by Steinman R. M. & Z. A. Cohn, the nuclei of DCs and macrophages are almost indistinguishable [172]. They are large and contorted in shape. In both the macrophages and the dendritic cells most of the heterochromatin is arranged along the nuclear envelope as a thin rim (Figures 8.4a and 8.5a–c). The nucleolus, when seen, is small and contains typical fibrous and granular components [172]. However, the monocyte-derived DCs differ from the physiological spleen DCs by the more rounded shape of

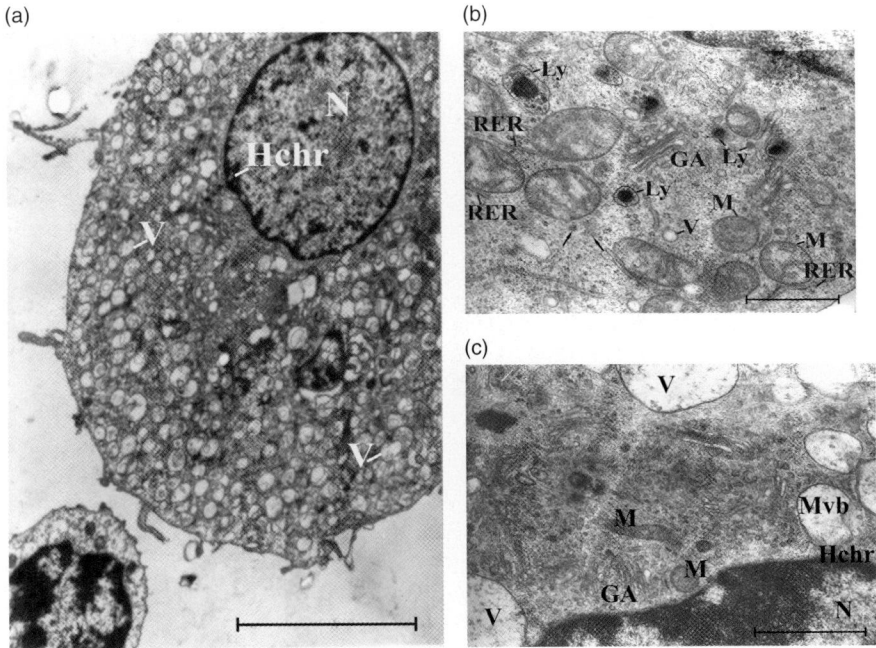

Figure 8.4. Electron micrographs of human monocyte-derived DCs sectioned in the plane of the adherent DC monolayer. Hchr – heterochromatin, N-nucleus, M-mitochondria, V-vesicles and vacuoles, RER-rough endoplasmic reticulum, GA-Golgi apparatus, Ly-lysosomes. Mvb-multivesicular bodies. Both free polysomes and membrane-bound (on the rough endoplasmic reticulum membrane) ribosomes are evident indicated by arrows on the figure **b**. **a** × 2000, **b** and **c** × 5000 Scale bar: a– 5; b,c −1 μm

the nucleus and its lateral position which is closer to one side of the membrane (Figures 8.4a and 8.5a). The cytoplasm of DCs contains large round-shaped mitochondria with well-developed cristae (Figure 8.4b–c). In macrophages, mitochondria are numerous as in the DCs but their diameters are small and the cristae less well developed when compared with the DCs [172]. Short slips of rough endoplasmic reticulum are present in DCs, generally in close association with the mitochondria (Figure 8.4b). Immature DCs also have a well developed Golgi apparatus, just as macrophages do (Figures 8.4b, c and 8.5a, c). Lysosomes (membrane-bound electron dense granules) are present in DCs, although less prominent than in macrophages (Figures 8.4b, c and 8.5a–c). Ribosomes are numerous in both cell types; they occur usually as attached to rough endoplasmic reticulum or as free polysomes scattered in cytoplasm (Figures 8.4b and 8.5c) [172]. Electron microscopy with higher magnification reveals different membrane microstructures on the DC surfaces (Figure 8.6). Most of them are villus-like structures (Figure 8.6a) but globular membrane protrusions are also detectable (Figure 8.6b). They potentially participate in endocytosis or intercellular contacts.

It should be stressed that DC morphology changes during their differentiation and depends on their functional condition [65]. For example, in blood DC precursors and immature DCs circulate, lacking prominent DC morphology [65]. They are much smaller, have large irregular-shaped nuclei and lack membrane protrusions. When they transit from the blood stream into tissues they become interstitial DCs and develop long membrane processes (branches). Langerhans cells (LCs) may be considered as a special

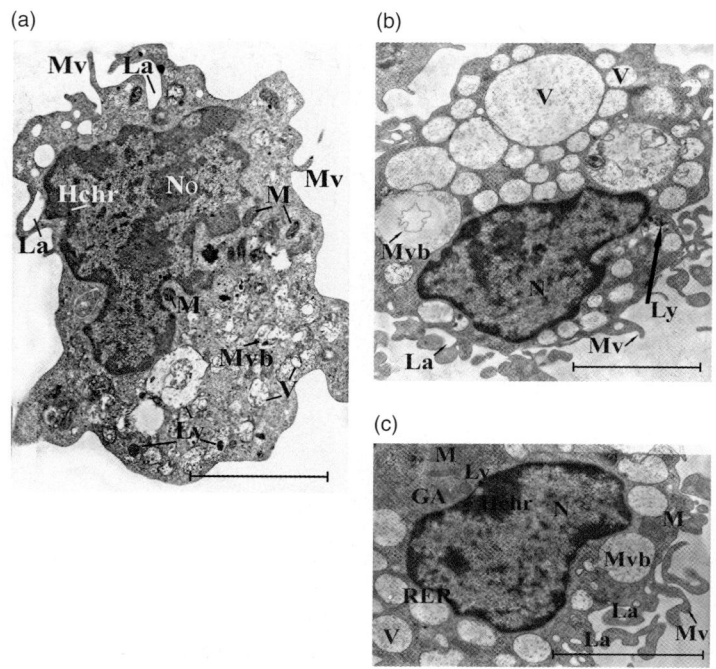

Figure 8.5. Electron micrographs of human macrophages sectioned in the plane of the adherent cell monolayer. Hchr – heterochromatin, N-nucleus, No-nucleolus, M-mitochondria, V-vesicles and vacuoles, RER-rough endoplasmic reticulum, GA-Golgi apparatus, Ly-lysosomes, La-lacunae, Mv- microvilli, Mvb-multivesicular bodies. Scale bar: 5 μm

epithelium-associated DC type although they probably have another origin than other interstitial DCs [65]. The interstitial DCs actively capture antigens and thus, they have prominent lysosomes and endosomes. Although they are poorly phagocytic cells compared with the macrophages [65].

In their next study R. Steinmann and M. D. Witmer purified a mouse spleen DC fraction on the basis of their low density and other properties differing from macrophages [173]. Just as macrophages, the DCs adhered to glass during a 0.5–1 hour incubation but in contrast to them they became floating cells after a

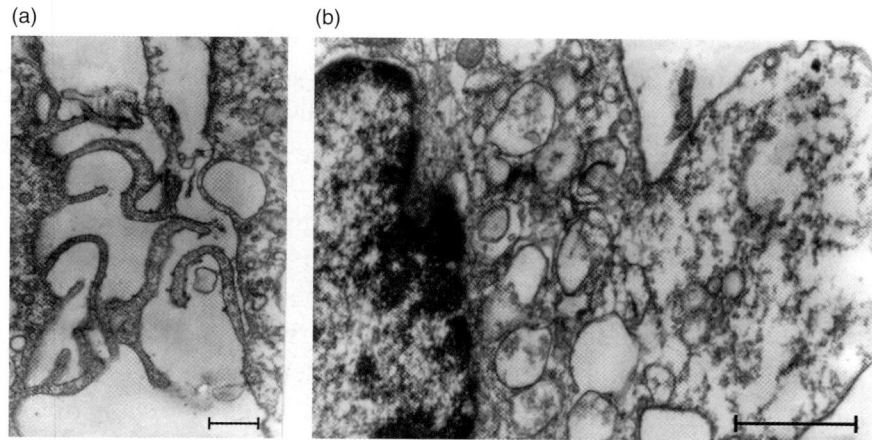

Figure 8.6. Electron micrographs of different structures formed by cytoplasmic membrane of DCs. Scale bar: 1 μm

night's cultivation. The remaining contaminating macrophages were removed using their capability to rosette sheep erythrocytes opsonized with antibodies [173].

The investigators found DCs to be the major stimulating cell type in the allogeneic mixed leukocyte reaction (allo-MLR) [173]. The authors concluded that DCs were at least 100 times more effective in stimulating cells than other major APCs (B-lymphocytes and macrophages). Subsequent studies revealed their potency to stimulate autologous T-lymphocytes in antigen-specific systems [75]. It should be stressed, however, that mature and immature DCs differ in their capabilities to present antigens and to stimulate lymphocyte proliferation [65]. It is mainly caused by the increase of MHC and costimulation molecule expression on the surface of mature DCs. It makes them better T-cell stimulators.

The functional criterion of DC definition is considered as the most important even today. For example, plasmacytoid DCs (pDCs) do not resemble, in their morphology, conventional DCs at all [107]. They have plasma cell features but they do actively present antigens when activated. Thus, there is not a clear morphological DC criterion. We do have a functional criterion but it is not enough for DC identification and definition because there are other APC types. Activated B-cells may be as effective or even better T-cell stimulators in allo-MLR than DCs [65, 112]. Moreover, immature DCs are poor APCs compared with mature ones. It makes the functional criterion insufficient.

Numerous scientific studies lead to the following concept of immature and mature DC functions [65]. Immature DCs are sentinels localized in tissues. They capture antigens of pathogenic microbes and viruses and process them. DCs sense pathogens using a set of Toll-like receptors (TLRs) binding conserved pathogen-associated molecular patterns (PAMPs). After antigen capture and subsequent processing they begin to mature. They lose their ability to capture and process antigens but increase MHC and costimulation molecule expression. DC maturation is induced by numerous bacterial and viral factors (components of bacterial cell wall, viral RNA, etc.) and also by pro-inflammatory cytokines produced in response to pathogens. Maturing DCs migrate from tissues into the afferent lymph where they become migrating veiled cells [65]. Initial DC-T-cell interactions in lymph nodes are mediated by adhesion molecules and semaphorins such as neuropilin-1 [133]. The spontaneous clustering of DCs with T lymphocytes may be observed during culture in vitro at 37°C (Figure 8.7). The initial interactions are followed by an engagement of the TCR by MHC-peptide complexes (signal 1) and the interaction of CD28 with CD80 and CD86 (B7-1 and B7-2) (signal 2). Both signals are necessary for the effective initiation and sustaining of T-cell immunity. Additional molecules are then up-regulated on both cell types that determine the nature of the ensuing T-cell response. Up-regulated molecules include semaphorins such as SEM4-A and members of the B7, CD28, TNF (4-1BBL, OX40L, CD40L, etc.) and TNFR (4-1BB, OX40, CD40, etc.) families of costimulatory molecules [133]. The interaction of DCs with T cells (mainly through the binding of CD40 to CD40L on the T-cell surface) leads to a full maturation of DCs. They become interdigitating DCs within draining lymph nodes. The survival and proliferation signals are also provided to activated T cells through costimulatory molecules such as OX40 and 4-1BB, which are cross-linked by ligands expressed on activated DCs (OX40L and 4-1BBL) [60, 133].

Interdigitating DCs are also found in tonsils and spleen white pulp. They have a prominent dendritic morphology with multiple long membrane protrusions like immature interstitial DCs but lose the capability for

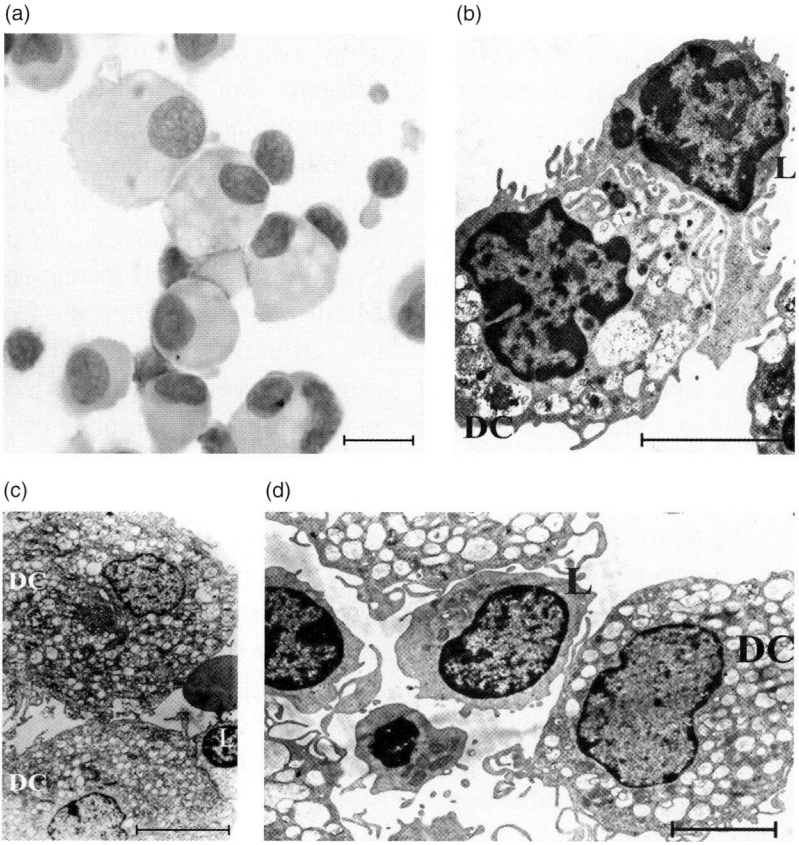

Figure 8.7. Spontaneous clustering of T cells with human monocyte-derived DCs during co-cultures *in vitro*. **a** Romanovsky-Giemsa azure-eosin staining, OMx900. **b-d** Electron micrographs of human sectioned cells. DC-dendritic cells, L-lymphocytes. Scale bar: a,b,d – 10; *c*-5 μm

endocytosis and thus, they reduce their lysosomal-endosomal compartment [65].

Mature DCs stably express MHC-peptide complexes on their surface [23]. In addition to increased costimulation molecule levels, they also express CD83 marker. CD83 is an immunoglobulin-like lectin receptor used for DC interactions with monocytes and some activated CD8$^+$ T lymphocytes [161]. It is necessary for the activation of CTLs by DCs [162]. Mature DCs express certain adhesion molecules such as CD54, providing effective interactions with T-cells, and chemokine receptors (CCR7) for constitutive lymph node chemokines which is necessary for their migration to the lymph nodes [154]. Only mature DCs secrete enough cytokines and chemokines, inducing T-cell chemotaxis and activation (fms-like tyrosine kinase-3 ligand (FLT3L), granulocyte-colony-stimulating factor (G-CSF), IL-1α, -1β, -2, -12, -6, CCL-2, -3, -4, -5, -17, -22 and macrophage inflammatory protein (MIP)-2) [26]. DCs can direct the fate of naïve CD4$^+$ T cells depending on the type of DC maturation stimulus (Figure 8.8) [133]. Following priming, CD4$^+$ T cells may differentiate towards the Th1 cells, which produce IFN-γ and support CD8$^+$ CTL responses or towards Th2 cells which secrete IL-4, -5, and -13, support humoral immunity and down-regulate Th1 responses. The direction of the Th polarization is determined by cytokines secreted by the stimulating DCs. The secreted cytokine profile of the DCs depends largely on the type of maturation

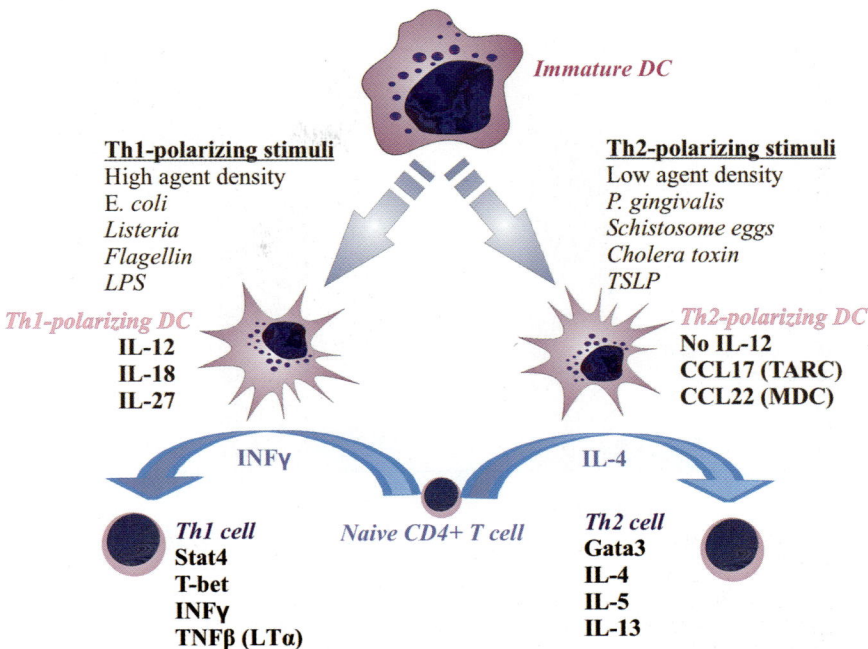

Figure 8.8. DCs direct Th polarization depending on the type of maturation stimuli. Abbreviations not mentioned in the text: MDC-macrophage-derived chemokine, TSLP – thymic stromal lymphopoietin and LTα – lymphotoxin α.

inducer (Figure 8.8). IL-12 is a key Th1-polarizing cytokine (Figure 8.8). DCs secrete biologically active IL-12p70 in response to the Th1-polarizing stimuli such as bacterial lipopolysaccharide (LPS) or flagellin [133]. According to our data (Figure 8.9) and studies by other groups, DCs that mature in the presence of bacterial LPS secrete much more pro-inflammatory cytokines (IL-1β, -6,-12, IFN-γ and TNF-α) than immature DCs [3, 190]. We have also shown that IL-2 and IL-10 levels do not change significantly during DC maturation but IL-4 production by mature DCs is lower than that of immature DCs (Figure 8.9). A monocyte-conditioned medium or cytokine combinations mimicking it – TNF-α and prostaglandin E2 (PGE2) which are generally applied to activate DC maturation, are not able to induce bioactive IL-12p70 secretion in contrast to that of LPS and other bacterial products [49, 69]. The Th1 differentiation programme is mediated largely by the transcription factors signal transducer and activator of transcription 4 (STAT4) and T-bet [133]. Th1 polarization can also be induced in the absence of IL-12p70 by mechanisms that are not entirely known but may be due in part to IL-12-related cytokines such as IL-27. Other DC maturation stimuli such as cholera toxin or schistosome eggs, can differentiate DCs that do not produce IL-12p70 and, in the presence of IL-4, induce naïve CD4$^+$ T cells to differentiate into IL-4-secreting Th2 cells [133]. It is not clear whether Th2 polarization is induced by specific DC cytokines or rather a default programme carried out in the absence of the Th1 polarization signal from the DCs. However, DC secretion of chemokines such as thymus and activation-regulated chemokine (TARC) and MDC can act to stimulate a Th2 response by preferentially attracting Th2 cells (Figure 8.8). The Th2 programme in CD4$^+$ T cells is dependent on transcription factors GATA-3 and c-Maf [133].

Recent studies have shown that the actual situation is much more complicated. The immature DCs, besides their sentinel

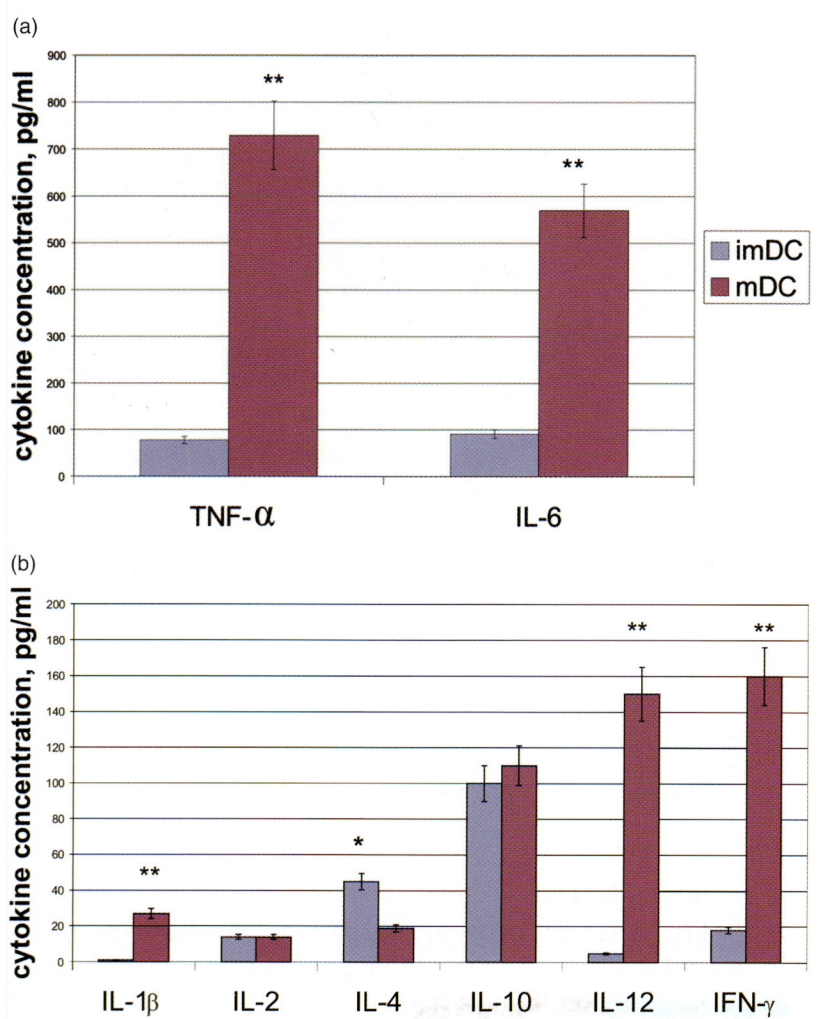

Figure 8.9. Secretion of cytokines by immature DCs (imDC) and DCs matured with bacterial LPS (mDC). **a** Levels of TNF-α and IL-6, **b** Levels of IL-1β, -2, -4, -12 and IFN-γ.
* $p < 0.05$; $^{**}p < 0.001$

functions (antigen capture and processing), fulfil other tasks. In the steady state most of the lymphoid organ DCs (in lymph nodes, spleen and thymus) are immature and capable to endocytize antigens and subsequently mature under appropriate stimuli [191]. Immature DCs constantly present MHC-self-peptide complexes on their surface but this presentation is only transient and they are rapidly degraded [192]. The major anti-inflammatory cytokine IL-10 suppresses DC maturation [190]. It is mainly secreted by monocytes, macrophages, certain T-regulatory (Treg) cells and DCs themselves

[33, 190]. When immature DCs encounter TLR ligands (such as LPS or other PAMPs) the transcription factor NF-κB is released and translocated to the nucleus where it activates gene transcription (Figure 8.10a). The MHC and costimulatory molecule (CD80, CD86) expression on the DC surface is up-regulated. DCs secrete pro-inflammatory cytokines and the soluble form of inhibitory immunoglobulin-like transcript 4 (sILT4) (Figure 8.10a). Autocrine cytokines as well as cytokines secreted by macrophages sensing microbes through interactions with their own TLRs synergistically act to stimulate DC

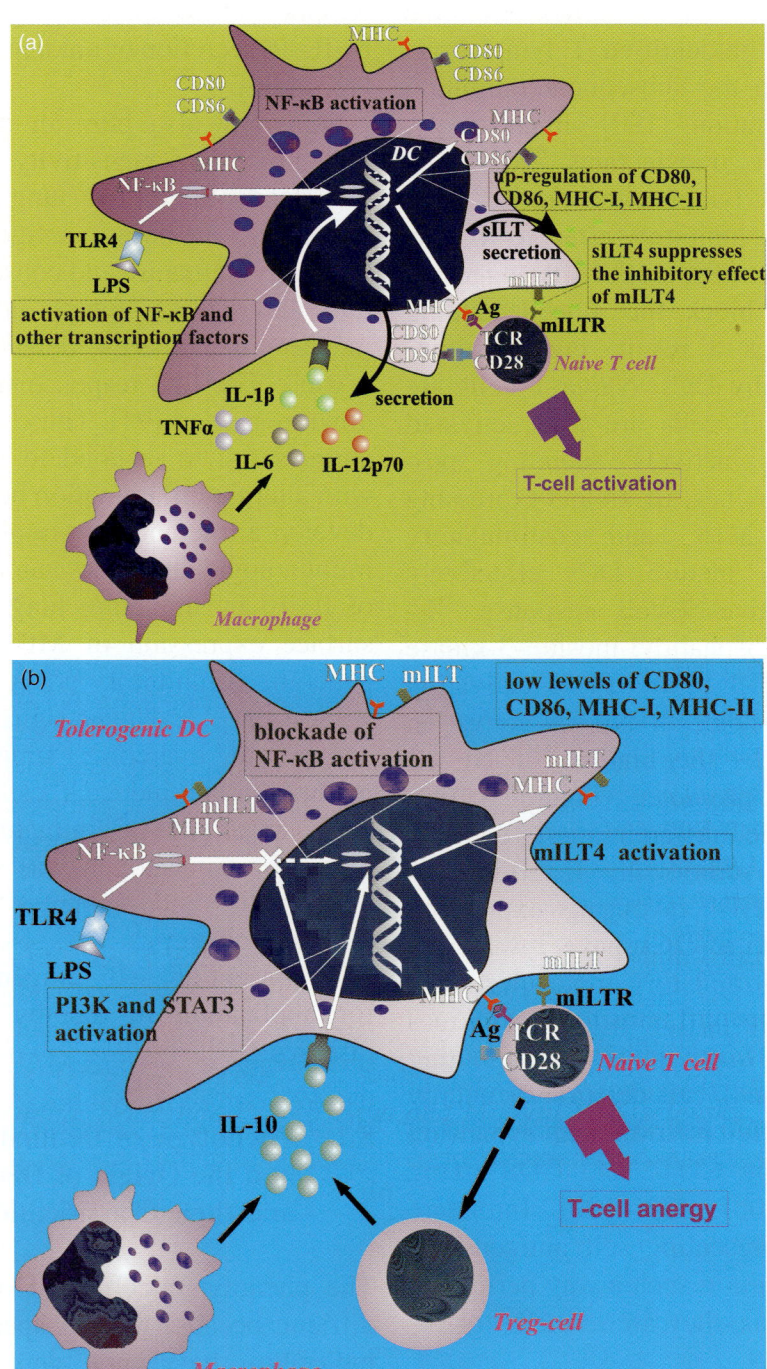

Figure 8.10. Differential effects of mature versus immature and/or IL-10-treated DCs on the T-cell immune response. **a** Mature DCs efficiently induce and sustain T-cell immunity. **b** Immature and/or IL-10 treated DCs down-regulate immune reactions by inducing development of Treg cells or causing anergy. mILT means membrane bound form of ILT4 and other members of the protein family (such as ILT3). mILTR is unidentified receptor molecule(s) on the T-cell surface recognizing ILT

maturation (Figure 8.10a). The interaction of membrane bound ILT4 (mILT4) on the DC surface with unidentified T lymphocyte receptors leads to the subsequent inhibition of T-cell proliferation [190]. Interestingly, murine fibroblast transfectants expressing ILT4 induced T lymphocyte proliferation, suggesting that the inhibitory effect of ILT4 is in fact DC-specific [190]. sILT4 is suggested to competitively block the T cell binding of mILT4 and as a result, favour stimulation of T cells by DCs. Naïve T cells are primed; memory T cells are also activated by mature DCs actively secreting pro-inflammatory cytokines, sILT4 and expressing high levels of MHC and costimulatory molecules. Thus, mature DCs effectively induce an adaptive T-cell response. IL-10 stimulates phosphatidyl-inositol-3-kinase (PI3K) and STAT3 [190]. PI3K activation results in the blockade of NF-κB activation and STAT3 blocks the binding of NF-κB to the IL12p40 promoter (Figure 8.10b). Consequently, the differentiation of Th1 cells is inhibited. Additionally, IL-10 inhibits production of sILT4 favouring expression of mILT4. Immature DCs have low levels of MHC and costimulatory molecules, they do not secrete pro-inflammatory cytokines (Figure 8.10 b). Immature DCs presenting self antigens cause T cell deletion or anergy or induce the differentiation and expansion of IL-10-producing $CD4^+$ and $CD8^+$ Treg cells (Figure 8.10b) [133, 190]. Immature DCs constantly presenting self antigens are believed to maintain in such a way peripheral self tolerance. Thus, they are termed "tolerogenic" DCs.

There are other factors that induce and/or maintain tolerogenic DC phenotype [133, 190]. Besides IL-10, other modulating factors such as transforming growth factor (TGF)-β, vitamin D3 and corticosteroids may render DCs tolerogenic. Treg cells are also capable to cause differentiation of tolerogenic DCs, either through engagement of CD86 and CD80 costimulatory molecules with the cytotoxic T-lymphocyte-associated antigen 4 (CTLA-4) or by IL-10 secretion or unidentified mechanisms [133, 190].

DCs may also play an important role in preventing hypersensitivity to allergens. In the steady state, the lung DCs constantly encounter air-borne antigens but remain relatively immature and constitutively migrate into the regional lymph nodes where they induce either anergy, deletion of T cells or a weak Th2-like response that is eventually down-regulated [94]. Thus, most humans and animals fail to respond to inhaled allergens with allergic inflammation because they either develop a tolerance or simply fail to respond immunologically. The autocrine production of IL-10 by immature lung DCs can inhibit surface expression of MHC-II and exert a generalized inhibitory effect on T-cell proliferation [94]. A danger signal must be strong enough to overcome suppression of DC maturation and induce T-cell response.

An injection of immature DCs pulsed with a certain antigen was shown to induce Treg cells and suppress antigen-specific immune responses [18, 44, 45]. Immature DCs presenting self antigens are suggested for application in therapy of autoimmune diseases [18].

8.2. Phenotype of Dendritic Cells and the Origin of Dendritic Cells and their Classification

The phenotypic definition of DCs is rather difficult because the DC-specific cell surface molecules have not yet been identified [65, 101]. DCs are usually defined as Lin^-MHCII^+-cells because they do not have cell surface lineage-specific antigens, which are expressed by B lymphocytes (CD19, CD20 and CD24), T lymphocytes (CD3), and NK cells (CD16, CD56 and CD57). However, DCs and their precursors may have variable levels of the LPS receptor component CD14 (CD14$^{low/dim/high}$), which is considered to be specifically expressed by monocytes/macrophages (CD14^{high}) [34, 65, 180]. DCs constantly possess a high density of MHC-II molecules. There are several studies characterizing blood DC subtypes which carry CD16 (FcγRIII) – a cell surface antigen specific for NK cells, neutrophils and monocytes/macrophages [101, 159].

Immature blood DCs almost completely lack the costimulation molecules CD86 and CD80 but they may have low levels of CD40 [65]. LCs were shown to express CD40 and low levels of CD86, CD80. Upon their maturation DCs rapidly up-regulate the surface expression of MHC classes I and II as well as of costimulatory molecules [65]. Variable (high on activation) levels of costimulation molecules are detected on the cell surface of other APCs (B-cells, macrophages). Thus, costimulatory molecules expression is not suitable for DC definition. Another cell surface antigen associated with DC maturation is CD83 [65]. It should be stressed that CD83 expression is not restricted to mature DCs. The receptor was found on unidentified brain cells [161], some on activated B-cells [65] and on a specialized subtype of helper NK cells with the following phenotype CD83^{+}/CCR7^{+}/CD56^{+}/CD25^{+} [102]. The NK subtype migrates to the lymph nodes, responding to constitutive chemokines CCL19 and CCL21. Thus, CD83 marker expression is not sufficient for identification of the mature DCs in lymph nodes.

Today it is clear that DCs originate from bone marrow precursors [65]. However, there are numerous contradictory data concerning classification of whole DC-type and subtypes such as lymphoid or myeloid lineages [7]. This fact and the existence of multiple DC subtypes make their phenotypic definition even more complicated.

Interstitial DCs and LCs are traditionally considered as myeloid ones and indeed evidence generated by different experimental approaches supports the concept [94]. LCs differ from interstitial DCs by E-cadherin expression and by the presence of Birbeck's granules – unique intracellular organelles taking part in endocytosis [61, 94]. LCs also express CD1a molecules participating in non-peptide antigen presentation [74, 94, 113]. The CD1 surface protein family is related to MHC class I molecules. They also form complexes with β2-microglobulin but in contrast to MHC-I, they serve for the presentation of non-peptide antigens. TGF-β is required for LC differentiation. Other DC types can develop in the absence of TGF-β. CD1a is also expressed by thymocytes [149].

LCs capture antigens via a lectin-type receptor – langerin (CD207) [61, 113]. Langerin is localized on the cell surface as well as inside the cell in close association with Birbeck's granules. Interstitial DCs utilize another set of lectins for endocytosis: mannose macrophage receptor (MMR) (CD206) (also expressed by macrophages) and dendritic-cell-specific-intercellular-adhesion-molecule-grabbing-nonintegrin (DC-SIGN) (CD209) (expressed by macrophages as well) [61, 62, 113]. DEC-205 (CD205) lectin is expressed by both interstitial DCs and LCs and also by thymus epithelial cells [113].

The myeloid origin of these DC subtypes is proved by studies *in vitro* in which murine or human monocytes or intermediate myeloid precursors that retained the capacity to generate macrophages, gave rise to cells resembling interstitial DCs or LCs [7]. Precursors with the dual potential of differentiation either into DCs or macrophages were identified in mouse bone marrow [111]. Randolph G. J. et al. have demonstrated DC differentiation from monocytes capturing zymosan molecules in a model of transendothelial trafficking [143]. The model imitates monocyte migration from the tissues into the lymph nodes. Afterwards, *in vivo* differentiation of dermal CD11b^{+}, F4/80^{-} phagocytic cells (considered to be monocytes) into DCs upon migration to the lymph nodes has been reported [144]. At last, a recent study by Leon B. et al. undoubtedly proved monocytes to be immediate DC precursors *in vivo* [92]. They injected purified monocytes intravenously into irradiated mice and observed the regeneration of all spleen DC subtypes.

CD11c$^+$ myeloid blood DCs, which express myeloid cell-specific cell surface molecules such as CD13 and CD33, are supposed to be immediate precursors of tissue mDC [94]. Blood mDCs have monocytoid morphology. Analogous cells were identified in murine blood [130].

The major part of human blood mDCs (mDC1) strongly expresses CD11c (CD11c^{high}) and CD1c (blood dendritic cell antigen-(BDCA)-1) [46]. They also carry on their cell surface low levels of IL-3 receptor (R) (CD123), which is regarded as a prominent feature of plasmacytoid DCs (pDCs). mDC1s express myeloid antigens CD13, CD33, Fc-receptors (CD32, CD64 and FcεRI). Moreover, they have the following phenotypic characteristics: CD4$^+$, Lin (CD3, CD16, CD19, CD20, CD56)$^-$, CD2$^+$, CD45RO$^+$, CD141 (BDCA-3)^{low}, CD303 (BDCA-2)$^-$, CD304 (BDCA-4/neuropilin-1)$^-$. A small proportion of mDC1s expresses CD14 and CD11b. CD1c-antigen is also found on CD1a$^+$ DCs, generated *in vitro* from monocytes and CD34$^+$-precursors, LCs and on some of the small resting blood B lymphocytes [46]. mDC1s spontaneously mature upon one day's cultivation in the presence of IL-3 and begin to express the pDC-specific surface antigen CD304 (BDCA-4/neuropilin-1) [46].

The minor mDC population (mDC2) resembles mDC1s in their monocytoid morphology but differ in the phenotype [46]. They strongly express CD141 (BDCA-3). Besides, they are CD4$^+$, Lin (CD3, CD16, CD19, CD20, CD56)$^-$, CD11c^{dim}, CD45RO$^+$, CD123$^-$,

CD2$^-$, CD303 (BDCA-2)$^-$, CD304 (BDCA-4/neuropilin-1)$^-$. As with CD1c$^+$-mDC1s, they have myeloid cell surface antigens CD13 and CD33 but they lack Fc-receptors (CD32, CD64 and FcεRI). A low level of CD141 is detected on monocytes, pDCs and mDC1s. This antigen is absent on the surface of CD1a$^+$ DCs generated *in vitro* from monocytes and CD34$^+$-precurssors. It is interesting that the level of expression of the main "mDC2-specific" surface antigen CD141 significantly increases on the surface of mDC1s and pDCs upon their spontaneous maturation after one day's cultivation in the presence of IL-3 *in vitro* [46]. Thus, this surface antigen is not specific for mDC2.

Many studies support the concept of the dual (myeloid-lymphoid) origin of DCs [7, 94]. Thymic DCs participating in the negative selection of T lymphocytes are traditionally considered as lymphoid cells [6]. The earliest murine thymic precursors, namely CD4^{low}-cells, which generate T, B and NK cells but not myeloid cells were assayed for their capacity to generate DCs upon intrathymic transfer into irradiated mice [5, 195]. These experiments showed that CD4^{low}-precursors could reconstitute fully the thymic population of DCs expressing CD8α in mice and led to the concept of lymphoid DCs [5]. Equivalent results were obtained in studies using human early thymic precursors [36, 81, 103, 145] and lymphoid bone marrow precursors [58]. Wu L. et al. showed that CD4^{low}-precursors reconstitute CD8α$^+$ DCs but not CD8α$^-$ DCs upon intravenous injection into irradiated mice [196]. The data lead to the hypothesis that mouse CD8α$^+$ DCs were lymphoid cells and CD8α$^-$ DCs were myeloid ones. However, the hypothesis was not supported by further studies. First of all, CD4^{low}-precursors were demonstrated to generate both murine DC subpopulations (CD8α$^+$ and CD8α$^-$ DCs) [104, 197]. Other studies showed that CD8α$^+$ and CD8α$^-$ DCs could be derived from either myeloid (such as monocytes) or lymphoid precursors [92, 183]. Thus, the concept must be revised. CD8α expression is not enough for the precise definition of mouse DC lineages (myeloid or lymphoid).

pDCs have a particular place among other DCs [107]. In human blood there were identified pDC precursors (pre-pDCs) as immature CD11c⁻ cells [63]. Pre-pDCs express CD4 and lack TCR-α, -β, -γ and -δ chains and CD3. They do not have B-cell (CD19, CD21) and myeloid cell-specific (CD13, CD14, CD33) cell surface antigens. Pre-pDCs, purified from human blood, express CD303 (BDCA-2) and CD304 (BDCA-4/neuropilin-1) [46]. CD303 is a lectin molecule used for antigen capture [47]. pDCs completely lose the lectin from their surface upon spontaneous maturation after 2 days cultivation in the presence of IL-3 [46]. CD304 (BDCA-4/neuropilin-1) is also present on the surface of mature mDC1 (as mentioned earlier). This semaphorin is important in the initial DC-T-cell interactions in lymph nodes (as mentioned above). Furthermore, neuropilin-1 is a neuron receptor governing axon growth as well as a receptor of endothelial cells and some tumour cells for vascular endothelium growth factor [48]. CD304 is also expressed by follicular memory Th cells [48].

Pre-pDCs mature into potent APCs upon cultivation in the presence of IL-3 and CD40L [63]. They also mature and secrete large amounts of IFN-α/β in response to viral or bacterial infection [79].

pDCs were identified not only in blood but also in lymphoid tissues (lymph nodes, tonsils, spleen, thymus, bone marrow and Peyer's patches) [107]. They also accumulate in sites of inflammation.

pDCs have absolutely a different set of TLRs than mDCs. mDCs express TLR-1, -2,-3,-4,-5,-7 and -8 and pDCs have only TLR-7 and -9 [68, 85]. TLR-7 binds viral single-stranded RNA and TLR-9 interacts with microbial DNA containing non-methylated CpG-sequences [107]. Thus, they may respond and induce subsequent T-cell reactions in response to the different types of pathogens.

Pre-pDCs were also identified in murine blood [129]. At approximately the same time, several research groups found in murine spleen, lymph nodes and thymus cells (CD11c^{lo-int}, B220$^+$) analogous to human pDCs, which secreted IFN-α/β [8, 13, 124, 130]. B220 (Lyb-5, CD45, common leukocyte antigen) is a tyrosine phosphatase expressed by almost all types of leucocytes [149]. It is especially interesting that in contrast to human pDCs, mouse pDCs express low levels of the myeloid cell-specific cell surface antigen CD11c.

The origin of pDCs is unclear. In contrast to mDCs, they express high levels of IL-3R (CD123) and need IL-3 for their differentiation, not GM-CSF [62]. Moreover, thymic pre-pDCs express pre-TCR-α, which associates with pre-TCR-β to form pre-TCR [146]. The transfection of CD34$^+$CD38$^-$ precursors from foetal liver with inhibitors of DNA-binding (Id)-2 and Id-3 blocked their differentiation into pDCs, B and T lymphocytes but not into NK and myeloid cells [170].

However, there is experimental evidence supporting the concept of the myeloid origin of pDCs. DCs, which expressed high levels of IL3R, were obtained from CD34$^+$ precursors, caring M-CSF receptor [132].

Comeau M. R. et al. have shown recently that CD123^{bright} blood pDCs might be subdivided into subtypes, differing by their functional and phenotypic characteristics, more or less lymphoid or myeloid [32]. They suggest that pDCs is a population(s) of lymphoid cells undergoing conversion to myeloid lineage.

The identification of a new DC subtype possessing mDC as well as NK-cell features has made the DC story even more puzzling. The DC subtype has been characterized in mice by several independent laboratories

[24, 71, 141, 160, 178]. The authors term the cell type as CD11c$^+$ CD11b$^+$ NK cells [160] or NK-DCs [71, 141] or IFN-producing killer-DCs [24, 178]. However, it is very likely that they are all talking about the same cell type. The cells express myeloid markers (CD11c and CD11b), NK-cell surface antigens (NK1.1, Dx5, NKG2D, Ly49) as well as common leukocyte antigen B220 (CD45). This DC subtype was found in normal mouse spleen, liver, lymph nodes and thymus [141]. They infiltrate tumours, accounting for up to 20% of CD11c$^+$-cells [178]. NK-DCs are capable of lysing NK-sensitive tumour-cell lines both *in vitro* and *in vivo* [24, 141, 178]. Depending on the stimulus applied (different types of CpG-oligonucleotides), they secrete significant levels of IFN-α/β, IL-12 and IFN-γ (through the autocrine action of IL-12) [24, 141]. Actually, they secrete more IFN-γ than typical NK cells [141, 178]. Tumour cell lysis depends on TRAIL-molecule (TNF-related apoptosis-inducing ligand) expression by NK-DCs [178]. After tumour cell lysis NK-DCs up-regulate MHC-II and costimulation molecules on their surface and become active APCs [24, 141]. NK1.1$^+$ CD11c$^+$B220$^+$ NK-DCs are capable of presenting *in vivo* antigen (ovalbumin peptide) even better than common spleen NK1.1$^-$ CD11c$^+$B220$^-$ DCs [141].

The field of NK-DC study is largely unexplored. Thus, there are uncertainties whether to classify some subtypes as NK cells or NK-DCs. For an example, Fujii S. et al. described the CD11c$^+$Dx5$^+$ cell population secreting IFN-γ in response to glycolypids α-galactosylceramide and α-C-galactosylceramide [57]. By formal criteria, the cells should be classified as NK-DCs but the authors consider them to be NK subtype.

An analogous cell type has not yet been identified in humans [168]. However, there are reports concluding that human NK cells have capacities to effectively present antigens themselves [64]. Un-activated human NK cells have low levels of MHC-II on their surface. The MHC-II surface level is greatly up-regulated and costimulation molecule expression is gained after NK-cell activation in the presence of IL-2 or target-cell lysis (NK-sensitive tumour-cell lines and influenza-virus-infected cells). Strikingly, MHC-II (HLA-DR, -DP, -DQ) and costimulatory (CD80, CD86, OX40L) molecules were expressed by all NK-cell clones, independently from the type of NK-receptor expressed [64]. Activated NK cells proved to be active APCs and effectively initiated primary immune reactions. NK cells expressing MHC-II and costimulation molecules were also identified *in vivo* in inflamed tonsils and samples from deciduae obtained from cytomegalovirus-infected mothers [64]. The data obtained by the group challenges the results of studies using a murine model and raises the question of whether mouse NK-DCs is a DC subtype or a NK subtype or they are simply NK cells converting to APCs? The recent study by Chen L. et al. [25] obviously excludes the possibility of mouse NK-cells differentiation into NK-DCs. Although, NK-DCs are able to generate conventional DCs and perhaps are at the intermediate stage of their development. The authors have shown that NK1.1$^+$CD11c$^+$-NK-DCs differentiate into NK1.1$^-$ DCs with concomitant MHC-II up-regulation. However, NK1.1$^+$CD11c$^-$-NK cells did not reconstitute NK1.1$^+$CD11c$^+$-NK-DCs upon adoptive transfer into irradiated mice. Chen L. et al. considered that possible NK-DC precursors might be Ly6C$^+$ monocytes because they generated NK1.1$^+$CD11c$^+$ as well as NK1.1$^-$CD11c$^+$ cells.

Thus, we may draw the following conclusions:

1. There are several types of DCs differing in many features. No common DC-specific markers have yet been identified. However, all DC subtypes (in an activated state) strongly express MHC-II molecules. Major DC subtypes

do not express/or have low levels of lineage-specific cell surface antigens of other immune cell types.

2. Different DC subtypes may be identified using complexes of specific markers. However, it should be stressed that the usage of single markers might be misleading because antigens expressed exclusively by a DC subtype have not been found (perhaps, the exception is langerin expressed by LCs). Usually, all these markers are expressed by other DC subtypes, monocytes/macrophages (related to mDCs) as well as by completely different cell types including neurons. The morphological and functional criteria must also be taken into account. The existence of multiple DC subtypes may be explained by their functional specialization for recognition and their further induction of specific immune responses against different types of pathogens (Th1 against intracellular microbes, Th2 during helminthic infections, etc.).

3. The origin of certain DC subtypes (pDCs, thymic DCs, CD8α^+ murine DCs, NK-DCs) has not yet been completely discovered.

8.3. Generation of Dendritic Cells *In Vitro* and a Comparison with Dendritic Cells *In Vivo*

In vitro assays helped tremendously in elucidating the DC differentiation pathways and factors indispensable for their development.

8.3.1. Generation of Human Dendritic Cells

In vitro studies of the differentiation of human DCs have been greatly influenced by the aim of optimizing culture systems to allow an efficient production of DCs for use in cancer immunotherapy.

First of all, DCs may be obtained directly from human blood by gradient centrifugation [73]. However, one leukopheresis procedure gives only 5×10^6 DCs.

Two main protocols to generate DCs, from either monocytes or CD34$^+$ precursors, have been described and generally involve a first differentiation phase followed by a maturation step [7].

8.3.1.1. Monocyte-Derived Dendritic Cells

GENERATION OF DENDRITIC CELLS IN THE PRESENCE OF GM-CSF AND IL-4
Today, mature DCs are usually obtained from CD14$^+$ monocytes using a well-known two-stage method [150, 152]. During the first stage, monocytes generate immature DCs after a 5–7 day cultivation in the presence of GM-CSF and IL-4. Immature monocyte-derived DCs have great capacities for antigen capture [152]. During the second step, DCs mature in response to the inflammatory factors (TNF-α, LPS, IFN-γ, CD40L, etc.)

Importantly, the functional repertoire of DCs derived from monocytes by standard protocol appears to be significantly restricted in comparison to their physiological counterparts. Perhaps, their major limitation is their low capacity for migration. It was shown that most of the DCs were unable to leave the site of injection and reach the lymph nodes upon the intradermal injection [116]. Moreover, they were not able to stimulate NK and CD4$^+$Th2 cells [182] and poorly stimulated humoral immunity [42]. Clearly it is very important because NK cells play a major role in anti-cancer and anti-viral immune responses by eliminating cells that are deficient in MHC-I-expression.

It is suggested that the cause of monocyte-derived DC functional restrictions is the absence of phospholipase A2 (PLA2) [182]. This is an enzyme that cleaves membrane phospholipids generating arachidonic acid and takes part in the synthesis of thrombocyte activation factor (TAF). Enzyme synthesis is inhibited by IL-4. Thus, DCs differentiating in the presence of IL-4 are unable to produce TAF as well as other arachidonic acid derivatives (prostaglandins, leukotrienes and lipoxins), which play an important role in leukocyte migration, NK-cell activation and Th2-cell differentiation.

Importantly, DCs generated by standard protocol are unstable and revert to monocytes/macrophages upon withdrawal of the cytokines [150]. Moreover, the reversal of TNF-α-mediated maturation of monocyte-derived DCs occurred when TNF-α was removed [125]. This fact, besides their functional deficiencies mentioned above, might have important implications regarding their use in cancer immunotherapy and suggests that monocyte-derived DCs might not have a physiological counterpart. However, we cannot exclude the possibility of DC conversion to monocytes/macrophages *in vivo*. As mentioned above, monocytes are able to generate DCs *in vivo* [92, 144].

It is interesting to note a recent study by Roy K. C. et al. [151]. They obtained DCs from monocytes in the presence of only IL-4 without the addition of GM-CSF. The morphology, phenotype and phagocytic activity of the DCs did not differ from DCs generated by the standard method. However, they did not express CD1a. DCs produced in the presence of only IL-4 produced more IL-12, in response to CD40L or the combination of LPS with IFN-γ, than conventional monocyte-derived DCs. They stimulated Th1-response in allo-MLR more potently. However, the method gave fewer cells than the standard protocol.

We generated DCs by the standard method of cultivation of peripheral blood monocytes in the presence of IL-4 and GM-CSF during 6 days [150, 152]. The DC morphology was typical for immature monocyte-derived DCs [82]. DCs floated or loosely adhered to plastic (Figure 8.11a). They were large, irregularly shaped cells with laterally positioned nuclei and an abundant foamy (highly vacuolated) cytoplasm (Figure 8.11b–d). Immature DCs had basophilic lightly stained cytoplasm with a more intense staining in the centre of the cells (Figure 8.11b). Their phenotype was also typical for immature DCs. They greatly expressed CD86, had variable levels of CD40 and did not express or had low levels of CD83, CD14 and CD80.

Analogous results were obtained by numerous scientists who generated DCs from peripheral blood monocytes in the presence of IL-4 and GM-CSF [66, 116, 140, 184]. The authors of the studies described immature monocyte-derived DCs as large floating or adherent irregular-shaped cells, which significantly expressed CD86 (53%–100%) and HLA-DR (80%–100%), did not express or have low levels of CD14 (0%–14%) as well as CD83 (0%–23%). In most of the studies, DCs expressed another costimulation molecule (CD80) weaker than that of CD86. According to different data its expression varied significantly and was detected on 2%–87% of the immature DCs.

The maturation of DCs occurred after the cultivation with TNF-α. Their maturation manifested, primarily, in appearance on their surface of CD80 costimulatory molecules and marker of mature DCs CD83 (Figures 8.12 and 8.13). Besides, cells up-regulated the CD40 and CD86 expression (Figure 8.12). Most of the mature DCs were floating cells and exhibited prominent membrane protrusions (Figure 8.14) but usually mature DC cultures combined adherent and non-adherent cells. Percentages of adherent and non-adherent cells varied significantly between experiments applying blood samples from different donors. The levels of CD83 and costimulatory molecule expression were similar in both adherent and non-adherent DC fractions. Different authors contradict each other in their descriptions of mature monocyte-derived CD83⁺DCs and describe

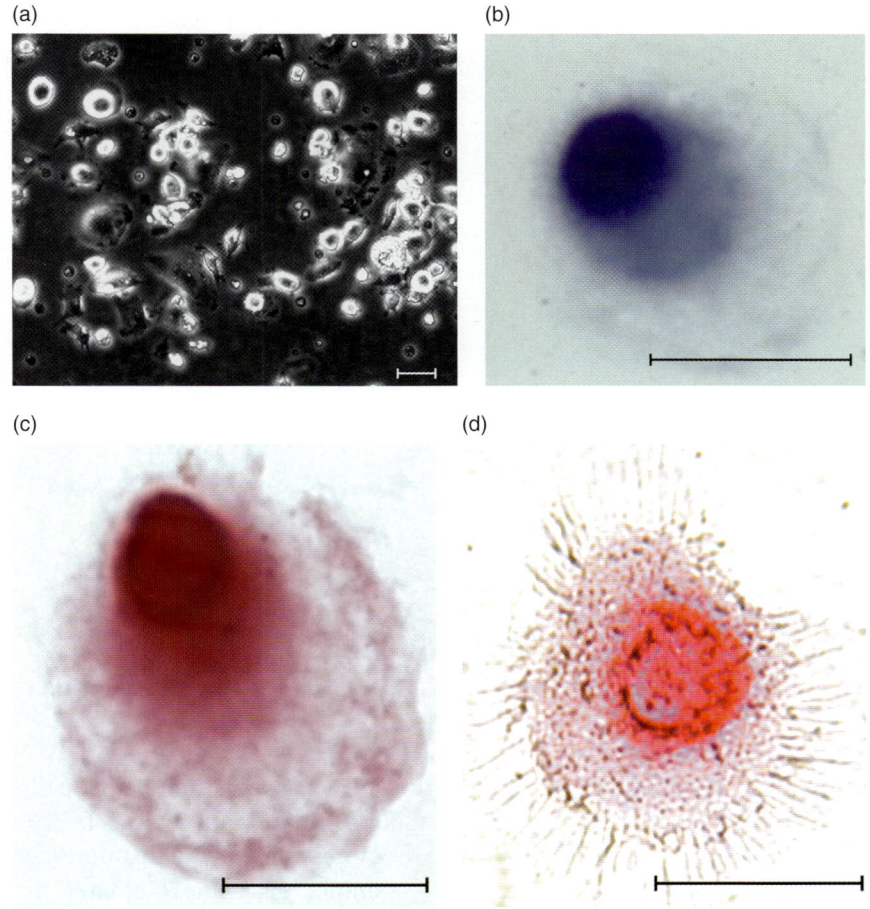

Figure 8.11. Human immature monocyte-derived DCs. **a** Phase-contrast micrographs in dark field, OMx400. Scale bar: 20 μm. **b** Romanovsky-Giemsa azure-eosin staining, **c** and **d** Ziehl fuchsin staining, Scale bar: 10 μm, OMx900

them either as non-adherent cells [134] or even as firmly adherent cells [204].

We also used LPS from different species of gram-negative bacteria as an inducer of DC maturation [27]. Immature human DCs were shown to be very labile in their routes of differentiation. In response to LPS, they turned into a mixed population of CD14+ macrophages and DCs at different stages of maturation (Figure 8.15). Macrophages are of great importance for anti-bacterial immune response. A minor part of the cells became fully mature CD83+ DCs. A major part of the DCs was on an intermediate level of maturation. They expressed high levels of costimulation molecules but did not have a CD83-marker. Interestingly, LPS was a poorer CD83 and CD80 inducer than TNF-α. However, it was as good or superior to the TNF-α in the up-regulation of CD86 costimulatory molecule expression. Strikingly, the best inducers of DC maturation (LPS from *Escherichia coli* and *Shigella sonnei*) turned out to up-regulate CD14 expression to the highest levels in mixed macrophage/DC populations. This fact obviously evidences the absolute necessity of the receptor molecules for the optimal activation of cells by LPS. It is possible that CD14+ macrophages actively secrete pro-inflammatory cytokines in response to LPS, assisting in such a way the maturation of CD14− DCs. Altogether, they could be producers of soluble CD14, which

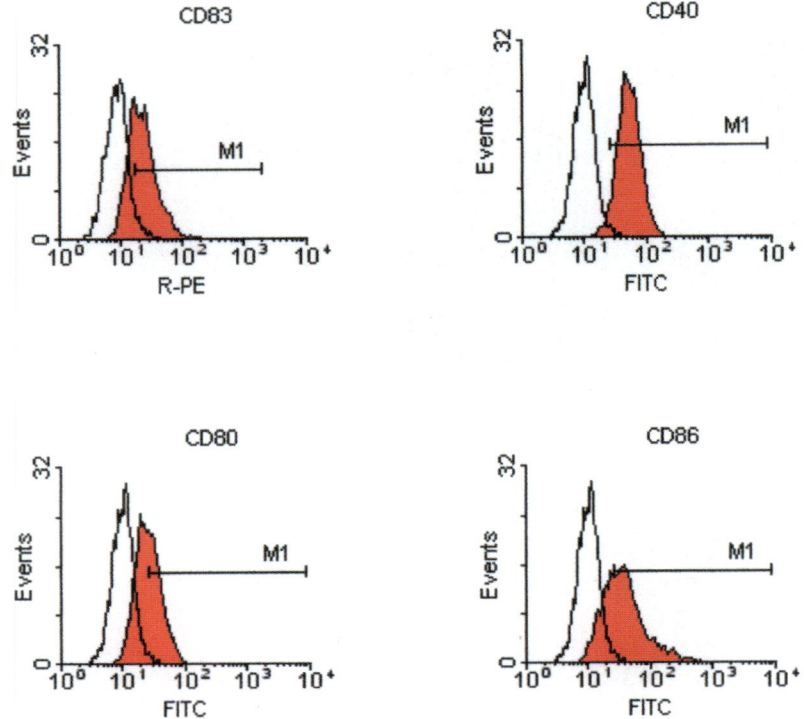

Figure 8.12. Phenotypic features of DCs matured with TNF-α. Events-number of cells, FITC, R-PE – logarithms of fluorescence intensity corresponding to fluorescent dyes FITC (fluorescein isothiocyanate) and PE (phycoerythrin). M1 – marker, comprising cells with fluorescence greater than in isotypic control. Isotypic control is delineated by a simple black line. Coloured histograms show samples labelled with antibodies to cell surface antigens

might be necessary for LPS binding by CD14⁻ DCs [187].

Costimulation molecule (CD80 and CD86) expression was significantly up-regulated on all the cells of the mixed leukocyte population obtained under LPS action including CD14⁺ macrophages. It is conceivable that all the cells from mixed population have good capacities for antigen presentation. It is well known that macrophages are capable of

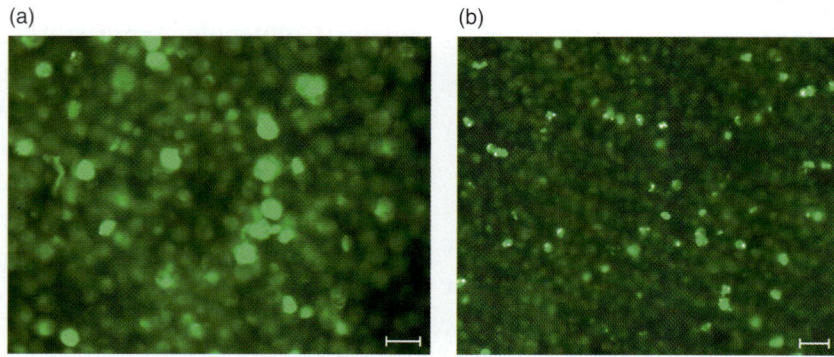

Figure 8.13. Expression of costimulatory molecule CD80 and marker of mature DCs CD83 by DCs, which matured upon 2 days cultivation in the presence of TNF-α. Micrographs of DCs labelled with FITC-conjugates of antibodies to **a** CD80 (OMx400) or **b** CD83 (OMx200), Scale bar: a 15, b 30 μm

(a)   (b)

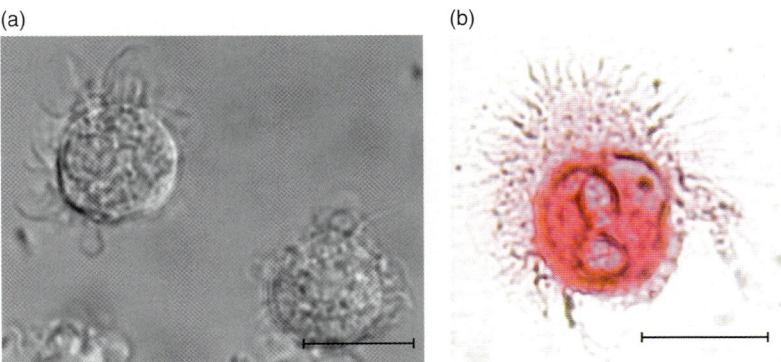

Figure 8.14. Micrographs of human monocyte-derived DCs, which matured upon 2 days cultivation in the presence of TNF-α. **a** Phase-contrast microscopy in bright field of floating mature DCs, OM × 400. **b** Ziehl fuchsin staining, OM × 900, Scale bar: 10 μm

differentiating into mature DCs [134]. We suggest that activated macrophages, developing from immature DCs under LPS action, are capable of generating mature DCs in certain conditions.

We observed the development of cells expressing the marker of mature DCs (CD83) as well as monocyte/macrophage-specific cell surface antigen (CD14) upon LPS stimulation of immature DCs (Figure 8.16). Cells coexpressing CD14 and CD83 are probably intermediates capable of differentiating either to macrophages or to mature DCs, depending

on the conditions. Lyakh L. A. et al. generated mature DCs from monocytes under serum-free conditions in the presence of GM-CSF, LPS and other maturation factors and identified cells with similar phenotype (CD14$^+$, CD83$^+$) [84, 100]. Another research group detected transient CD83 expression on LPS-stimulated monocytes and macrophages [20]. Chomarat P. et al. showed the importance of pro-inflammatory cytokine IL-6/TNF-α balance in determining the differentiation fates of monocytes and macrophages [30]. IL-6 up-regulates the expression of

(a)   (b)

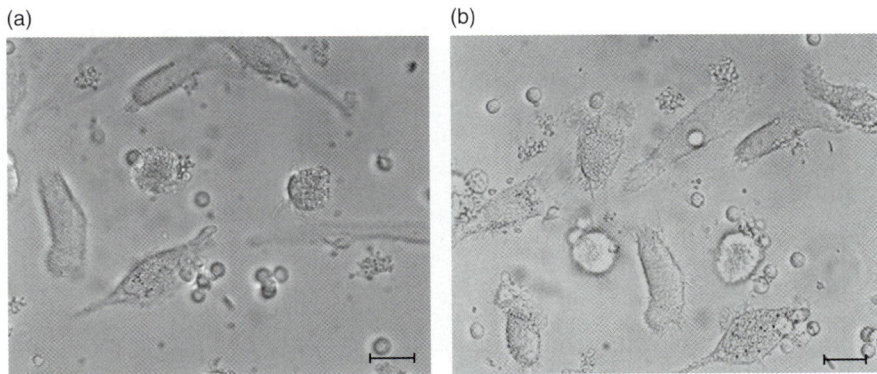

Figure 8.15. Mixed population of floating DCs and highly adherent macrophages obtained from immature human monocyte-derived DCs upon culturing in the presence of *E. coli* LPS.
a Phase-contrast micrograph in bright field of adherent macrophages and floating DCs.
b Phase-contrast micrograph in bright field focusing on the adherent macrophages, OM × 400, Scale bar: 10 μm. Notice contaminating lymphocytes

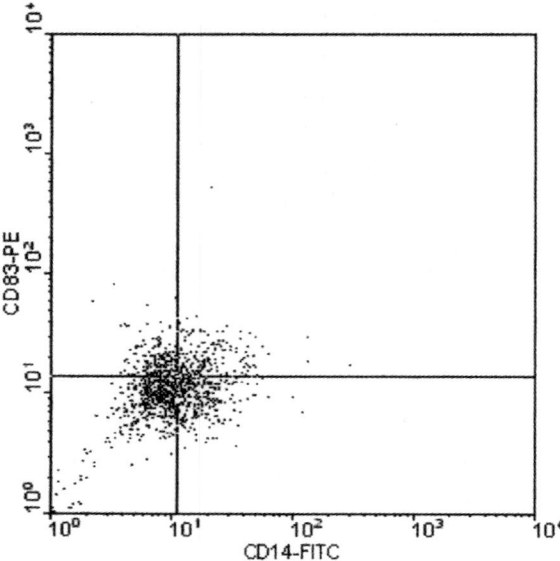

Figure 8.16. Expression of CD83 (marker of mature DCs) and CD14 (component of LPS receptor, monocyte/macrophage marker) by mixed leukocyte population obtained from immature DCs upon stimulation with LPS. Immature DCs were stimulated with *E. coli* LPS (1 μ*g/ml*) during 1 day. Cells were labelled simultaneously with specific antibodies to CD83 (PE-conjugated) and CD14 (FITC-conjugated). CD14-FITC and CD83-PE - logarithms of fluorescence intensity corresponding to fluorescent dyes FITC and PE. Quadrant was set using isotypic control

M-CSF receptor and facilitates M-CSF internalization, resulting in a predominant generation of macrophages from monocytes and probably from immature DCs, whereas, TNF-α down-regulates M-CSFR expression and skews monocyte differentiation from macrophages to mature DCs and prevents the conversion of immature DCs into macrophages.

Altogether, there are numerous contradictions concerning LPS potency as an inducer of DC maturation in comparison to pro-inflammatory factors [31, 134]. According to Nakamura I. et al., the maturation state of mouse DCs activated by LPS was instable [123]. DCs reached the maximal level of costimulatory molecule expression and the maximal T-cell activation potency after 6 hours incubation with LPS. However, in a 48 hour period they returned to an immature state. Interestingly, they even completely restored their endocytic capacities. Another research group obtained practically a homogenous and stable human mature DC population under LPS stimulation [134]. However, they remarked on the instability of mature DCs with intermediate levels of CD83 expression. Such cells, depending on the conditions, generated either completely mature DCs or macrophages. Thus, the stability of mature DCs is probably determined not by the nature of the stimuli applied but by the degree of maturation state achieved by DCs in a study.

Maturation of DCs in response to LPS depends on their ability to produce pro-inflammatory factors under its action. Besides pro-inflammatory cytokines, LPS induces the secretion of anti-inflammatory cytokine IL-10 [33]. IL-10 suppresses pro-inflammatory cytokine secretion. It helps the organism to regulate inflammatory reactions and DC maturation. The presence of LPS during monocyte differentiation into DCs leads to the generation of immature DCs, which are unresponsive to LPS stimulation and fail to mature under its action [148, 199]. However, such DCs mature in the presence of exogenous TNF-α and PGE-2 [148]. DCs generated from monocytes derived from different donors differ in their capabilities to mature in response to LPS [148]. Thus, many different factors, including cell concentration, period of incubation, etc., may influence DC maturation in response to LPS. It explains the contradictions of different authors considering LPS potency as a DC maturation factor.

GENERATION OF DENDRITIC CELLS FROM MONOCYTES IN THE PRESENCE OF GM-CSF AND IFN-α/β DCs may be generated from peripheral blood monocytes in the presence of GM-CSF and IFN-α and/or −β (IFN-DCs)

[155]. Under the action of the cytokine combination, monocytes differentiated into floating DCs during 3 days. The DCs had higher levels of costimulatory molecules (CD80, CD86, CD40) as well as adhesion (CD54) and HLA-DR (MHC-II) molecules, than that of DCs derived in the presence of the standard cytokine combination (IL-4 and GM-CSF). About 30%–40% of cells expressed CD83 and thus they were mature DCs. IFN-DCs also were more potent stimulators in allo-MLR. T cells stimulated by IFN-DCs in allo-MLR secreted significantly more IFN-γ than T cells activated by conventional monocyte-derived DCs. Thus, IFN-DCs polarize T cells towards Th1-type immune reactions. IFN-α/β induced IL-15 secretion by DCs. The cytokine is of great importance for APC-T-cell interactions, the induction of Th1-immune response and the viability of memory T cells. The full maturation of the DCs was achieved under LPS action during 2 days.

Besides, autologous IFN-DCs pulsed with inactivated HIV-1 (human immunodeficiency virus) particles, induced a much more potent proliferative response than DCs generated by standard protocol [155]. SCID-mice (severe-combined-immunodeficiency-syndrome) were reconstructed with human leukocytes and autologous IFN-DCs pulsed with inactivated HIV-1. Potent primary immune reactions developed, which manifested in viral antigen-specific antibody production.

IFN-DCs, like NK-DCs, expressed TRAIL and killed Jurkat tumour cells sensitive to TRAIL-induced apoptosis. TRAIL expression by DCs may have dual functions. First of all, TRAIL may induce the death of virus-infected or tumour cells sensitive to TRAIL-induced apoptosis. Secondly, it may induce apoptosis in DCs themselves after the fulfilment of their functions. A significant proportion of IFN-DCs (40%) bound annexin-GFP (green fluorescent protein) conjugated on the 5th day of incubation, revealing their early apoptotic state. On the 6th day their quantities significantly diminished.

The authors suggested that monocytes *in vivo* differentiated into DCs during infections in response to IFN-α/β secreted by pDCs [155].

GENERATION OF DENDRITIC CELLS FROM MONOCYTES IN THE PRESENCE OF IL-4 AND IL-3
IL-3 is a key cytokine for pDC generation from pre-pDCs having high levels of IL-3R. However, monocytes do express low levels of the receptor. Ebner S. et al. obtained DCs from human monocytes in the presence of IL-3 (instead of GM-CSF) and IL-4 [50]. The yield of the cells was as high as in the standard protocol. DC morphology and their phenotype (CD markers and TLRs) were similar to DCs derived by the standard method. However, the cells, like the DCs obtained with IL-4 alone (mentioned above), did not express CD1a. The DCs generated in the presence of IL-3 and IL-4 secreted less IL-12 and induced IL-4 and IL-5 secretion by naïve CD4$^+$ T cells in allo-MLR, thus, governing the induction of Th2-type reactions in contrast to DCs derived by the standard protocol.

8.3.1.2. Generation of Dendritic Cells from CD34$^+$ Precursors In Vitro
DCs may be derived from CD34$^+$ bone-marrow or blood precursors [21, 22]. The differentiation of DCs occurred after a rather long (about 2 weeks) incubation in the presence of GM-CSF and TNF-α [21]. The yield of the cells was increased by the addition of stem cell factor (SCF) or FLT3L [22].

Such cultures generated mixed populations of immature DCs resembling LCs and interstitial DCs. During culturing, two independent intermediate DC types developed: CD14$^+$ pre-DCs and CD1a$^+$ pre-DCs. In further incubation, CD14$^+$ CD1a$^-$ cells differentiated into DCs, which did not express E-cadherin. They resembled immature dermal interstitial DCs or mature lymphoid organ interdigitating DCs. In the presence of M-CSF, the intermediates generated macrophages. This fact pointed to their myeloid origin.

CD14$^-$ CD1a$^+$intermediates differentiated into LC-like DCs expressing E-cadherin and langerin.

LC-like DCs were also obtained from CD11b$^-$ fraction of CD14$^+$ CD1a$^-$ intermediates by the addition of TGF-β [76]. LC-like DCs differentiated also from monocytes or CD11c$^+$ blood mDCs *in vitro* in the presence of GM-CSF, IL-4 and TGF-β [7]. Maturation of the cells was achieved by the addition of IL-1 and TNF-α.

We obtained immature DCs from human bone-marrow precursors by culturing in the presence of IL-4 and GM-CSF or their combination with TNF-α [166]. The yields of DCs were significantly improved by the addition of TNF-α to the cell culture medium cell. The DCs resembled monocyte-derived immature DCs (Figure 8.17a–d). We observed mitotic cells (Figure 8.17f) as well as DCs with two nuclei (Figure 8.17e) in the cell cultures. Some contaminating macrophage-like cells were also evident (Figure 8.17a and f). The profile of costimulatory molecule expression on the DC surface largely correlated with the immature monocyte-derived DCs.

Several studies showed CD34$^+$ progenitor-derived DCs to be more potent CTL activators than monocyte-derived DCs [52, 118].

8.3.1.3. Differentiation of Dendritic Cells from Multipotent Lymphoid Precursors In Vitro

CD34$^+$CD10$^+$Lin$^-$ bone-marrow progenitors endowed with T-, B- and NK-cell but not myeloid differentiation capacity, produced DCs after culture with IL-1β,-7, GM-CSF, SCF and FLT3L [58]. Interestingly, CD34$^+$CD1a$^-$ lymphoid-committed thymic precursors generated DCs after culture with IL-7, TNF-α, SCF and FLT3L in the absence of GM-CSF. However, this cytokine improved the yield of DCs [36, 81]. Nevertheless, it was reported that CD34$^+$CD1a$^-$ thymic precursors

generated monocytes when cultured with M-CSF, indicating that they retained some myeloid capacity [36]. This result might support the theory that human thymic non-plasmacytoid CD11c$^+$ DCs are myeloid-derived. In this sense, a thymic CD11b$^+$ DC subset expressing the myeloid markers M-CSFR, CD14, CD33 and CD64 has been described [7]. Moreover, a common differentiation pathway for DCs and monocytes from thymic CD34$^+$CD1a$^-$ precursors, independent of T-cell differentiation pathway, has been identified [7].

8.3.1.4. Differentiation of Plasmacytoid Dendritic Cells In Vitro

Blom B. et al. obtained pDCs from blood CD34$^+$CD45RA$^-$CD123$^-$-cells after culture in the presence of FLT3L [14]. Their maturation into antigen-presenting DCs was induced with IL-3 and CD40L [63] or IL-3 and TNF-α [83]. Whereas, the IL-3 and IL-4 combination induced apoptosis in pDCs indicating their differential requirements compared with mDCs [83].

8.3.2. Generation of Mouse Dendritic Cells

8.3.2.1. Differentiation of Murine Dendritic Cells from Bone-Marrow Progenitors In Vitro

Murine DCs are usually obtained by culturing mouse bone marrow in the presence of GM-CSF or its combination with IL-4 [99, 105]. However, it should be noticed, that this method yields impure DC populations (70%–95% purity depending on a method applied for DC generation and time of incubation), which also comprises granulocyte and macrophage contaminations [99]. Following subsequent DC maturation in the presence of TNF-α, or other inducers (LPS, CD40L), a phenotypically homogenous population of mature

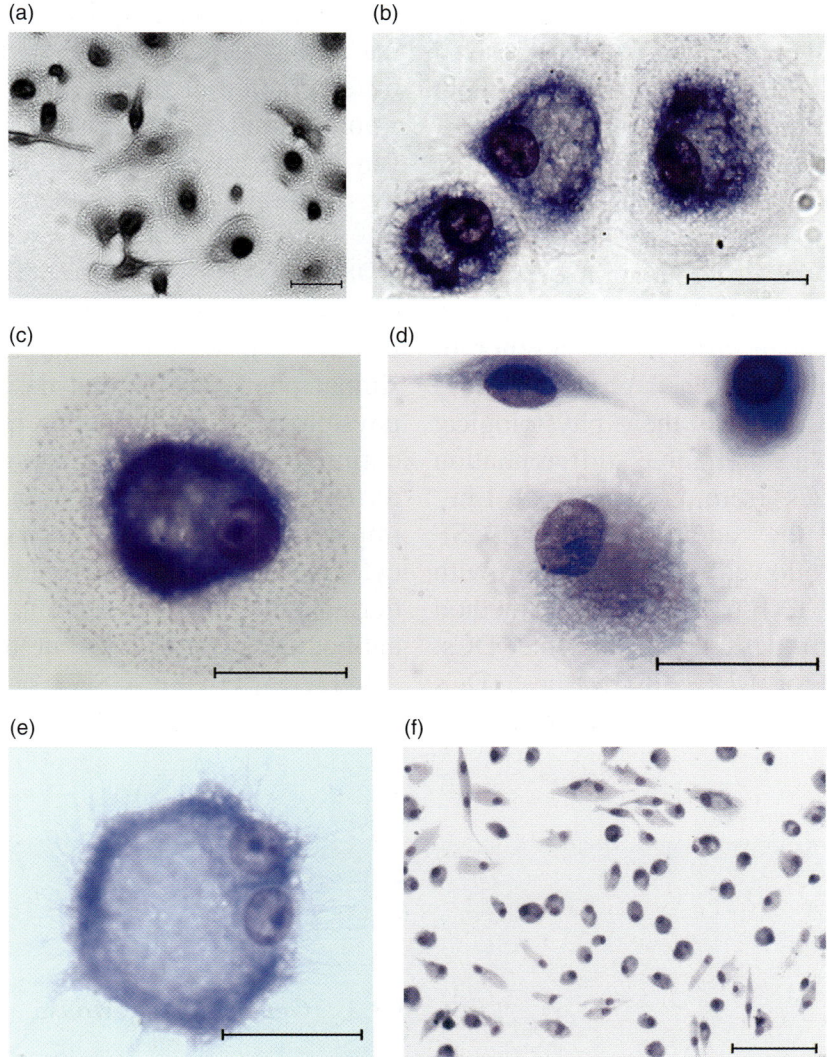

Figure 8.17. Micrographs of human bone-marrow-derived immature DCs. **a** Phase-contrast micrograph in bright field of fixed but uncoloured cells, OM × 400, Scale bar: 10 μm. **b–f** Romanovsky-Giemsa azure-eosin staining **b–e** OM × 900, Scale bar: 10 μm f OM × 200, Scale bar: 50 μm

DCs develops. The DCs express significantly costimulatory (CD80, CD86 and CD40) and MHC-II molecules but do not have CD8α.

In contrast, when bone-marrow Lin⁻ cells were incubated with GM-CSF, SCF and TNF-α, followed by maturation with GM-CSF and TNF-α, two mature DC subtypes with different phenotypes were generated [201]. Both were CD11c⁺, MHC-II^{high}, CD86^{high}, CD40⁺ and negative for CD8α and DEC-205 (an endocytic receptor expressed by mouse interstitial DCs and LCs). The populations differed in their expression of E-cadherin, M-CSFR and non-specific esterase (NSE). E-cadherin⁻M-CSFR⁺NSE⁺ DCs developed from CD11c⁺CD11b⁺ immature DCs, which also generated macrophages when cultured with M-CSF. This result indicates that CD11c⁺CD11b⁺ immature DCs are myeloid intermediates. By contrast,

E-cadherin⁺M-CSF⁻NSE⁻ DCs, displaying characteristics of epidermal LCs, were derived from CD11c⁺CD11b⁻ immature DCs without the capacity to differentiate into macrophages.

The generation of LC-like DCs from CD11c⁺CD11b⁻ intermediates is not dependent on the presence of TGF-β1, which is required for the differentiation of LCs *in vivo* [15]. It is conceivable that the process of LC generation *in vitro* in the absence of TGF-β1 is incomplete. Their phenotype does not fully correspond to their physiological counterparts. An alternative differentiation protocol for LCs from bone-marrow Lin⁻ cells requires the addition of GM-CSF and TGF-β1 followed by maturation with GM-CSF and TNF-α [202]. The method gives E-cadherin⁺DEC-205⁺ LC-like DCs. The expression of DEC-205 by these DCs could correspond to a more mature and/or

physiological phenotype and might reflect the requirements for TGF-β1 for the *in vivo* differentiation of LCs.

Interestingly, culture of bone-marrow Lin⁻ cells with FLT3L alone followed by maturation with either LPS or IFN-α, generated both CD8α⁻CD11b^hi and CD8α⁺CD11b^low DCs [17]. The data suggest that FLT3L is a key cytokine to drive the *in vitro* differentiation of DCs with a similar phenotype to that described for their physiological counterparts. However, when defining the cytokine requirements of DC differentiation and maturation pathways it is important to take into account that certain cytokines can be produced endogenously during culture. In this sense it was shown that antibodies against IL-6 but not IL-2, -3,-4, -7, -11, 15, G-CSF, CSF-1 or TGF-β1 could block FLT3L-driven differentiation of DCs

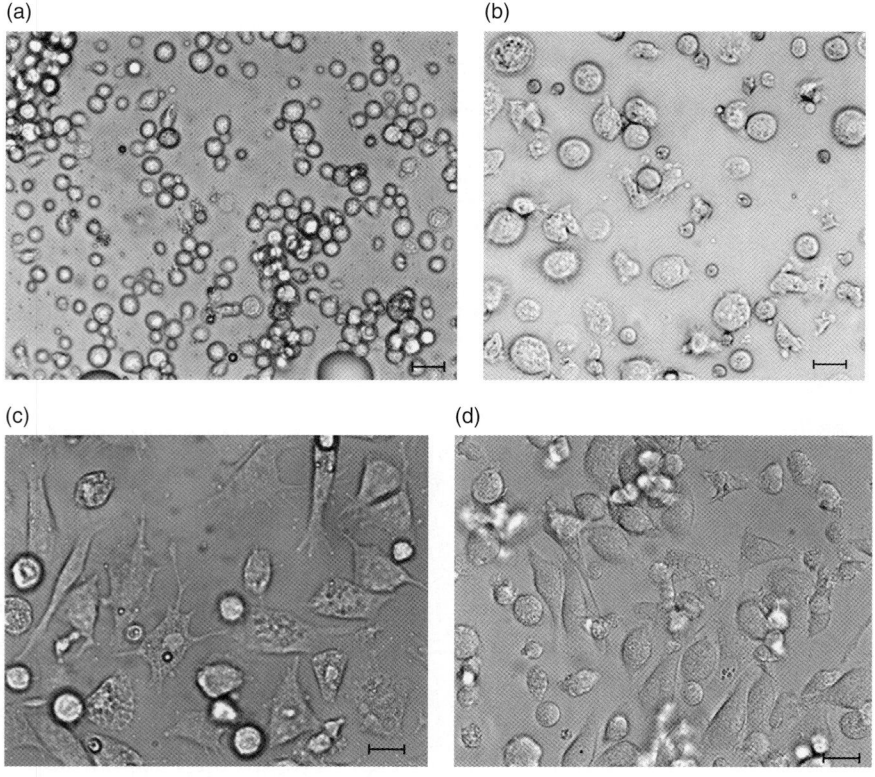

Figure 8.18. Generation of mouse DCs from bone-marrow precursors. Phase-contrast micrographs in bright field of different stages of DC generation. **a** Bone-marrow cells. (First day). Scale bar: 20 μm **b** Third day. **c** Fifth day. **d** Seventh day of incubation. Scale bar: 10 μm

revealing an essential role for IL-6 in the FLT3L-mediated generation of $CD8\alpha^-CD11b^{hi}$ and $CD8\alpha^+CD11b^{low}$ DCs [7, 17].

We obtained mouse DCs from bone-marrow progenitors by culture in the presence of murine recombinant GM-CSF and IL-4 during 7 days [105]. We followed the process of DC generation from small bone marrow precursors (first day) to immature DCs (seventh day) [3, 91] (Figure 8.18). As a result the cultures produced typical mouse DCs – large irregular-shaped cells, which floated or loosely adhered to plastic (Figures 8.18d and 8.19a). They showed high phagocytic capacities for bacterial cells (Figure 8.19d and e). Their phenotype was the following: MHC-II^+, $CD14^{low}$, $CD80^+$, $CD86^{low}$, $CD83^-$, $CD40^{low}$ (Figure 8.20) and fully corresponded to reference data [99, 105].

Maturation of mouse DCs was induced with LPS or TNF-α. As noticed by other authors, TNF-α was a less efficient maturation inducer of mouse bone-marrow derived dendritic cells than bacterial LPS [99]. Even on the third day of incubation with the cytokine, some DCs remained adherent cells although they exhibited prominent membrane protrusions (Figure 8.21 a–e). The expression of costimulatory and MHC-II molecules was stimulated moderately by the addition of TNF-α. Mature DCs down-regulated the phagocytosis of bacteria (Figure 8.21f).

Bacterial LPS proved to be a much better inducer of DC maturation. DC proliferation was down-regulated. They became floating stellate cells showing numerous membrane

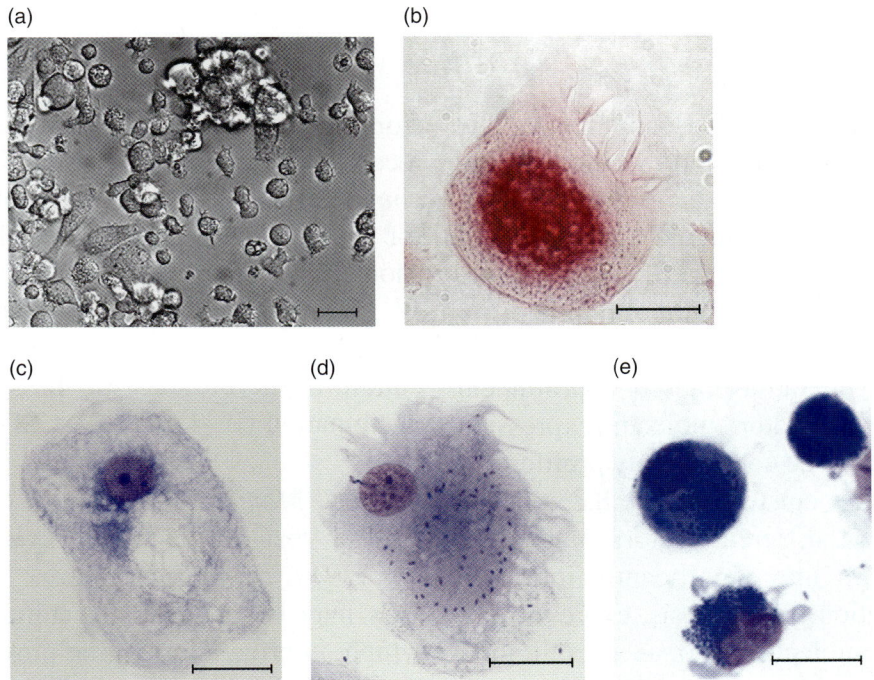

Figure 8.19. Micrographs of mouse immature bone-marrow-derived DCs. **a** Phase-contrast microscopy in bright field of mouse immature DCs on the 7th day of culture in the presence of IL-4 and GM-CSF, OM × 400. **b** Ziehl fuchsin staining, OM × 900. **c** Romanovsky-Giemsa azure-eosin staining, OM × 900. **d** and **e** Immature mouse bone-marrow-derived DCs, which phagocityzed *S. aureus* cells during 1 **d** or 3 **e** hours of coincubation. Romanovsky-Giemsa azure-eosin staining, OM × 900. Scale bar:a – 20; b,c,d - 10 μm

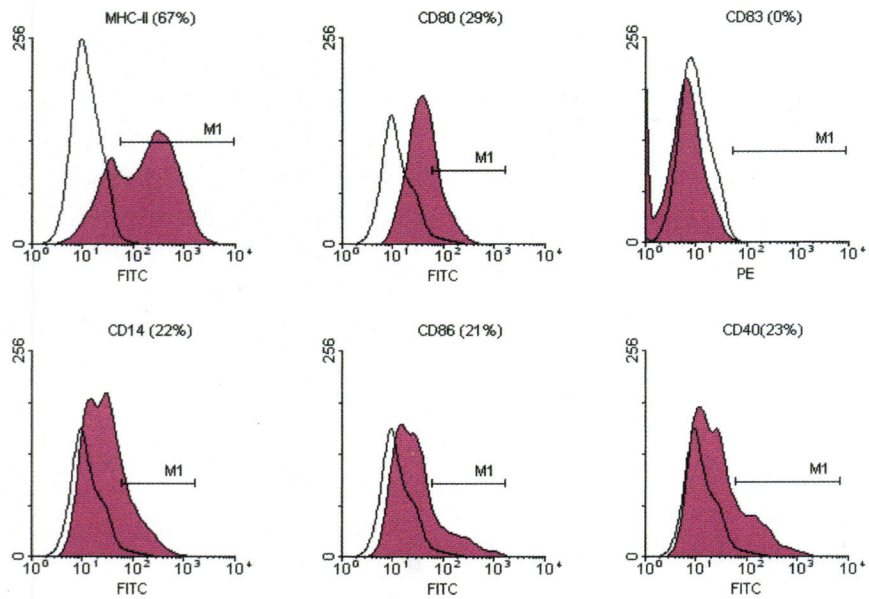

Figure 8.20. Phenotype of mouse immature bone-marrow-derived DCs. Events–number of cells, FITC, PE – logarithms of fluorescence intensity corresponding to fluorescent dyes FITC (fluorescein isothiocyanate) and PE (phycoerythrin). M1 – marker, comprising cells with fluorescence greater than in isotypic control. Isotypic control is delineated by a simple black line. Coloured histograms show samples labelled with antibodies to cell surface antigens

protrusions (Figure 8.22). Costimulatory and MHC-II molecule expression was prominently up-regulated. Interestingly, mouse DCs, like human DCs, up-regulated the CD14 expression in response to LPS.

The presence in the medium of immunosuppressive ganglioside GM1 during the last three days of DC generation caused a prominent decrease in costimulatory molecule expression on their surface. The cells actively proliferated and formed large clusters (Figure 8.23). Thus, the presence of different factors in the DC culture medium may significantly influence their proliferation, endocytosis, expression of costimulatory molecules and, as a result, their capacities for antigen-presentation.

8.3.2.2. Generation of Dendritic Cells from Mouse Monocytes

Although human monocytes are the most common source for further DC generation, a detailed protocol for murine DC generation from monocytes has been described only recently by Leon B. et al. [92]. The method is completely analogous to the protocol applied for human DC generation. However, we should also remark on a study by Schreus M. W. J. et al., who obtained DCs from uncharacterized murine adhering mononuclear cells by culture in the presence of the same cytokine combination (IL-4 and GM-CSF) [163].

8.3.2.3. Mouse Dendritic Cell Generation from Multipotent Thymic Lymphoid Precursors

DCs may be obtained by culture of CD4^{low} lymphoid progenitors in the presence of IL-1, -3, -7, TNF-α, SCF and FLT3L without GM-CSF required for myeloid precursor development [156]. In contrast to physiological thymus DCs the cells derived *in vitro* did not express CD8α. This fact probably reflects requirements for other unidentified factors for physiological DC differentiation.

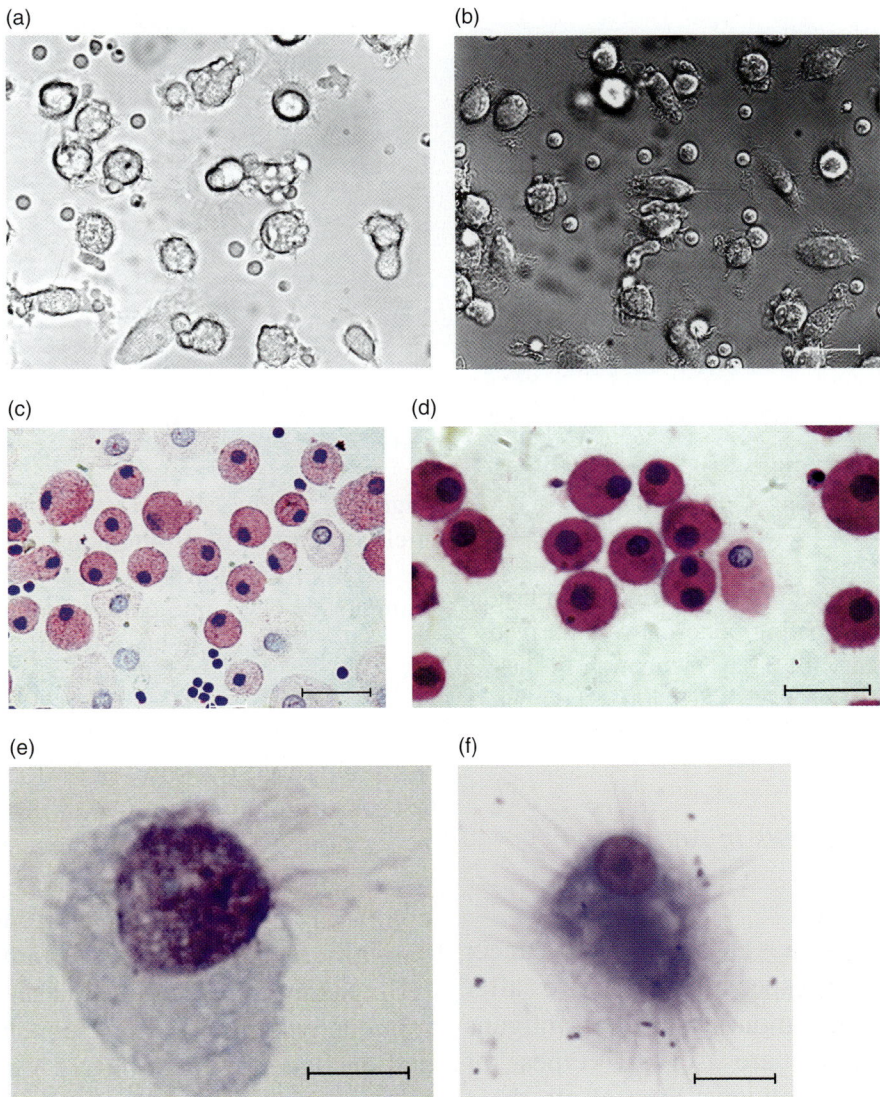

Figure 8.21. Mouse bone-marrow-derived DCs matured with TNF-α. 1 **a** or 3 **b–f** days of incubation with the cytokine. **a** and **b** Phase-contrast micrographs, OM × 400. **c** Brachet staining revealing cellular RNA, OM × 900. **d** Shabadash periodic acid-Schiff staining, OM × 900. **e** Romanovsky-Giemsa azure-eosin staining, OM × 900. **f** DCs phagocityzing *S. aureus* cells during an hour coincubation. Romanovsky-Giemsa azure-eosin staining, OM × 900.
Scale bar: a, b, c, d, - 20; e, f - **10** μm

8.4. Application of Dendritic Cells in Medical Practice

Vaccination provides the most effective and low-cost method for infectious disease prophylaxis. However, today we lack effective vaccines for many dangerous human infectious diseases including AIDS, hepatitis C, tuberculosis and malaria. In the opinion of Ralph M. Steinman, founder of the DC study field, and his colleague Melissa Pope, research in the field may be effectively applied for the development of more effective vaccines as well as for the generation of anti-tumour vaccines [174].

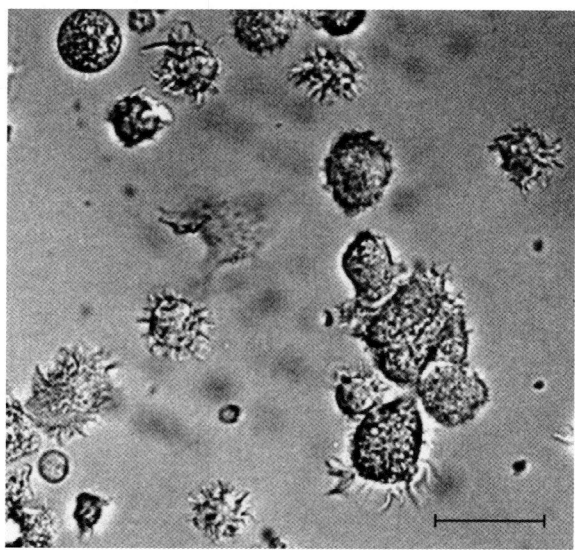

Figure 8.22. Phase-contrast micrograph in bright field of mouse floating bone-marrow-derived DCs matured with 2 day incubation in the presence of *E. coli* LPS, OMx400, Scale bar: **20** μm.

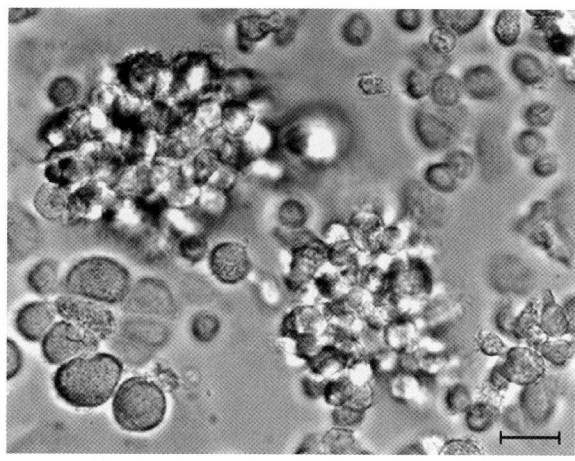

Figure 8.23. Phase-contrast micrographs in bright field of clusters of proliferating mouse immature DCs formed in response to addition of ganglioside GM1 into culture medium, OMx400, Scale bar: 20 μm.

8.4.1. Dendritic Cells in Anti-cancer Therapy

The idea to use DCs as anti-cancer vaccines became especially attractive after the discovery of tumour-associated antigens [77, 135]. There are several types of tumour-associated antigens. First of all, there are antigens of oncogenic viruses such as hepatitis B and C viruses, papilloma virus, etc. Secondly, there are mutated proteins generated as a result of somatic mutations. Of special interest, tumours often express certain proteins expressed in embryos but not in normal adult organisms (α-fetoprotein, telomerase, CEA-carcinoembryonic antigen, etc.). Also, some of the normal tissue antigens are hyperexpressed by tumours (melanoma and prostate-cancer antigens). Certain tumour-specific peptide epitopes may be derived from self antigens such as the commonly expressed ceramide synthase Lass5 [186]. They are not presented by normal cells and appear only at the surface of tumour cells with impaired function of transporter associated with antigen processing (TAP). Such peptides act as immunogenic neoantigens and may be exploited for immune intervention against processing-deficient tumours. Thus, it is commonly agreed that many tumours express antigens recognized by the immune system [56]. Nevertheless, in most cases an adequate immune response does not develop. Tumours and oncogenic viruses have a variety of ways to escape immune reactions. Most tumour antigens, perhaps except for viral ones, are poorly immunogenic. Tumour cells and virus-infected cells are generally MHC-I-deficient. In many cases, tumour cells secrete immuno-suppressive factors or factors suppressing APC development such as gangliosides and prostanoids [19, 108, 137, 165, 167, 169, 193].

Today, mature DCs are believed to be the most effective anti-cancer vaccines (Figure 8.24) [43]. A study using murine models has shown that immunization with mature DCs pulsed with a tumour antigen effectively protected mice against further challenge with lowly immunogenic tumour (all mice in the experimental group survived) [26]. Immature DCs pulsed with the same

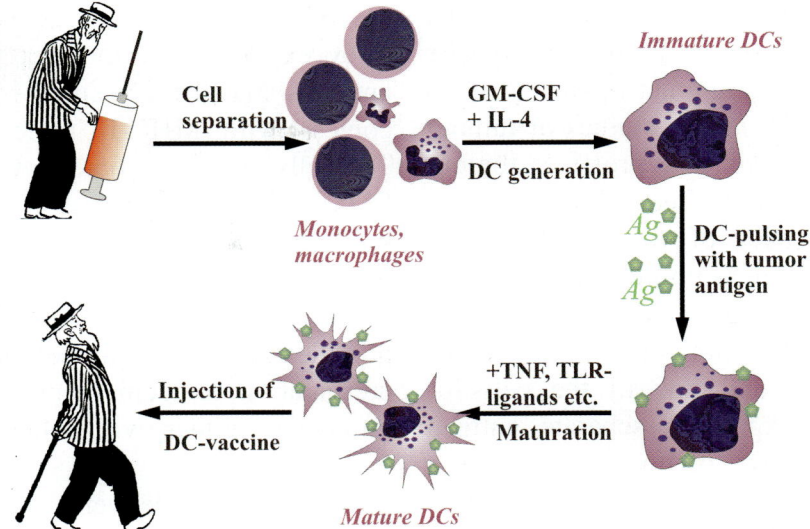

Figure 8.24. Anti-cancer DC-vaccines. Autologous DCs for vaccination purposes are usually generated using a patient's peripheral blood monocytes by the method described above [150, 152]. They are loaded (pulsed) with tumour antigens, matured with different stimuli and reintroduced back to the patient

antigen were completely ineffective (all the mice died). DCs pulsed with an antigen in the presence of factors inducing their maturation (TNF-α IL-1β, LPS, monocyte-conditioned medium, etc.) can effectively present antigens and induce T-cell response. This fact was proved by a number of studies *in vitro*, experiments applying the mouse model; even several healthy volunteers took part in the tests [26, 42, 105, 128]. When DC vaccines were tested with the participation of healthy volunteers, it was shown that the T-cell immune response developed rapidly during 7 days but CD4+ as well as CD8+ T-cell reactions peaked only 1–3 months after immunization [42]. T-cell memory was generated. However, the authors remarked that a natural viral infection induced more robust immune reactions and long-lasting memory.

It should be stressed once more that immunization with immature DCs pulsed with an antigen does not induce an effective immune response and even suppresses it or blocks the development of immune reactions [18, 44, 45, 114]. For example, the injection of immature DCs pulsed with an influenza-virus

matrix peptide lead to the development of a tolerance towards the antigen in a group of healthy volunteers [44]. Jonuleit H. et al. compared directly the effectiveness of mature and immature tumour peptide-pulsed DCs in patients with metastatic melanoma [78]. They injected DCs into lymph nodes. Only mature DCs induced a melanoma-specific CTL response. As shown by another research group, only mature DCs are capable of migrating effectively from the site of the injection into the lymph nodes [189].

Nevertheless, there is a report of a positive clinical response in a patient with a fibrosarcoma treated by a subcutaneous injection of DCs pulsed with a tumour lysate in the absence of any maturation inducers [59]. Unfortunately, the phenotype of the DCs was not determined. We cannot exclude the possibility of DC maturation under the action of unidentified factors in tumour lysate (viruses and heat shock proteins [28]).

Besides DC type the source of tumour antigens and routes of DC delivery obviously play an important role in vaccine efficacy. Several types of antigen (peptides, proteins, cell lysates, RNA, DNA and viral vectors, heat shock proteins and apoptotic bodies) were successfully tested in animal models [10]. In clinical studies, the major sources of tumour antigens are peptides and proteins, tumour lysates are used less frequently [43, 80]. The major drawback of vaccines based on peptides and proteins is implicated by the fact that not all tumour antigens have yet been identified. Moreover, tumour cell populations are heterogenous and not all the cells of a tumour may express a separate antigen [43]. Tumour lysate obviously contains a wide spectrum of different antigens including unidentified ones. Nevertheless, there is a risk of an autoimmune condition developing upon immunization with DCs pulsed with a total tumour lysate [80]. Reassuringly, until now, no autoimmune reactions upon immunization with tumour lysate-pulsed DCs have been observed [43].

Recently, the application of DCs transfected with total tumour RNA for the treatment of metastatic lung and colon cancer has been reported [121]. The DCs induced CTLs able to specifically lyse tumours. Another example of RNA-transfected DC-vaccines is a clinical experience of Vieweg and colleagues in which patients with prostate cancer vaccinated with DCs transfected with mRNA encoding tumour antigens such as PSA and patients with renal cancer vaccinated with DCs transfected with unfractionated tumour-derived mRNA developed tumour antigen–specific $CD8^+$ T-cell responses [67, 176]. The hallmark of the early clinical experience from this group is that virtually all vaccinated patients responded immunologically with the induction of measurable T-cell responses. Furthermore, clinically related responses such as the reduction in PSA levels were often seen in the vaccinated patients in the prostate cancer trials [67].

In the opinion of O'Neill D. W. et al. DCs pulsed with either tumour lysates, killed tumour cells or tumour proteins proved to be the most effective in cancer therapy [133]. They explain it by the fact that exogenous antigens may be presented by DCs both in context with MHC-II molecules to $CD4^+$ Th cells and in context with MHC-I to $CD8^+$ CTLs in a process of so-called cross-presentation. This process is considered to be DC-specific. Thus, in this case CTLs obtain help from Th cells. Whereas RNA provides antigenic epitopes only for MHC-I presentation, antigenic peptides are presented in context either with MHC-I or MHC-II molecules.

The way of delivery may significantly influence DC migration and immunogenicity. Morse M. A. et al. have demonstrated that human DCs successfully reached lymphatic nodes upon intradermal but not intravenous injection [117]. A recent study by Mullins D. W. et al. has fully supported their results [120]. However, Fong L. et al. have demonstrated that antigen-specific reactions developed upon intravenous as well as intradermal injection of human DCs [55]. Upon intravenous injection a more effective specific-antibody response developed. A comparative study based on the murine model suggested that DCs injected intravenously are less immunogenic than ones delivered intra-dermally [90]. Some groups injected DCs directly into lymph nodes and induced the development of prominent immune reactions towards tumour antigens [55, 73]. However, the technique is rather difficult.

In recent years a number of early phase clinical trials have been performed and have demonstrated the safety and feasibility of DC immunotherapy [43, 60, 77, 119, 126, 128, 133, 203]. Let us cite a few examples.

Hsu F. J. et al. treated 4 patients suffering from follicular lymphoma with injections of blood DCs pulsed with tumour-specific idiotypic antibodies [73]. Tumour regression was observed in 3 patients.

Nestle F. O. et al. used monocyte-derived DCs for the treatment of metastatic melanoma

[127]. As a source of antigens they utilized either melanoma peptides or tumour lysate. They injected DCs into the undamaged lymph nodes of 16 patients. 11 patients showed a delayed type hypersensitivity (DTH) reaction in response to peptide-pulsed DCs. Objective tumour regression was observed in 5 of them. In another study, 11 patients with IVth stage metastatic melanoma were treated with mature DCs pulsed with melanoma peptide MAGE-3A1 [181]. Each of the patients received 3 subcutaneous and 2 intravenous DC-vaccine injections. Antigen-specific immune reactions developed and MAGE-3A1-specific CTLs expanded. In 6 patients regression of separate metastases was observed. Interestingly, non-regressing metastases did not express MAGE-3 mRNA. These promising results inspired randomized phase III clinical trials of autologous DC vaccines in comparison to standard chemotherapy implying dacarbazine (DTIC) for treatment of patients with metastatic melanoma [158]. As vaccines, the researchers utilized autologous monocyte-derived DCs pulsed with peptides from melanocyte-specific proteins (tyrosinase, MAGE-1, -3, Melan-A analogue, etc) after their maturation in the presence of the combination of pro-inflammatory factors TNF-α, IL-1β,-6 and PGE-2. Unfortunately, neither protocol of treatment gave any significant positive results. An objective response was observed in 3 of the 55 patients (5.5%) in the case of standard DTIC therapy and in 2 of the 53 patients (3.8%) of the group vaccinated with autologous DCs. However, the authors noted that in comparison to standard chemotherapy, the DC-vaccination significantly increased the complete life expectancy in subgroups of patients with unimpaired general health status (Karnofsky=100) or HLA-A2+/HLA-B44-gaplotypes. The following factors may explain the low efficacy of their DC-vaccine. First of all, the conditions for DC maturation were not optimal [60]. The authors used the combination of pro-inflammatory factors without

the addition of TLR-agonists, which are important for complete DC maturation and IL-12 secretion (discussed below). Furthermore, they used for DC-pulsing peptides, which have numerous disadvantages, as discussed earlier.

Promising results were obtained in trials of autologous DC vaccines for the treatment of metastatic forms of prostate, kidney, breast, colon, thyroid gland and uterus cancer and myeloma [42, 73, 76, 122].

We tested the DC-vaccine efficacy in cancer treatment using mouse models of B16 melanoma and Ehrlich carcinoma. Every 2 weeks mice were immunized with an injection of different quantities of autologous DCs pulsed with tumour lysate. Finally, they received 3 injections of syngeneic DC-vaccine. After immunization some mice were sacrificed. Lymphocytes were separated from their spleens. We determined their cytotoxic activity towards tumour cell lines used for immunization as well as towards unrelated immortalized cell lines. As a control we used lymphocytes obtained from unvaccinated animals. Lymphocytes obtained from immunized mice showed statistically a significant increase of their killer activity towards tumour cell lines used for the immunization in comparison to the lymphocytes of intact animals. However, we did not observe any increase of lymphocyte cytotoxic activity towards the unrelated CaO-1 ovarian cancer tumour cell line. These experimental data show that DC-vaccination leads to an increase of specific cytotoxicity towards tumour cell lines used for DC pulsing. It was found that the optimal dose of DCs utilized for vaccination was 1×10^6 cells per mouse. A further increase in the quantity of DCs used for vaccination did not improve the cytotoxic activity of lymphocytes. The maximal cytotoxic activity was observed after 2–3 injections of the vaccine. When the optimal vaccine dose and number of vaccinations were determined we designated a protocol of mouse immunization. Mice were immunized with 3 injections of 1×10^6 autologous tumour lysate-pulsed DCs. Two weeks after the final immunization, the mice were challenged with different doses of tumour cells (B16 melanoma or Ehrlich carcinoma). Tumour nodules developed much later in vaccinated animals than in unvaccinated mice. They lived significantly longer than animals in the control group which did not receive the vaccine. However, all the animals, including vaccinated ones finally developed tumours and died. Vaccine efficiency dramatically lowered with an increase of a tumour cell infecting dose. The best vaccine efficiency was observed only when we applied the lowest infecting dose leading to the development of tumour nodules and final death in 100% of challenged unvaccinated animals (control group) – 5×10^4 tumour cells for a mouse.

DC anti-cancer vaccines do not provoke any negative side effects. In some cases they gave certain, although not very prominent, positive clinical effects. It is encouraging because all the studies until now have been conducted with the participation of incurable patients with metastatic cancer after the failure of all generally used therapies. It is tempting to assume that DC-vaccines might be much more effective for the treatment of cancer patients with less severe disease after maximal cytoreduction by surgery or chemotherapy. In support though, anti-cancer DC-vaccines proved their efficiency in preventing liver carcinoma recurrence in mice [72].

8.4.2. Application of DC-Vaccines for Infectious Disease Prophylaxis

Presently, anti-infectious DC-vaccines are not used in clinical practice. However, there is experimental evidence suggesting them as an effective and safe method for infectious disease prophylaxis. Encouraging results were obtained in assays applying models *in vitro*, studies based on animal models and even

clinical trials with the participation of human volunteers [1, 2, 9, 16, 97, 106, 138, 147, 164, 175, 188, 194].

There are reports of protective DC-vaccine effects against *Chlamydia trachomatis* infection. Su H. et al. showed that mouse DCs phagocytized killed bacteria; secreted IL-12p40 and presented bacterial antigens to CD4$^+$ T cells [175]. Moreover, mice immunized with DCs pulsed with killed *C. trachomatis* bacteria developed an effective protective immunity towards the genital tract infection. At the same time, Shaw J. et al. demonstrated that immunization of mice with syngeneic DCs pulsed with recombinant major membrane protein of *C.trachomatis* did not raise a protective immune response [164]. Moreover, DCs unexpectedly stimulated an unfavourable Th2-type immune response instead of a protective Th1-type immune response. However, the same DCs *in vitro* secreted IL-12 and stimulated proliferation of CD4$^+$ T cells. The authors suggested that the nature of an antigen used for the pulsing of DCs influenced the type of the immune response induced. The same conclusions were drawn by Rey-Ladino J. et al. [147]. They showed that DCs pulsed with viable *C. trachomatis* had high levels of MHC-II, CD80, CD86, CD40 and ICAM (intracellular adhesion molecule)-1 and produced significant amounts of IL-12 and TNF-α. The DCs effectively activated CD4$^+$ T cells. In contrast, DCs pulsed with the inactivated microbes showed low levels of CD40 and CD86 costimulatory molecules but had higher levels of MHC-II, ICAM-I and CD80. Such DCs secreted less pro-inflammatory cytokines. The DCs pulsed with the viable bacteria had more prominent protective effects.

Worgall S. et al. demonstrated that 45% of mice immunized with DCs pulsed with *Pseudomonas aerogenosa* survived longer than 14 days after the challenge with the bacteria [194]. At the same time, all unvaccinated animals and mice who obtained DCs activated by LPS from *E. coli* died during 72 hours. The protection was provided by CD4$^+$ T cell response because vaccination protected CD8(-/-), but not CD4(-/-) mice.

Bacci A. et al. used RNA from *Candida albicans* to generate a DC-vaccine [9]. The RNA-transfected DCs expressed fungal mannoproteins on their surface, up-regulated expression of MHC-II and costimulatory molecules, secreted IL-12 and induced anti-fungal specific protective Th1 type immune resistance in mice [9, 138].

Analogous DC-vaccines were shown to induce an effective protective immunity in cases of protozoan infections with *Toxoplasma gondii* [16] and *Leishmania major* [188] as well as in cases of spiro-chetoses induced by *Borrelia burgdorferi* in mouse models [106]. The anti-infectious DC-vaccine also proved to be effective against viral infection of mice with the lymphocytic choriomeningitis virus (LCMV) [97].

Several research groups tried to apply DCs as more effective anti-tuberculosis vaccines. Demangel C. et al. introduced DCs infected with Bacillus Chalmette Guerin (BCG) into the mouse trachea [40]. As expected, the infected DCs appropriately matured *in vitro* and induced, the specific Th1-type immune response in the draining lymph nodes. However, the response was not higher than that induced by simple subcutaneous BCG vaccination. In their subsequent study, Demangel C. et al. utilized DCs producing more Th1-polarizing cytokine IL-12 because of the activation through CD40 binding to CD40L [41]. The CD40-stimulated BCG-infected mouse DCs displayed an increased capacity to release bioactive IL-12 and activate IFN-γ-producing T cells *in vitro*. However, although mice immunized with the DC vaccine demonstrated increased levels of type 1 cytokine production *in vivo*, the response did not increase lung resistance to intrapulmonary infection with the virulent *Mycobacterium tuberculosis*. Feng C. G. et al. employed, for mouse DC infection, a viral construct expressing the mycobacterial CD8$^+$ T cell peptide epitope [51]. The construct-infected DCs were more effective than BCG-infected DCs in activating antigen-specific CD8$^+$ T cells to secrete IFN-γ *in vitro* suggesting that the use of such peptide constructs might eventually be useful in genetic vaccines against *M. tuberculosis*.

We undertook a series of studies in order to determine the protective effect of DC-vaccines against *Klebsiella pneumoniae* (K2 strain) lethal infection employing a mouse model. The vaccine showed a very high protective efficiency. Depending on the immunization protocols and dose of bacteria per injection, 83%–100% of vaccinated animals survived, whereas in the control group of unvaccinated animals almost all the mice (80%–100%) died.

Akbar S. M. et al. have demonstrated a very high efficacy of vaccines based on DCs pulsed with the recombinant hepatitis B-virus antigen (HBsAg) in comparison to HBsAg-vaccination in the mouse model of chronic hepatitis B [1]. Subsequently they have shown the safety and efficiency of this approach for the treatment of humans with chronic hepatitis B [2]. This method might also be effectively used for the vaccination of non-responders to the HBsAg-vaccination.

Lu W. et al. showed, first in rhesus macaques infected with SIV (simian immun-odeficiency virus) [95] and subsequently in patients chronically infected with HIV [96], that DC vaccination induced robust T-cell responses in most vaccinees and that this correlated with a marked reduction in viral titres.

Thus, DC-vaccines might be of great help in protection against and even in treatment of infectious diseases that are not effectively prevented by contemporary vaccines.

8.4.3. New Approaches in Dendritic Cell-Based Vaccination

As discussed earlier, DC-based vaccines are safe and seem to have a great potential for protection against infectious diseases and probably even in cancer treatment. However, DC-vaccines are often not as effective as they should be. First of all, anti-cancer DC-vaccines turned out to be not as effective as we had hoped. Thus, there are numerous projects intending to improve DC-vaccine efficacy or develop new DC-based strategies.

Improving the maturation protocol is obviously a central challenge. The most widely used maturation protocol for the human monocyte-derived DCs consists of four reagents: TNF, IL-1β, IL-6, and PGE2, also known as monocyte-conditioned media mimic or cytokine cocktail. A recent phase III clinical trial (discussed earlier) failed to show that vaccinating melanoma patients with cytokine cocktail–matured DCs provided any benefit over standard DTIC chemotherapy [158]. It is not inconceivable that the suboptimal nature of the maturation conditions and hence the suboptimal immunogenicity of the DCs was a primary reason for the failure. It is tempting to speculate that the main culprit in the cytokine cocktail formula was PGE2. The rationale for including PGE2 in the maturation protocol is to endow the *ex vivo*–generated DCs with the capacity to migrate [98, 157] but PGE_2 in the context of the tumour microenvironment can mediate Th2 polarization and promote the differentiation of DCs secreting the immunosuppressive cytokine IL-10 [115]. Therefore, the key negative impact of PGE2 on the function of *ex vivo*–generated DCs is probably that PGE2 abolishes both the responsiveness of mature DCs to stimulation through CD40 and their ability to synthesize IL-12 when they reach the lymph node and encounter cognate T cells [157]. Sporri and Reis e Sousa have shown that the optimal activation of DCs requires TLR signalling, which this maturation protocol does not provide [171]. Moreover, a recent study comparing several maturation protocols found that cytokine cocktail–matured DCs were most effective,

even more than immature DCs, at expanding a population of immunosuppressive Treg cells expressing the forkhead box transcription factor FOXP3 [11].

As mentioned earlier, DC-vaccines should induce a CTL response as well as a Th response necessary for the effective initiation of CTL reactions [133]. Thus, when using peptides as a source of antigens for DC pulsing, investigators should use such peptides or their combinations that are presented to both CD8+ and CD4+ T cells. When peptides are used as antigens their compatibility with the patient's allelic types of MHC molecules must be taken into account as well. This problem is eliminated by using proteins, tumour lysates or killed tumour cells for DC pulsing. The cross-presentation involving presentation of exogenous antigens in the context with both MHC-I and –II molecules to CD8+ as well as to CD4+ T cells can be stimulated by the binding of TLR ligands to their specific TLRs on the DC surface [38]. The process of cross-presentation is also stimulated by the targeting of antigens to Fc-receptors using their complexes with antigen-specific antibodies [142].

The process of DC-vaccine preparation *in vitro* is difficult and expensive. Therefore, many scientists attempt to recruit DCs, load them with an antigen and induce their maturation *in vivo*. Chemokines, such as MIP-3β, may be used to attract DCs to the site of antigen injection [87]. *Ex vivo* derived immature DCs can be induced to mature *in situ* by a preceding injection of TLR agonists [122]. DCs that matured *in situ* were shown to be better inducers of anti-tumour immune response than those that matured *in vitro* [122]. This approach seems to be preferable to DC maturation *in vitro* because certain important cytokines, such as IL-12, are secreted only transiently after DC contact with inducers of maturation and then DCs are "exhausted" and are unable to secrete more IL-12 in response to interaction with antigen-specific T cells. Besides, the TLR-ligand treatment of sites of immature DC-injection may improve their survival and migration to lymph nodes. CpG-oligodeoxiribonucleotides, either injected at the same time with a protein antigen or conjugated with it, can induce DC maturation *in situ* [29, 110]. Belli F. et al. showed that the immunization of metastatic melanoma patients with the autologous tumour-derived heat shock protein gp-96-peptide complexes induced DC maturation *in situ*, initiated immune reactions and even led to positive clinical responses [12].

Kumagi T. et al. demonstrated that the injection of immature DCs into mouse tumour nodules necrotized by ethanol injection led to their regression and prolonged survival of the animals [86]. The authors associate the effect with anti-cancer immunity developing in response to necrotized tumour antigenic material processed by the DCs. The decrease of tumour size associated with massive leukocyte infiltration was observed by Triozzi P. L. et al., who injected immature DCs into metastatic nodules of cancer patients [184].

In addition, several rapid 2–3 day "fast-DC" protocols have been developed that generate DCs able to stimulate T-cell responses *in vitro* as effectively as DCs generated by standard protocols, which usually require 7–9 days of culture [39, 89, 155]. In a recently published clinical trial, HER2/neu-positive breast cancer patients vaccinated with peptide-loaded DCs generated in a 2 day culture of monocytes incubated with IFN-γ and LPS induced HER2/neu-specific CD4$^+$ and CD8$^+$ T cell responses and measurable decreases in tumour volume [35]. Importantly, *in vitro* analysis suggests that DCs generated in such a manner are mature, as judged by phenotypic analysis, and transiently secrete IL-12 but are not "exhausted" because they are able to respond to CD40 signalling by producing more IL-12 [35].

Some tumour cells, for example neuroblastoma and melanoma, hyperexpress gangliosides (non-peptide antigens). As it was demonstrated by Wu D. Y. et al., DCs were capable to present melanoma-specific ganglioside GD3 to NKT cells [198]. The data may be used for the development of an effective anti-tumour therapy.

The efficacy of DC-vaccines may be increased by the blocking of inhibitory molecules such as CTLA-4 (cytotoxic T lymphocyte-associated antigen) on the T-cell surface or by inhibiting Treg cells. It was shown that effects from anti-tumour vaccines, including DCs pulsed with tumour peptides, increased if CTLA-4 was blocked by inhibitory antibodies [70, 139, 185]. However, the approach induced severe autoimmune disorders in experimental animals and cancer patients. Treg cells may be inhibited or depleted by using cytotoxic antibody-conjugates to CD25 (IL-2R subunit constantly expressed by Treg cells) or IL-2-conjugates with cytotoxic molecules [133]. Tanaka H. et al. showed that lowly immunogenic mouse tumours decreased in size but did not completely disappear after the depletion of CD4$^+$CD25$^+$ Treg cells [179]. The immune responses to mature antigen-loaded DCs were enhanced in mice depleted from CD4$^+$CD25$^+$ Treg cells [131]. In a recent phase I/II clinical trial, Dannull et al. were able to show that partial removal of Treg cells can further increase DC-vaccine–induced immune responses in cancer patients [37]. The combination of Treg-cell depletion with CTLA-4 blockade synergistically enhances immune responses to an anti-tumour vaccine [177].

In conclusion, investigations of DCs and their interactions with other immune cells are of the greatest importance for developing effective DC-based vaccines as well as for improving the efficiency of conventional vaccines and vaccination protocols.

References

[1] Akbar S. M., Furukawa S., Hasebe A., Horiike N., Michitaka K., Onji M. (2004) Production and efficacy of dendritic cell-based vaccine for murine chronic hepatitis B virus carrier. Int. J. Mol. Med. 14: 295–299.

[2] Akbar S. M., Furukawa S., Onji M., Murata Y., Niva T., Kanno S., Murakami H., Horiike N. (2004) Safety and efficacy of hepatitis B surface antigen-pulsed dendritic cells in human volunteers. Hepatol. Res. 29: 136–141.

[3] Akhmatova N. K., Lebedinskaya O. V., Kiselevsky M. V., Makashin A. I., Semenova I. B., Kurbatova E. A., Egorova N. B., Semenov B. F. (2005) Influence of dendritic cells generated using immunomodulators of microbial origin on proliferative and cytotoxic activities of lymphocytes. JMEI 6: 58–62.

[4] Akhmatova N. K., Semenova I. B., Kurbatova E. A., Lebedinskaya O. V., Egorova N. B., Shubina I. J., Kiselevsky M. V. (2006) Phagocytic activity of dendritic cells generated from mouse bone marrow. Vestnik Ural'skoy medecinskoy akademicheskoi nauki. 1: 14–18 (Original text in Russian).

[5] Ardavin C., Wu L., Li C. L., Shortman K. (1993) Thymic dendritic cells and T cells develop simultaneously in the thymus from a common precursor population. Nature 362: 761–763.

[6] Ardavin C. (1997) Thymic dendritic cells. Immunol. Today 180: 350–361.

[7] Ardavin C., Martinez del Hoyo G., Martin P., Anjuere F., Arias C. F., Marin A. R., Ruiz S., Parrillas V., Hernandes H. (2001) Origin and differentiation of dendritic cells. Trends Immunol. 22: 691–700.

[8] Asselin-Paturel C., Boonstra A., Dalod M., Durand I., Yessand N., Dezutter-Dambuyant C., Vicari A., O'Garra A., Biron C., Briere F., Trinchieri G. (2001) Mouse type I IFN-producing cells are immature APCs with plasmacytoid morphology. Nat. Immunol. 2: 1144–1150.

[9] Bacci A., Montagnoli C., Perruccio K., Bozza S. Gaziano R., Pitzurra L., Velardi A., Fe' d'Ostiani C., Cutler J. E., Romani L. (2002) Dendritic cells pulsed with fungal RNA induce protective immunity to Candida albicans in hematopoietic transplantation. J. Immunol. 168: 2904–2913.

[10] Banchereau J., Steinman R. M. (1998) Dendritic cells and the control of immunity. Nature 392: 245–252.

[11] Banerjee D. K., Dhodapkar M. V., Matayeva E., Steinman R. M., Dhodapkar K. M. (2006) Expansion of FOXP3high regulatory T cells by human dendritic cells (DCs) in vitro and after injection of cytokine-matured DCs in myeloma patients. Blood 108: 2655–2661.

[12] Belli F., Testori A., Rivoltini L., Maio M., Andreola G., Sertoli M. R., Gallino G., Piris A., Cattelan A., Lazzari I., Carrabba M., Scita G., Santantonio C., Pilla L., Tragni G., Lombardo C., Arienti F., Marchiano A., Queirolo P., Bertolini F., Cova A., Lamaj E., Ascani L., Camerini R., Corsi M., Cascinelli N., Lewis J. J., Srivastava P., Parmiani G. (2002) Vaccination of metastatic melanoma patients with autologous tumor-derived heat shock protein gp96-peptide complexes: clinical and immunologic findings. J. Clin. Oncol. 20: 4169–4180.

[13] Bjorck P. (2001) Isolation and characterization of plasmacytoid dendritic cells from Flt3 ligand and granulocyte–macrophage colony-stimulating factor-treated mice. Blood 98: 3520–3526.

[14] Blom B., Ho S., Antonenko S., Liu Y. J. (2000) Generation of interferon-α-producing predendritic cell (Pre-DC)2 from human CD34+ hematopoietic stem cells. J. Exp. Med. 192: 1785–1795.

[15] Borkowskki T. A., Letterio J. J., Farr A. G., Udey M. C. (1996) A role for endogenous transforming growth factor β1 in Langerhans-cell biology: the skin of transforming growth factor β1 null mice is devoid of epidermal Langerhans cells. J. Exp. Med. 184: 2417–2422.

[16] Bourguin I., Moser M., Buzoni-Gatel D., Tielemans F., Bout D., Urbain J., Leo O. (1998) Murine dendritic cells pulsed in vitro with Toxoplasma gondii antigens induce protective immunity in vivo. Infect Immun. 66: 4867–4874.

[17] Brasel K., De Smedt T., Smith J. L., Maliszewski C. R. (2000) Generation of murine dendritic cells from flt3-ligand-supplemented bone marrow cultures. Blood 96: 3029–3039.

[18] Bruder D., Westendorf A. M., Hansen W., Prettin S., Grubber A. D., Qian Y., von Boehmer H., Mahnke K., Buer J. (2005) T-cell stimulation by steady-state dendritic cells

prevents autoimmune diabetes. Diabetes 54: 3395–3401.

[19] Caldwell S., Heitger A., Shen W., Liu Y., Taylor B., Ladisch S. (2003) Mechanisms of ganglioside inhibition of APC function. J. Immunol. 171: 1676–1683.

[20] Cao W., Lee S. H., Lu J. (2005) CD83 is preformed inside monocytes, macrophages and dendritic cells, but it is only stably expressed on activated dendritic cells. Biochem. J. 385: 85–93.

[21] Caux C., Massacrier C., Dezutter-Dambuyant C., Vanbervilet B., Jaquet C., Schmitt D., Banchereau J. (1995) Human dendritic Langerhans cells generated *in vitro* from CD34$^+$ progenitors can prime naive CD4$^+$ T cells and process soluble antigen. J. Immunol. 155: 5427–5435.

[22] Caux C., Vanbervilet B., Massacrier C., Dezutter-Dambuyant C., de Saint-Vis B., Jaquet C., Yoneda K., Imamura S., Schmitt D., Banchereau J. (1996) CD34$^+$ hematopoietic progenitors from human cord blood differentiate along two independent dendritic cell pathways in response to GM-CSF + TNFα. J. Exp. Med. 184: 695–706.

[23] Cella M., Engering A., Pinet V., Pietras T., Lanzavecchia A. (1997) Inflammatory stimuli induce accumulation of MHC class II complexes on dendritic cells. Nature 388: 782–787.

[24] Chan C. W., Crafton E., Fan H. N., Flook J., Yoshimura K., Skarica M., Brokstedt D., Dubensky T. W., Stins M. F., Lanier L. L., Pardoll D. M., Housseau F. (2006) Interferon-producing killer dendritic cells provide a link between innate and adaptive immunity. Nat. Med. 12: 207–213.

[25] Chen L., Calomeni E., Wen J., Ozato K., Shen R., Gao J.-X. (2007) Natural killer dendritic cells are an intermediate of developing dendritic cells. J. Leukoc. Biol. 81: 1422–1433.

[26] Chen Z., Dehm S., Bonham K., Kamencic H., Juurlink B., Zhang X., Gordon J. R., Xiang J. S. (2001) DNA array and biological characterization of the impact of the maturation status of mouse dendritic cells on their phenotype and antitumor vaccination efficacy. Cell Immunol. 214: 60–71.

[27] Chikileva I. O., Khalturina E. O., Mazurov D. V., Lvov V. A., Shmigol V. I., Aparin P. G., Shingarova L. N., Vasilenko R. N., Abramov V. M.,

Danenko F. V., Kiselevsky M. V. (2003) Effect of different types of bacterial lipopolysaccharide on the differentiation of human dendritic cells. Mol. Med. 3: 54–58 (Original text in Russian).

[28] Cho B. K. (2000) A proposed mechanism for the induction of cytotoxic T lymphocyte production by heat shock fusion proteins. Immunity 12: 263–272.

[29] Cho H. J., Takabayashi K., Cheng P. M., Nguyen M. D., Corr M., Tuck S., Raz E. (2000) Immunostimulatory DNA-based vaccines induce cytotoxic lymphocyte activity by a T-helper cell-independent mechanism. Nat. Biotechnol. 18: 509–514.

[30] Chomarat P., Dantin C., Bennett L., Banchereau J., Palucka A. K. (2003) TNF skews monocyte differentiation from macrophages to dendritic cells. J. Immunol. 171: 2262–2269.

[31] Colic M., Mojsilovic S., Pavlovic B., Vucicevic D., Majstrovic I., Bufan B., Stojic-Vukanic Z., Vasiljic S., Vucevic D., Gasic S., Balint B. (2004) Comparison of two different protocols for the induction of maturation of human dendritic cells *in vitro*. Vojnosanit. Pregl. 61: 471–478.

[32] Comeau M. R., Van der Vuurst de Vries A.-R., Maliszewski C. R., Galibert L. (2002) CD123^{bright} plasmacitoid predendritic cells: progenitors undergoing cell fate conversion ? J. Immunol. 169: 75–83.

[33] Corinti S., Albanesi C., La Sala A., Pastore S., Girolomoni G. (2001) Regulatory activity of autocrine IL-10 on dendritic cell functions. J. Immunol. 166: 4312–4318.

[34] Crawford K., Gabuzda D., Pantazopoulos V., Xu J., Clement C., Reinherz E., Alper C. A. (1999) Circulating CD2$^+$ monocytes are dendritic cells. J. Immunol. 163: 5920–5928.

[35] Czerniecki B. J., Koski G. K., Koldovsky U., Xu S., Cohen P. A., Mick R., Nisenbaum H., Pasha T., Xu M., Fox K. R., Weinstein S., Orel S. G., Vonderheide R., Coukos G., DeMichele A., Araujo L., Spitz F. R., Rosen M., Levine B. L., June C., Zhang P. J. (2007) Targeting HER-2/neu in early breast cancer development using dendritic cells with staged interleukin-12 burst secretion. Cancer Res. 67: 1842–1852.

[36] Dalloul A. H., Patry C., Salamero J., Canque B., Grassi F., Schmitt C. (1999) Functional and phenotypic analysis of thymic CD34$^+$CD1a$^-$

progenitor-derived dendritic cells: predominance of CD1a$^+$ differentiation pathway. J. Immunol. 162: 5821–5828.

[37] Dannull J., Su Z., Rizzieri D., Yang B. K., Coleman D., Yancey D., Zhang A., Dahm P., Chao N., Gilboa E., Vieweg J. (2005) Enhancement of vaccine-mediated antitumor immunity in cancer patients after depletion of regulatory T cells. J. Clin. Invest. 115: 3623–33.

[38] Datta S. K., Redecke V., Prilliman K. R., Takabayashi K., Corr M., Tallant T., DiDonato J., Dziraski J., Akira S., Schoenberger S. P., Raz E. (2003) A subset of Toll-like receptor ligands induces cross-presentation by bone marrow-derived dendritic cells. J. Immunol. 170: 4102–4110.

[39] Dauer M., Obermaier B., Herten J., Haerle C., Pohl K., Rothenfusser S., Schnurr M., Endres S., Eigler A. (2003) Mature dendritic cells derived from human monocytes within 48 hours: a novel strategy for dendritic cell differentiation from blood precursors. J. Immunol. 170: 4069–4076.

[40] Demangel C., Bean A. G., Martin E., Feng C. G., Kamath A. T., Britton W. J. (1999) Protection against aerosol *Mycobacterium tuberculosis* infection using *Mycobacterium bovis Bacillus Calmette Guerin*-infected dendritic cells. Eur. J. Immunol. 29: 1972–1979.

[41] Demangel C., Palendira U., Feng C. G., Heath A. W., Bean A. G., Britton W. J. (2001) Stimulation of dendritic cells via CD40 enhances immune responses to *Mycobacterium tuberculosis* infection. Infect. Immunol. 69: 2456–2461.

[42] Dhodapkar M. V., Steinman R. M., Sapp M., Desai H., Fossella C., Krasovsky J., Donahoe S. M., Dunbar P. R., Cerundolo V., Nixon D. F., Bhardwaj N. (1999) Rapid generation of broad T-cell immunity in humans after a single injection of mature dendritic cells. J. Clin. Invest. 104: 173–180.

[43] Dhodapkar M. V., Bhardwaj N. (2000) Active immunization of humans with dendritic cells. J. Clin. Immunol. 20: 167–173.

[44] Dhodapkar M. V., Steinman R. M., Krasovsky J., Munz C., Bhardwaj N. (2001) Antigen-specific inhibition of effector T cell function in humans after injection of immature dendritic cells. J. Exp. Med. 193: 233–238.

[45] Dhodapkar M. V., Steinman R. M. (2002) Antigen-bearing immature dendritic cells induce peptide specific CD8$^+$ regulatory T cells *in vivo* in humans. Blood 100: 174–177.

[46] Dzionek A., Fuchs A., Schmidt P., Cremer S., Zysk M., Miltenyi S., Buck D. W., Schmitz J. (2000) BDCA2, BDCA3, and BDCA4: three markers for distinct subsets of dendritic cells in human peripheral blood. J. Immunol. 165: 6037–6046.

[47] Dzionek A., Sohma Y., Nagafune J., Cella M., Colonna M., Facchetti F., Günther G., Johnston I., Lanzavecchia A., Nagasaka T., Okada T., Vermi W., Winkels G., Yamamoto T., Zysk M., Yamaguchi Y., Schmitz J. (2001) BDCA-2, a novel plasmacytoid dendritic cell-specific type II C-type lectin, mediates antigen capture and is a potent inhibitor of interferon α/ß induction. J. Exp. Med. 194: 1823–1834.

[48] Dzionek A., Inagaki Y., Okawa K., Nagafune J., Rock J., Sohma Y., Winkels G., Zysk M., Yamaguchi Y., Schmitz J. (2002) Plasmacytoid dendritic cells: from specific surface markers to specific cellular functions. Hum. Immunol. 63: 1133–1148.

[49] Ebner S., Ratzinger G., Krosbacher B., Schmuth M., Weiss A., Reider D., Kroczek R. A., Herold M., Heufler C., Fritsch P., Romani N. (2001) Production of IL-12 by human monocyte-derived dendritic cells is optimal when the stimulus is given at the onset of maturation and is further enhanced by IL-4. J. Immunol. 166: 633–641.

[50] Ebner S., Hofer S., Nguyen V. A., Furhapter C., Herold M., Fritsch P., Heufler C., Romani N. (2002) A novel role for IL-3: human monocytes cultured in the presence of IL-3 and IL-4 differentiate into dendritic cells that produce less IL-12 and shift Th cell responses toward a Th2 cytokine pattern. J. Immunol. 168: 6199–6207.

[51] Feng C. G., Demangel C., Kamath A. T., Macdonald M., Britton W. J. (2001) Dendritic cells infected with *Mycobacterium bovis Calmette Guerin* activate CD8$^+$ T cells with specificity for a novel mycobacterial epitope. Int. Immunol. 13: 451–458.

[52] Ferlazzo G., Wesa A., Wei W. Z., Guli A. (1999) Dendritic cells generated from CD34+ progenitor cells or from monocytes differ in their ability to activate antigen-specific CD8+ T cells. J. Immunol. 163: 3597.

[53] Ferlazzo G., Münz C. (2004) NK cell compartments and their activation by dendritic cells. J. Immunol. 172: 1333–1339.

[54] Ferlazzo G., Pack M., Thomas D., Paludan C., Schmid D., Strowig T., Bougras G., Muller W. A., Moretta L., Münz C. (2004) Distinct roles of IL-12 and IL-15 in human natural killer cell activation by dendritic cells from secondary lymphoid organs. Proc. Natl. Acad. Sci. U.S.A. 101: 16606–16611.

[55] Fong L., Brockstedt D., Benike C., Engeman E. G. (2001) Dendritic cells injected via different routes induce immunity in cancer patients. J. Immunol. 166: 4254–4259.

[56] Foss F. M. (2002) Immunologic mechanisms of antitumor activity. Semin Oncol. 29: 5–11.

[57] Fujii S., Shimizu K., Hemmi H., Fukui M., Bonito A. J., Chen G., Franck R. W., Tsuji M., Steinman R. M. (2006) Glycolipid α-C-galactosylceramide is a distinct inducer of dendritic cell function during innate and adaptive immune responses of mice. Proc. Natl. Acad. Sci. U.S.A. 103: 11252–11257.

[58] Galy A., Travis M., Cen D., Chen B. (1995) Human T, B, natural killer, and dendritic cells arise from a common bone marrow progenitor cell subset. Immunity 3: 459–473.

[59] Geiger J., Hutchinson R., Hohenkirk L., McKenna E., Chang A., Mule J. (2000) Treatment of solid tumors in children with tumor-lysate-pulsed dendritic cells. Lancet 356: 1163–1165.

[60] Gilboa E. (2007) DC-based cancer vaccines. J. Clin. Invest. 117: 1195–1203.

[61] Girolomoni G., Caux C., Dezutter-Dambuyant C., Lebecque C., Ricciardi-Castagnoli P. (2002) Langerhans cells: still a fundamental paradigm for studying the immunobiology of dendritic cells. Trends Immunol. 23: 6–8.

[62] Granelli-Piperno A., Pritsker A., Pack M., Shimelovich I., Arrighi J.-F., Park C. G., Trumpfheller C., Piguet V., Moran T. M., Steinman R. M. (2005) Dendritic cell-specific intercellular adhesion molecule 3-grabbing nonintegrin/CD209 is abundant on macrophages in the normal human lymph node and is not required for dendritic cell stimulation of the mixed leucocyte reaction. J. Immunol. 175: 4265–4273.

[63] Grouard G., Rissoan M.-C., Filgueira L., Durand I., Banchereau J., Liu Y.-J. (1997) The enigmatic plasmacytoid T cells develop into dendritic cells with IL-3 and CD40 ligand. J. Exp. Med. 185: 1101–1111.

[64] Hanna J., Gonen-Gros T., Fitchett J., Rowe T., Daniels M., Arnon T. I., Gazit R., Joseph A., Schjetne K. W., Steinle A., Porgador A., Mevorach D., Goldman-Wohl D., Yagel S., LaBarre M. J., Buckner J. H., Mandelboim O. (2004) Novel APC-like properties of human NK cells directly regulate T cell activation. J. Clin. Invest. 114: 1612–1623.

[65] Hart D. N. J. (1997) Dendritic cells: unique leukocyte populations which control the primary immune response. Blood 90: 3245–3287.

[66] Hasebe H., Nagayama H., Sato K., Enomoto M., Takeda Y., Takahashi T. A., Hasumi K., Eriguchi M. (2000) Dysfunctional regulation of the development of monocyte-derived dendritic cells in cancer patients. Biomed. Pharmacother. 54: 291–298.

[67] Heiser A., Coleman D., Dannull J., Yancey D., Maurice M. A., Lallas C. D., Dahm P., Niedzwiecki D., Gilboa E., Vieweg J. (2002) Autologous dendritic cells transfected with prostate-specific antigen RNA stimulate CTL responses against metastatic prostate tumors. J. Clin. Invest. 109: 409–417.

[68] Hemmi H., Kaisho T., Takeuchi O., Sato S., Sanjo H., Hoshino K., Horiuchi T., Tomizawa H., Takeda K., Akira S. (2002) Small antiviral compounds activate immune cells via the TLR7 MyD88-dependent signaling pathway. Nat. Immunol. 3: 196–200.

[69] Hochrein H., O'Keeffe M., Luft T., Vandenabele S., Grumont R. J., Maraskovsky E., Shortman K. (2000) Interleukin(IL)-4 is a major regulatory cytokine governing bioactive IL-12 production by mouse and human dendritic cells. J. Exp. Med. 192: 823–834.

[70] Hodi F. S., Mihm M. C., Soiffer R. J., Haluska F. G., Butler M., Seiden M. V., Davis T., Henry-Spires R., MacRae S., Willman A., Padera R., Jaklitsch M. T., Shankar S., Chen T. C., Korman A., Allison J. P., Dranoff G. (2003) Biologic activity of cytotoxic T lymphocyte-associated antigen 4 antibody blockade in previously vaccinated melanoma and ovarian carcinoma patients. Proc. Natl. Acad. Sci. U.S.A. 100: 4712–4717.

[71] Homann D., Jahreis A., Wolfe T., Hughes A., Coon B., van Stipdonk M. J., Prilliman K. R., Schoenberger S. P., von Herrath M. G. (2002) CD40L blockade prevents autoimmune diabetes

152   I.O. Chikileva et al.

by induction of bitypic NK/DC regulatory cells. Immunity 16: 403–415.

[72] Homma S., Toda G., Gong J., Kufe D., Ohno T. (2001) Preventive antitumor activity against hepatocellular carcinoma (HCC) induced by immunization with fusions of dendritic cells and HCC cells in mice. J. Gastroenterol. 36: 764–771.

[73] Hsu F. J., Benike C., Fagnoni F., Liles T. M., Czerwinski D., Taidi B., Englemann E. G., Levy R. (1996) Vaccination of patients with B-cell lymphoma using autologous antigen-pulsed dendritic cells. Nature 392: 245–252.

[74] Hunger R. E., Sieling P. A., Ochoa M. T., Sugaya M., Burdick A. E., Rea T. H., Brennan P. J., Belisle J. T., Blauvelt A., Porcelli S. A., Modlin R. L. (2004) Langerhans cells utilize CD1a and langerin to efficiently present nonpeptide antigens to T cells. J. Clin. Invest. 113: 701–708.

[75] Inaba K., Steinman R. M. (1986) Accessory cell – T lymphocyte interactions. Antigen dependent and independent clustering. J. Exp. Med. 163: 247–261.

[76] Jaksits S., Kriehuber E., Charbonnier A. S., Rappersberger K., Stingl G., Maurer D. (1999) CD34+ cell-derived CD14+ precursor cells develop into Langerhans cells in a TGF-β 1-dependent manner. J. Immunol. 163: 4869–4877.

[77] Jefford M., Maraskovsky E., Cebon J., Davis I. D. (2001) The use of dendritic cells in cancer therapy. Lancet Oncol. 2: 343–353.

[78] Jonuleit H., Giesecke-Tuettenberg A., Tuting T., Thurner-Schuler B., Stuge T. B., Paragnik L., Kandemir A., Lee P. P., Knop J., Enk A. H. (2001) A comparison of two types of dendritic cell as adjuvants for the induction of melanoma-specific T-cell responses in humans following intranodal injection. Int. J. Cancer 93: 243–251.

[79] Kadowaki N., Antonenko S., Lau J. Y.-N., Liu Y.-J. (2000) Natural interferon-α/β-producing cells link innate and adaptive immunity. J. Exp. Med. 192: 219–226.

[80] Keller R. (2001) Dendritic cells: their significance in health and disease. Immunol. Lett. 78: 113–122.

[81] Kelly K. A., Lucas K., Hochrein H., Metcalf D., Wu L., Shortman K. (2001) Development of dendritic cells in culture from human and murine thymic precursor cells. Cell Mol. Biol. (Noisy-le-grand). 47: 43–54.

[82] Khalturina E. O., Lebedinskaya O. V., Shubina I. J., Donenko F. V., Raihlin N. T., Kiselevsky M. V. (2004) Morphological features and immunophenotype of human monocyte-derived dendritic cells. Morphology 3: 89–92.

[83] Kohrgruber N., Halanek N., Groger M., Winter D., Rappersberger K., Schmitt-Egenolf M., Stingl G., Maurer D. (1999) Survival, maturation and function of CD11c− and CD11c+ peripheral blood dendritic cells are differentially regulated by cytokines. J. Immunol. 163: 3250–3259.

[84] Koski G. K., Lyakh L. A., Rice N. R. (2001) Rapid lipopolysaccharide-induced differentiation of CD14(+) monocytes into CD83(+) dendritic cells is modulated under serum-free conditions by exogenously added IFN-γ and endogenously produced IL-10. Eur. J. Immunol. 31: 3773–3781.

[85] Krug A., Towarowski A., Britsch S., Rothenfusser S., Hornung V., Bals R., Giese T., Engelmann H., Endres S., Krieg A. M., Hartmann G. (2001) Toll-like receptor expression reveals CpG DNA as a unique microbial stimulus for plasmacytoid dendritic cells which synergizes with CD40 ligand to induce high amounts of IL-12. Eur. J. Immunol. 31: 3026–3037.

[86] Kumagi T., Akbar S. M., Horiike N., Onji M. (2003) Increased survival and decreased tumor size due to intratumoral injection of ethanol followed by administration of immature dendritic cells. Int. J. Oncol. 23: 949–955.

[87] Kumamoto T., Huang E. K., Paek H. J., Morita A., Matsue H., Valentini R. F., Takashima A. (2002) Induction of tumor-specific protective immunity by *in situ* Langerhans cell vaccine. Nat. Biotechnol. 20: 64–69.

[88] Langerhans P. (1868) Ueber die nerven der menschlichen haut. Archiv für pathologische Anatomie und Physiologie, und für Klinische Medicin. Berlin 44: 325–337.

[89] Lapenta C., Santini S. M., Spada M., Donati S., Urbani F., Accapezzato D., Franceschini D., Andreotti M., Barnaba V., Belardelli F. (2006) IFN-alpha-conditioned dendritic cells are highly efficient in inducing cross-priming CD8(+) T cells against exogenous viral antigens. Eur. J. Immunol. 36: 2046–2060.

[90] Lappin M. B., Weiss J. M., Delattre V., Mai B., Dittmar H., Maier C., Manke K.,

Grabbe S., Martin S., Simon J. C. (1999) Analysis of mouse dendritic cell migration *in vivo* upon subcutaneous and intravenous injection. Immunology 98: 181–188.

[91] Lebedinskaya O. V., Akhmatova N. K., Kiselevsky M. V. (2005) The comparative characteristics of morphological and phenotypic features of mouse dendritic cells generated from bone-marrow precursors or embryonic liver. Materials of Russian Scientific Conference "Actual problems of theoretical and clinical medicine". Perm'; GOU VPO PGMA Roszdrava: 21–24.

[92] Leon B., Martinez del Hoyo G., Parrillas V., Hernandez Vargas H., Sanchez-Mateos P., Longo N., Lopez-Bravo M., Ardavin C. (2004) Dendritic cell differentiation potential of mouse monocytes: monocytes represent immediate precursors of $CD8^-$ and $CD8^+$ splenic dendritic cells. Blood 103: 2668–2676.

[93] Levine T. P., Chain B. M. (1992) Endocytosis by antigen presenting cells : dendritic cells are as endocytically active as other antigen presenting cells. Proc. Natl. Acad. Sci. U.S.A. 89: 8342–8346.

[94] Lipscomb M. F., Masten B. J. (2002) Dendritic cells: immune regulators in health and disease. Physiol. Rev. 82: 97–130.

[95] Lu W., Wu X., Lu Y., Guo W., Andrieu J. M. (2003) Therapeutic dendritic-cell vaccine for simian AIDS. Nat. Med. 9: 27–32.

[96] Lu W., Arraes L. C., Ferreira W. T., Andrieu J. M. (2004) Therapeutic dendritic-cell vaccine for chronic HIV-1 infection. Nat. Med. 10: 1359–1365.

[97] Ludewig B., Ehl S., Karrer U., Odermatt B., Hengartner H., Zinkernagel R. (1998) Dendritic cells efficiently induce protective antiviral immunity. J. Virol. 72: 3812–3818.

[98] Luft T., Jefford M., Luetjens P., Toy T., Hochrein H., Masterman K.-A., Maliszewski C., Shortman K., Cebon J., Maraskovsky E. (2002) Functionally distinct dendritic cell (DC) populations induced by physiologic stimuli: prostaglandin E2 regulates the migratory capacity of specific DC subsets. Blood 100: 1362–1372.

[99] Lutz M. B., Kukutsch N., Oglivie A. L., Rössner S., Koch F., Romani N., Schuler G. (1999) An advanced culture method for generating large quantities of highly pure dendritic cells from mouse bone marrow. J. Immunol. Methods 223: 77–92.

[100] Lyakh L. A., Koski G. K., Telford W., Gress R. E., Cohen P. A., Rice N. R. (2000) Bacterial lipopolysaccharide, TNF-α, and calcium ionophore under serum-free conditions promote rapid dendritic cell-like differentiation in $CD14^+$ monocytes through distinct pathways that activate NF-κB. J. Immunol. 165: 3647–55.

[101] MacDonald K. P. A., Munster D. J., Clark G. J., Dzionek A., Schmitz J., Hart D. N. J. (2002) Characterization of human blood dendritic cell subsets. Blood 100: 4512–4520.

[102] Mailliard R. B., Alber S. M., Shen H., Watkins S. C., Kirkwood J. M., Herberman R. B., Kalinski P. (2005) IL-18-induced $CD83^+C$ $CCR7^+$ NK helper cells. J. Exp. Med. 202: 941–953.

[103] Marquez C., Trigueros C., Fernandez E., Toribio M. L. (1995) The development of T and non-T cell lineages from $CD34^+$ human thymic precursors can be traced by the differential expression of CD44. J. Exp. Med. 181: 475–483.

[104] Martin P., del Hoyo G. M., Anjuerre F., Ruiz S. R., Arias S. F., Marin A. R., Ardavin C. (2000) Concept of lymphoid versus myeloid dendritic cell lineages revisited: booth $CD8\alpha^+$ and $CD8\alpha^-$ dendritic cells are generated from $CD4^{low}$ lymphoid-committed precursors. Blood 96: 2511–2519.

[105] Mayordomo J. I., Zorina T., Storkus W. J., Zitvogel L., Celluzzi C., Falo L. D., Melief C. J., Ildstad S. T., Kast W. M., Deleo A. B. (1995) Bone marrow-derived dendritic cells pulsed with synthetic tumour peptides elicit protective and therapeutic antitumour immunity. Nat Med. 12: 1297–1302.

[106] Mbow M., Zeidner N., Panella N., Titus R., Piesman J. (1997) Borrelia burgdoferi-pulsed dendritic cells induce a protective immune response against tick-transmitted spirochets. Infect. Immunol . 65: 3386–3390.

[107] McKenna K., Beignon A.-S., Bhardwaj N. (2005) Plasmacytoid dendritic cells: linking innate and adaptive immunity. J. Virol. 79: 17–27.

[108] Menetrier-Caux C., Thomachot M. C., Alberti L., Montamin G., Blay J. Y. (2001) IL-4 prevents the blockade of dendritic cell differentiation induced by tumor cells. Cancer Res. 61: 3096–3104.

[109] Menges M., Baumeister T., Rössner S., Stoitzner P., Romani N., Gessner A., Lutz M. B.

(2005) IL-4 supports the generation of a dendritic cell subset from murine bone marrow with altered endocytosis capacity. J. Leucoc. Biol. 77: 535–543.

[110] Merad M., Sugie T., Engleman E. G., Fong L. (2002) In vivo manipulation of dendritic cells to induce therapeutic immunity. Blood 99: 1676–1682.

[111] Metcalf D. (1997) Murine hematopoietic stem cells committed to macrophage dendritic cell formation: stimulation by Flk2 ligand with enhancement by regulators using the gp130 receptor chain. Proc. Natl. Acad. Sci. U.S.A. 94: 11552–11556.

[112] Metlay J. P., Puré E., Steinman R. M. (1989) Distinct features of dendritic cells and anti-Ig activated B cells as stimulators of the primary mixed leukocyte reaction. J. Exp. Med. 169: 239–254.

[113] Mizumoto N., Takashima A. (2004) CD1a and langerin: acting as more than Langerhans cell markers. J. Clin. Invest. 113: 658–660.

[114] Morel P. A., Feili-Hariri M. (2001) How do dendritic cells prevent autoimmunity? Trends Immunol. 22: 546–547.

[115] Morelli A. E., Thomson A. W. (2003) Dendritic cells under the spell of prostaglandins. Trends Immunol. 24: 108–111.

[116] Morse M. A., Vredenburgh J. J., Lyerly H. K. (1999) A comparative study of the generation of dendritic cells from mobilized peripheral blood progenitor cells of patients undergoing high dose chemotherapy. J. Hematother. Stem Cell Res. 8: 577–584.

[117] Morse M. A., Coleman R. E., Akabani G., Niehaus N., Coleman D., Lyerly H. K. (1999) Migration of human dendritic cells after injection in patients with metastatic malignancies. Cancer Res. 59: 56–58.

[118] Mortarini R., Anichini A. (1997) Autologous dendritic cells derived from CD34+ progenitors and from monocytes are not functionally equivalent antigen-presenting cells in the induction of melan-A/MART-127–35-specific CTLs from peripheral blood lymphocytes of melanoma patients with low frequency of CTL precursors. Cancer Res. 57: 5534.

[119] Mosca P. J., Lyerly H. K., Clay T. M., Morse M. A., Lyerly H. K. (2007) Dendritic cell vaccines. Front Biosci. 12: 4050–4060.

[120] Mullins D. W., Sheasley S. L., Ream R. M., Bullock T. N., Fu Y. X., Engelhard V. H. (2003) Route of immunization with peptide- pulsed dendritic cells controls the distribution of memory and effector T-cells in lymphoid tissues and determines the pattern of regional tumor control. J. Exp. Med. 198: 1023–1034.

[121] Nair S. K., Morse M., Boczkowski D., Cumming R. I., Vasovic L., Gilboa E., Lyerly H. K. (2002) Induction of tumor-specific cytotoxic T lymphocytes in cancer patients by autologous tumor RNA-transfected dendritic cells. Ann. Surg. 235: 540–549.

[122] Nair S., McLaughlin C., Weizer A., Su Z., Boczkowski D., Dannull J., Vieweg J., Gilboa E. (2003) Injection of immature dendritic cells into adjuvant-treated skin obviates the need for ex vivo maturation. J. Immunol. 171: 6272–6285.

[123] Nakamura I., Kajino K., Bamba H., Itoh F., Takikita M., Ogasawara K. (2004) Phenotypic stability of mature dendritic cells tuned by TLR or CD40 to control the efficiency of cytotoxic T cell priming. Microbiol. Immunol. 48: 211–219.

[124] Nakano H., Yanagita M., Gunn M. D. (2001) CD11c$^+$B220$^+$Gr-1$^+$ cells in mouse lymph nodes and spleen display characteristics of plasmacytoid dendritic cells. J. Exp. Med. 194: 1171–1178.

[125] Nelson E. L., Strobl S., Subleski J., Prieto D., Kopp W. C., Nelson P. J. (1999) Cycling of human dendritic cell effector phenotypes in response to TNFα: modification of the current "maturation" paradigm and implications for in vivo immunoregulation. FASEB J. 13: 2021–2030.

[126] Nencioni A., Brossart P. (2004) Cellular immunotherapy with dendritic cells in cancer: current status. Stem Cells 22: 501–513.

[127] Nestle F. O., Alijagic S., Gilliet M., Sun Y., Grabbe S., Dummer R., Burg G., Schadendorf D. (1996) Vaccination of melanoma patients with peptide- or tumor lysate-pulsed dendritic cells. Nature Med. 2: 328–332.

[128] Nouri-Shirazi M., Banchereau J., Fay J., Palucka K. (2000) Dendritic cell based tumor vaccines. Immunol. Lett. 74: 5–10.

[129] O'Keefe M., Hochrein H., Vremec D., Pooley J., Evans R., Woulfe S., Shortman K. (2002) Effects of administration of progeniopoietin 1, Flt-3 ligand, granulocyte colony-stimulating factor, and pegylated granulocyte–macrophage colony-stimulating factor on

dendritic cell subsets in mice. Blood 99: 2122–2130.

[130] O'Keefe M., Hochrein H., Vremec D., Scott B., Hertzog P., Tatarczuch L., Shortman K. (2003) Dendritic cell precursor populations of mouse blood: identification of the murine homologues of human blood plasmacytoid pre-DC2 and CD11c$^+$ DC1 precursors. Blood 101: 1453–1459.

[131] Oldenhove G., de Heusch M., Urbain-Vansanten G., Urbain J., Maliszewski C., Leo O., Moser M. (2003) CD4$^+$CD25$^+$ regulatory T cells control T helper cell type 1 responses to foreign antigens induced by mature dendritic cells *in vivo*. J. Exp. Med. 198: 259–266.

[132] Olweus J., BitMansour A., Warnke R., Thompson P. A., Carballido J., Picker L. J., Lund-Johansen F. (1997) Dendritic cell ontogeny: a human dendritic cell lineage of myeloid origin. Proc. Natl. Acad. Sci. U.S.A. 94: 12551–12556.

[133] O'Neill D. W., Adams S., Bhardwaj N. (2004) Manipulating dendritic cell biology for the active immunotherapy of cancer. Blood 104: 2235–2246.

[134] Palucka K. A., Taquet N., Sanchez-Chapuis F., Gluckman J. C. (1998) Dendritic cells as the terminal stage of monocyte differentiation. J. Immunol. 160: 4587–4595.

[135] Parmiani G., Castelli C., Dalerba P., Mortarini R., Rivoltini L., Marincola F. M., Anichini A. (2002) Cancer immunotherapy with peptide-based vaccines: what have we achieved? Where are we going? J. Natl. Cancer Inst. 94: 805–818.

[136] Paschenkov M. V., Pinegin B. V. (2001) Major properties of dendritic cells. Immunology 22: 7–16 (Original text in Russian).

[137] Peguet-Navarro J., Sportouch M., Popa I., Berthier O., Schmitt D., Portoukalian J. (2003) Gangliosides from human melanoma tumors impair dendritic cell differentiation from monocytes and induce their apoptosis. J. Immunol. 170: 3488–3494.

[138] Perruccio K., Bozza S., Montagnoli C., Bellocchio S., Aversa F., Martelli M., Bistoni F., Velardi A., Romani L. (2004) Prospects for dendritic cell vaccination against fungal infections in hematopoetic transplantation. Blood Cell Mol. Dis. 33: 248–255.

[139] Phan G. Q., Yang J. C., Sherry R. M., Hwu P., Topalian S. L., Schwartzentruber D. J., Restifo N. P., Haworth L. R., Seipp C. A., Freezer L. J., Morton K. E., Mavroukakis S. A., Duray P. H., Steinberg S. M., Allison J. P., Davis T. A., Rosenberg S. A. (2003) Cancer regression and autoimmunity induced by cytotoxic T lymphocyte-associated antigen 4 blockade in patients with metastatic melanoma. Proc. Natl. Acad. Sci. U.S.A. 100: 8372–8377.

[140] Piemonti L., Monti P., Zerbi A., Balzano G., Allavena P., Di Carlo V. (2000) Generation and functional characterization of dendritic cells from patients with pancreatic carcinoma with special regard to clinical applicability. Cancer Immunol. Immunother. 49: 544–550.

[141] Pillarisetty V. G., Katz S. C., Bleier J. I., Shah A. B., DeMatteo R. P. (2005) Natural killer dendritic cells have both antigen presenting and lytic function in response to CpG produce IFN-γ via autocrine IL-12. J. Immunol. 174: 2612–2618.

[142] Rafiq Q., Bergtold A., Clynes R. (2002) Immune complex mediated antigen presentation induces tumor immunity. J. Clin. Invest. 110; 71–79.

[143] Randollph G. J., Beaulieu S., Lebecque S., Steinman R. M., Muller W. A. (1998) Differentiation of monocytes into dendritic cells in a model of transendothelial trafficking. Science 282: 480–483.

[144] Randollph G. J., Inaba K., Robbiani D. F., Steinman R. M., Muller W. A. (1999) Differentiation of phagocytic monocytes into lymph node dendritic cells *in vivo*. Immunity 11: 753–761.

[145] Res P. C., Martinez-Caseres E., Cristina Jaleco A., Staal F., Noteboom E., Weijer K., Spits H. (1996) CD34$^+$CD38^{dim} cells in the human thymus can differentiate into T, natural killer, and dendritic cells but are distinct from pluriopotent stem cells. Blood 87: 5196–5206.

[146] Res P. C., Couwenberg F., Vyth-Dreese F. A., Spits H. (1999) Expression of pTα mRNA in a committed dendritic cell precursor in the human thymus. Blood 94: 2647–2657.

[147] Rey-Ladino J., Koochesfahani K., Zaharik M., Shen C., Brunham R. (2005) A live and inactivated *Chlamydia trachomatis* mouse pneumonitis strain induces the maturation of dendritic cells that are phenotypically and immunologically distinct. Infect Immunol. 73: 1568–1577.

[148] Riesser C., Papesh C., Herold M., Böck G., Ramoner R., Klocker H., Bartsch G.,

Thurnher M. (1998) Differential deactivation of human dendritic cells by endotoxin desensitization: role of tumor necrosis factor-α and prostaglandin E2. Blood 91: 3112–3117.

[149] Roitt I., Brostoff J., Male D. (2000) Immunology. Fifth edition. Mir, Moscow.

[150] Romani N., Reider D., Heuer M., Ebner S., Kampgen E., Eibl B., Niederwieser D., Schuler G. (1996) Generation of mature dendritc cells from human blood: an improved method with special regard to clinical applicability. J. Immunol. Methods 196: 137–151.

[151] Roy K. C., Bandyopadhyay G., Rakashit S., Ray M., Bandyopadhyay S. (2004) IL-4 alone without the involvement of GM-CSF transforms human peripheral blood monocytes to a $CD1a^{dim}$, $CD83^+$ myeloid dendritic cell subset. J. Cell. Sci. 117: 3435–3445.

[152] Sallusto F., Lanzavecchia A. (1994) Efficient presentation of soluble antigen by cultured human dendritic cells is maintained by granulocyte–macrophage colony-stimulating factor plus interleukin-4 and down-regulated by tumor necrosis factor α. J. Exp. Med. 179: 1109–1118.

[153] Sallusto F., Nicolo C., De Maria R., Corinti S., Testi R. (1996) Ceramide inhibits antigen uptake and presentation by dendritic cells. J. Exp. Med. 184: 2411–2416.

[154] Sallusto F., Palermo B., Lenig D., Miettinen M., Matikainen S., Julkunen I., Forster R., Burgstahler R., Lipp M., Lanzavecchia A. (1999) Distinct patterns and kinetics of chemokine production regulate dendritic cell function. Eur. J. Immunol. 29: 1617–1625.

[155] Santini M. S., Lapenta C., Logozzi M., Parlato S., Spada M., Di Pucchio T., Bellardelli F. (2000) Type I interferon as a powerful adjuvant for monocyte-derived dendritic cell development and activity in vitro and in Hu-PBL-SCID mice. J. Exp. Med. 191: 1777–1788.

[156] Saunders D., Lukas K., Ismaili J., Wu L., Maraskovsky E., Dunn A., Shortman K. (1996) Dendritic cell development in culture from thymic precursor cells in the absence of granulocyte/macrophage colony stimulating factor. J. Exp. Med. 184: 2185–2196.

[157] Scandella E., Men Y., Gillessen S., Forster R., Groettrup M. (2002) Prostaglandin E2 is a key factor for CCR7 surface expression and migration of monocyte-derived dendritic cells. Blood 100: 1354–1361.

[158] Schadendorf D., Ugurel S., Schuler-Thurner B., Nestle F. O., Enk A., Bröcker E. B., Grabbe S., Rittgen W., Edler L., Sucker A., Zimpfer-Rechner C., Berger T., Kamarashev J., Burg G., Jonuleit H., Tüttenberg A., Becker J. C., Keikavoussi P., Kämpgen E., Schuler G. (2006) Dacarbazine (DTIC) versus vaccination with autologous peptide-pulsed dendritic cells (DC) in first-line treatment of patients with metastatic melanoma: a randomized phase III trial of the DC study group of the DeCOG. Ann Oncol. 17: 563–570.

[159] Schakel K., Mayer E., Federle C., Schmitz M., Riethmuller G., Rieber E. P. (1998) A novel dendritic cell population in human blood: one-step immunomagnetic isolation by a specific mAb (M-DC8) and in vitro priming of cytotoxic T lymphocytes. Eur. J. Immunol. 28: 4084–4093.

[160] Schleicher U., Hesse A., Bogdan C. (2005) Minute numbers of contaminant $CD8^+$ T cells or $CD11b^+CD11c^+$ NK cells are the source of IFN-γ in IL-12/IL-18-stimulated mouse macrophage populations. Blood 105: 1319–1328.

[161] Scholler N., Hayden-Ledbetter M., Hellström K.-E., Hellström I., Ledbetter J. A. (2001) CD83 is a sialic acid-binding Ig-like lectin (Siglec) adhesion receptor that binds monocytes and a subset of activated $CD8^+$ T cells. J. Immunol. 166: 3865–3872.

[162] Scholler N., Hayden-Ledbetter M., Dahlin A., Hellström I., Hellström K.-E., Ledbetter J. A. (2002) Cutting edge: CD83 regulates the development of cellular immunity. J. Immunol. 168: 2599–2602.

[163] Schreus M. W. J., Eggert A. A. O., De Boer A. J., Figdor C. G., Adema G. J. (1999) Generation and functional characterization of mouse monocyte-derived dendritic cells. Eur. J. Immunol. 29: 2835–2841.

[164] Shaw J., Grund V., Durling L., Crane D., Caldwell H. (2002) Dendritic cells pulsed with a recombinant chlamidial major outer membrane protein antigen elicit a CD4(+) type 2 rather than type 1 immune response that is not protective. Infect Immunol. 70: 1097–1105.

[165] Shen W., Ladisch S. (2002) Ganglioside GD1a impedes lipopolysaccharide-induced maturation of human dendritic cells. Cell Immunol. 220: 125–133.

[166] Shubina I. J., Lebedinskaya O. V., Akhmatova N. K., Kiselevsky M. V. (2005)

Potential sources of dendritic cells for generation of anti-cancer vaccines. Med. Immunol. 7: 15 (Original text in Russian).

[167] Shurin G. V., Shurin M. R., Bykovskaia S., Lotze M. T., Barksdale E. M. Jr. (2001) Neuroblastoma-derived gangliosides inhibit dendritic cell generation and function. Cancer Res. 61: 363–369.

[168] Smyth M. J. (2006) Imatinib mesylate – uncovering a fast track to adaptive immunity. N. Engl. J. Med. 354: 2282–2284.

[169] Sombroek M. J., Stam A. J., Masterson A. J., Lougheed S. M., Schakeel M. J., Meijer C. J., Pinedo H. M., van den Eertwegh A. J., Scheper R. J., de Gruijl T. D. (2002) Prostanoids play a major role in the primary tumor induced inhibition of dendritic cell differentiation. J. Immunol. 168: 4333–4343.

[170] Spits H., Cowenberg F., Bakker A. Q., Weijer K., Uittenbogaart C. H. (2000) Id2 and Id3 inhibit development of CD34$^+$ stem cells into predendritic cell (Pre-DC)2 but not into pre-DC1: evidence for a lymphoid origin of pre-DC2. J. Exp. Med. 192: 115–1784.

[171] Sporri R., Reis e Sousa C. (2005) Inflammatory mediators are insufficient for full dendritic cell activation and promote expansion of CD4+ T cell populations lacking helper function. Nat. Immunol. 6: 163–170.

[172] Steinman R. M., Cohn Z. A. (1973) Identification of a novel cell type in peripheral lymphoid organs of mice. I. Morphology, quantisation, tissue distribution. J. Exp. Med. 137: 1142–1162.

[173] Steinman R. M., Witmer M. D. (1978) Lymphoid dendritic cells are potent stimulators of the primary mixed leucocyte reaction in mice. Proc. Natl. Acad. Sci. U.S.A. 75: 5132–5136.

[174] Steinman R. M., Pope M. (2002) Exploiting dendritic cells to improve vaccine efficacy. J. Clin. Invest. 109: 1519–1526.

[175] Su H., Messer R., Whitmire W., Fischer E., Portis J., Caldwell H. (1998) Vaccination against chlamydial genital tract infection after immunization with dendritic cells pulsed ex vivo with nonviable Chlamydiae. J. Exp. Med. 7: 809–818.

[176] Su Z., Dannull J., Heiser A., Yancey D., Pruitt S., Madden J., Coleman D., Niedzwiecki D., Gilboa E., Vieweg J. (2003) Immunological and clinical responses in metastatic renal cancer patients vaccinated with tumor RNA-transfected dendritic cells. Cancer Res. 63: 2127–2133.

[177] Sutmuller R. P. M., van Duivenvoorde L. M., van Elsas A., Schumacher T. N. M., Wildenberg M. E., Allison J. P., Toes R. E. M., Offringa R., Melief C. J. M. (2001) Synergism of cytotoxic T lymphocyte-associated antigen 4 blockade and depletion of CD25$^+$ regulatory T cells in antitumor therapy reveals alternative pathways for suppression of autoreactive cytotoxic T lymphocyte responses. J. Exp. Med. 194: 823–832.

[178] Taieb J., Chaput N., Menard C., Apetoh L., Ullrich E., Bonmort M., Pequignot M., Casares N., Terme M., Flament C., Opolon P., Lecluse Y., Metivier D., Tomasello E., Vivier E., Ghiringhelli F., Martin F., Klatzmann D., Poynard T., Tursz T., Raposo G., Yagita H., Ryffel B., Kroemer G., Zitvogel L. (2006) A novel dendritic cell subset involved in tumor immunosurveillance. Nat. Med. 12: 214–219.

[179] Tanaka H., Tanaka J., Kjaergaard J., Shu S. (2002) Depletion of CD4$^+$CD25$^+$ regulatory cells augments the generation of specific immune T cells in tumor-draining lymph nodes. J. Immunother. 25: 207–217.

[180] Thomas R., Lipsky P. E. (1994) Human peripheral blood dendritic cell subsets. Isolation and characterization of precursor and mature antigen-presenting cells. J. Immunol. 153: 4016–4028.

[181] Thurner B., Haendle I., Roder C., Dieckmann D., Keikavoussi P., Jonuleit H., Bender A., Maszek C., Schreiner D., von den Driesh P., Brocker E. B., Steinman R. M., Enk A., Kampgen E., Schuler G. (1999) Vaccination with mage-3A1 peptide-pulsed mature, monocyte derived dendritic cells expands specific cytotoxic T cells and induces regression of some metastases in advanced stage IV melanoma. J. Exp. Med. 190: 1669–1678.

[182] Thurner M., Zelle-Rieser C., Ramoner R., Bartsch G., Holtl L. (2001) The disabled dendritic cell. FASEB J. 15: 1054–1061.

[183] Traver D., Akashi K., Manz M., Merad M., Miyamoto T., Engleman E. G., Weissman I. L. (2000) Development of CD8α-positive dendritic cells from a common myeloid progenitor. Science 290: 2152–2154.

[184] Triozzi P. L., Khurram R., Aldrich W. A., Walker M. J., Kim J. A., Jaynes S. (2000) Intratumoral injection of dendritic cells derived *in vitro* in patients with metastatic cancer. Cancer 89: 2646–2653.

[185] van Elsas A., Sutmuller R. P. M., Hurwitz A. A., Ziskin J., Villasenor J., Medema J.-P., Overwijk W. W., Restifo N. P., Melief C. J. M., Offringa R., Allson J. P. (2001) Elucidating the autoimmune and antitumor effector mechanisms of a treatment based on cytotoxic T-lymphocyte antigen-4 blockade in combination with a B16 melanoma vaccine: comparison of prophylaxis and therapy. J. Exp. Med. 194: 481–489.

[186] van Hall T., Wolpert E. Z., van Veelen P., Laban S., van der Veer M., Roseboom M., Bres S., Grufman P., de Ru A., Meiring H., de Jong A., Franken K., Teixeira A., Valentijn R., Drijfhout J. W, Koning F., Camps M., Ossendorp F., Karre K., Ljunggren H. G., Melief C. J., Offringa R. (2006) Selective cytotoxic T-lymphocyte targeting of tumor immune escape variants. Nat. Med. 12: 417–424.

[187] Verhasselt V., Buelens C., Willems F., De Groote D., Haeffner-Cavaillon N., Goldman M. (1997) Bacterial lipopolysaccharide stimulates the production of cytokines and the expression of costimulatory molecules by human peripheral blood dendritic cells: evidence for a soluble CD14-dependent pathway. J. Immunol. 158: 2919–2925.

[188] von Stebut E., Belkaid Y., Nguen B., Cushing M., Sacks D., Udey M. (2000) Leishmania major-infected murine langerhans cell-like dendritic cells from susceptible mice release IL-12 after infection and vaccinate against experimental cutaneous Leishmaniasis. Eur. J. Immunol. 30: 3498–3506.

[189] de Vries I. J. M., Krooshoop D. J. E. B., Scharenborg N. M., Lesterhuis W. J., Diepstra J. H. S., van Muijen G. N. P., Strijk S. P., Ruers T. J., Boerman O. C., Oyen W. J. G., Adema G. J., Punt C. J. A., Figdor C. G. (2003) Effective migration of antigen-pulsed dendritic cells to lymph nodes in melanoma patients is determined by their maturation state. Cancer Res. 63: 12–17.

[190] Wallet M. A., Sen P., Tisch R. (2005) Immunoregulation of dendritic cells. Clin. Med. Res. 3: 166–175.

[191] Wilson N. S., El-Sukkari D., Belz G. T., Smith C. M., Steptoe R. J., Heath W. R., Shortman K., Villadangos J. A. (2003) Most lymphoid organ dendritic cell types are phenotypically and functionally immature. Blood 102: 2187–2194.

[192] Wilson N. S., El-Sukkari D., Villadangos J. A. (2004) Dendritic cells constitutively present self antigens in their immature state *in vivo* and regulate antigen presentation by controlling the rates of MHC class II synthesis and endocytosis. Blood 103: 2187–2195.

[193] Wolfl M., Batten W. Y., Posovszky C., Bernhard H., Berthold F. (2002) Gangliosides inhibit the development from monocytes to dendritic cells. Clin. Exp. Immunol. 130: 441–448.

[194] Worgall S., Kikuchi T., Singh R., Martushova K., Lande L., Crystal R. (2001) Protection against pulmonary infection with Pseudomonas aerogenosa following immunization with *P. aerogenosa*-pulsed dendritic cells. Infect. Immunol. 69: 4521–4527.

[195] Wu L., Scollay R., Egerton M., Pearse M., Spangrude G. J., Shortman K. (1991) CD4 expressed on earliest T-lineage precursor cells in the adult murine thymus. Nature 349: 71–74.

[196] Wu L., Li C.-L., Shortman K. (1996) Thymic dendritic cell precursors: relationship to the T-lymphocyte lineage and phenotype of the dendritic cell progeny. J. Exp. Med. 184: 903–911.

[197] Wu L., D'Amico A., Hochrein H., O'Keefe M., Shortman K., Lucas K. (2001) Development of thymic and splenic dendritic cell populations from different hematopoietic precursors. Blood 98: 3376–3382.

[198] Wu D. Y., Segal N. H., Sidobre S., Kronenberg M., Chapman P. B. (2003) Cross-presentation of disialoganglioside GD3 to natural killer T cells. J. Exp. Med. 198: 173–181.

[199] Xie J., Qian J., Wang S., Freeman III M. E., Epstein J., Yi Q. (2003) Novel and detrimental effects of lipopolysaccharide on *in vitro* generation of immature dendritic cells: involvement of mitogen-activated protein kinase p38. J. Immunol. 171: 4792–4800.

[200] Yanagawa Y., Onoé K. (2003) CCR7 ligands induce rapid endocytosis in mature dendritic cells with concomitant up-regulation

of Cdc42 and Rac activities. Blood 101: 4923–4929.

[201] Zhang Y., Harada A., Wang J. B., Zhang Y. Y., Hashimoto S., Naito M., Matsushima K. (1998) Bifurcated dendritic cell differentiation *in vitro* from murine lineage phenotype negative c-kit$^+$ bone marrow hematopoietic progenitor cells. Blood 92: 118–128.

[202] Zhang Y., Zhang Y. Y., Ogata M., Chen P., Harada A., Hashimoto S., Matsushima K. (1999) Transforming growth factor β1 polarizes murine hematopoietic progenitor cells to generate Langerhans cell-like dendritic cells through a monocyte/macrophage differentiation pathway. Blood 93: 1208–1220.

[203] Zhong H., Shurin M. R., Han B. (2007) Optimizing dendritic cell-based immunotherapy for cancer. Expert Rev. Vaccines 6: 333–345.

[204] Zhou L.-J., Tedder T. F. (1996) CD14+ blood monocytes can differentiate into functionally mature CD83+ dendritic cells. Proc. Natl. Acad. Sci. U.S.A. 93: 2588–2592.

Index

3

3